Second Edition

Nursing Theories

CONCEPTUAL & PHILOSOPHICAL FOUNDATIONS

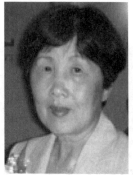

Hesook Suzie Kim, PhD, RN, has been professor of nursing at the University of Rhode Island since 1979 and Professor II at the Institute of Nursing Science, Faculty of Medicine, University of Oslo in Norway from 1992 to 2003. She is professor emerita of nursing at the University of Rhode Island, from which she retired in 2004, and currently holds the professorship at Buskerud University College in Norway. Dr. Kim had taught at the University of Rhode Island since 1973 and was dean of the College of Nursing there from 1983 to 1988. Her PhD is in sociology from Brown University, and her nursing degrees (BS and MS) are from Indiana University. She has published extensively in the area of nursing epistemology, theory development in nursing, the nature of nursing practice, and collaborative decision-making in nursing practice as well as in various areas of clinical nursing research. Most notably, Dr. Kim is the author of a seminal book on the metaparadigm of nursing originally published in 1983, entitled *The Nature of Theoretical Thinking in Nursing,* the second edition of which was published in 2000.

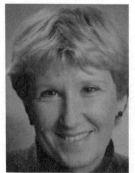

Ingrid Kollak, PhD, RN, has been professor of nursing science at the Alice Salomon University of Applied Sciences (ASFH) in Berlin since 1995. (Dr. Kollak was educated and worked as a nurse in Germany, where a registration system is not common.) She studied German, sociology, and pedagogy at the Ruhr University in Bochum and spent time studying and researching in France, Austria, and the U.S. between 1984 and 1993. Dr. Kollak gained her PhD in German and qualified as a teacher and as a nurse. She teaches in bachelor's and master's programs at ASFH and at Berlin's Humboldt University and is a member of the postgraduate research center Multimorbidity in Old Age and Special Care Problems, organized by five Berlin universities. Since 2002 Dr. Kollak has been coeditor of *Pflege und Gesellschaft (Nursing and Society),* the theoretical journal of the German Society of Nursing. She has published extensively on self-care, culture, and difference as well as language, communication, and specialist media.

Second Edition

Nursing Theories

CONCEPTUAL & PHILOSOPHICAL FOUNDATIONS

Hesook Suzie Kim, PhD, RN ■ **Ingrid Kollak,** PhD, RN

Editors

 Springer Publishing Company

10/06

Springer Publishing Company, Inc.
11 West 42nd Street
New York, NY 10036

Acquisitions Editor: Ruth Chasek
Production Editor: Sara Yoo
Cover design by Joanne Honigman

06 07 08 09 10 / 5 4 3 2 1

Library of Congress Cataloging-in-Publication Data

Nursing theories : conceptual and philosophical foundations / editors, Hesook Suzie Kim, Ingrid Kollak. — 2nd ed.
    p. ; cm.
  Includes bibliographical references and index.
  Summary: "This book is written for advanced nursing students. The second edition of Nursing Theories explores the conceptual and philosophical foundations of selected major nursing theories. The book is not a survey or evaluation of nursing theories, but is designed to assist students in understanding the core philosophical concepts behind nursing theories and how they can be applied to current nursing practice. New to this second edition: Essays warranted by developments in the science and research of nursing. Three chapters addressing: pragmatism, evidence-based nursing, biography. Newly authored chapters on systems and transcultural thoughts reflecting current thinking and new directions. Completely rewritten chapters on interaction and self-care to incorporate current debates"—Provided by the publisher.

  ISBN 0-8261-4005-X (soft cover)
  1. Nursing—Philosophy.
  [DNLM: 1. Nursing Theory. 2. Models, Nursing. 3. Philosophy, Nursing. WY 86 N97374 2006] I. Kim, Hesook Suzie. II. Kollak, Ingrid.

RT84.5.N8795 2006
610.73'01—dc22

2005013728

Printed in the United States of America by Sheridan Books, Inc.

To Our Students

Contents

Contributors

Friedrich Balke, PhD, holds a doctorate in philosophy from Ruhr-Universität Bochum and is an academic coordinator of the postgraduate research school at the University of Cologne in Germany. He has published widely on political philosophy, social and cultural theory, and contemporary French philosophy.

May Solveig Fagermoen, PhD, RN, is associate professor at the Institute of Nursing Science at the University of Oslo, Norway. She received her basic nursing education from Aker School of Nursing and nurse teacher's degree from the Norwegian School of Advanced Studies in Nursing. Dr. Fagermoen holds an MA in nursing from the University of Washington School of Nursing in Seattle and a PhD in nursing from University of Rhode Island, Kingston. She has published two books on teaching and learning in nursing, and has published widely in the area of nursing practice and qualitative nursing research.

Jacqueline D. Fortin, DNSc, RN, is associate professor emerita of nursing at the University of Rhode Island. She received a BS in nursing from the University of Rhode Island, an MS in nursing from Boston College, and a DNSc degree from Boston University. Dr. Fortin taught at the University of Rhode Island from 1974 to 2001, mostly in the College of Nursing's doctoral program since 1985. Her area of research was in postoperative pain.

Martina Hasseler, Dr. rer. Medic., is professor of nursing science in the bachelor of nursing degree course of the Protestant University of Applied Sciences, Berlin.

Her major fields of work and research are health and nursing policy, research into provision and its optimization, international comparison of health and care systems, and evidence-based nursing. Dr. Hasseler's recent publications are on health policy and its effects on day care, nursing needs and nursing-need constellations, reform of long-term-care insurance, evidence-based nursing, and prevention.

Heiko Kleve, PhD, has a diploma in social work/social pedagogy, and is a sociologist working also as a systems consultant (DGSF), a conflict mediator (FH), and a case manager/case management trainer (DGS/DBSH/DBfK). He is professor of the theory and history of social work at the Alice Salomon University of Applied Sciences in Berlin. His major fields of work and research are systems theory/constructivism, postmodernism, and the theory and methodology of social work. Dr. Kleve's recent publications are on social work studies, systems theory and postmodernism, including *Foundations and Applications of a Theory and Methods Program* (2003).

Penny Powers, PhD, RN, is professor and department head of graduate nursing programs at South Dakota State University College of Nursing in Brookings. She earned her PhD in nursing from the University of Washington, Seattle. Dr. Powers has worked as a medical and surgical nurse in Canada and the U.S. Her publications focus on power, oppression, empowerment, discourse analysis, and interpretive research methods.

Birgit Rommelspacher, Dr. phil., is a professor in psychology with emphasis on interculturality and gender studies at Alice Salomon University of Applied Sciences in Berlin since 1990. She studied psychology in Bonn, Münster, Cincinnati, Ohio in the US, and Munich, and philosophy and social-economic history in Munich. She received the Doctor of philosophy degree from Ludwig Maximilian University of Munich. She has numerous publications in the areas of culture, racism, and gender studies, among which are *Multicultural society-monocultural psychology? (Multikulturelle Gesellschaft-Monokulturelle Psychologie?), Dominant culture—Texts on strangeness and power (Dominanzkultur. Texte zu Fremdheit und Macht), and Acknowledgement and exclusion. Germany as a multicultural society (Anerkennung und Ausgrenzung. Deutschland als Multikulturelle Gesellschaft)* published in 2002.

Barbara Schulte-Steinicke, PhD, is a psychologist and is a guest lecturer at the Alice Salomon University of Applied Sciences in Berlin. Her major fields of work and research are personal health and biographical, creative, and therapeutic writing. She is currently in the process of initiating the first course of studies of biographical and creative writing in Germany. Dr. Schulte-Steinicke's recent publications include *Die deutsche Schreibkrise. Empirische Studien zum Schreiben in Deutschland* (with L. Werder, 2003); "Wissenschaftliches Schreiben—Ergebnisse einer empirischen Umfrage" (in *Jahrbuch für Akademisches Schreiben,* with L. Werder, 2004); "Erinnern, Schreiben, Bewahren. Kreatives Schreiben mit Seniorinnen und Senioren" (in *Pflege und Gesellschaft,* Vol. 1, 2004), and "Kreatives Schreiben zur psychologischen Selbsthilfe für seelische Gesundheit fördern" (in *Gesundheitspsychologische Perspektiven,* M. Rieländer, editor, to be published in 2004).

Donna Schwartz-Barcott, PhD, RN, is professor and director of graduate studies in nursing in the College of Nursing at the University of Rhode Island, Kingston. She holds a PhD in anthropology from the University of North Carolina and teaches courses in knowledge development in the client domain and inductive approaches to theory development in the doctoral program. Dr. Schwartz-Barcott and Dr. Kim developed the Hybrid Model of Concept Development to enhance the theoretical and empirical grounding of core concepts in nursing, which was published in *Concept Development in Nursing: Approaches and Applications,* edited by Rodgers and Knafl (1993, 2000). Dr. Schwartz-Barcott has coauthored several articles dealing with a variety of fieldwork approaches (e.g., ethnography and action research) to inductive theory development, including some newer strategies for enhancing the linkage between practice and theory development.

Björn Sjöström, PhD, RN, is professor of nursing at the University of Skövde in Sweden and is an adjunct professor at the University of Rhode Island College of Nursing. He received a PhD from Gothenburg University and also has been a faculty member there. His area of research is in pain and pain assessment, and he has applied phenomenography in various clinical nursing research projects. Dr. Sjöström has numerous publications on postoperative pain and pain assessment. He is currently a coordinator of a joint doctoral program in nursing between the University of Rhode Island and the University of Skövde.

Susanne Wied, MA, RN, has a master's degree in nursing education and a number of qualifications in communication skills, color therapies, and color testing. She conceived and coedited the first German nursing encyclopedia, *Pschyrembel Wörterbuch Pflege.* Ms. Weid researches, writes books, and gives interdisciplinary lectures about the scientifically based use of colors for a health-promoting caring environment. *Colorspace* will be published online at http://www.farbe-raum-gesundheit.de.

ABOUT THE TRANSLATORS

Several chapters in this book were originally written in German and were translated into English by the following individuals:

Ellen M. Klein received a BA in German and linguistics from the University of Michigan at Ann Arbor and an MA in German linguistics from the Free University of Berlin.

Gerald Nixon teaches translation and essay writing at Berlin's Free University. He received a BA in the study of modern languages in England.

Preface

The second edition of this book, like the first, provides a systematic, analytical treatise of nursing's major theoretical work through in-depth analyses of conceptual and philosophical ideas that underpin nursing theories and theoretical frameworks. It is written for advanced nursing students and others who need to understand these ideas and their relationship to theory development and to nursing practice. It is not a survey of nursing theories or an evaluation of nursing theories in terms of their theoretical structures and contents. Instead, readers will gain a deeper understanding of nursing theories through examining them in their conceptual and philosophical contexts. No nursing theory has been developed in a vacuum—each has rich and varied roots in Western philosophical traditions, and this book allows readers to step back and view this larger picture. The themes we have selected for inclusion are all familiar to students of nursing and may evoke different conceptual pictures for them. We believe this conceptual approach makes the book especially rich and interesting as well as challenging.

We hope that this book will be used as a companion to the original theoretical works for better understanding of not only the theories themselves but also of the essential questions about nursing theory development, such as how different conceptual and philosophical perspectives influence theoretical approaches to study key phenomena in nursing. We think this book initiates the third tier in the exposition of theoretical nursing: the first being the original theories proposed and advanced by various authors, and the second tier focusing on analysis and evaluation of nursing's conceptual frameworks and theories. This third tier focuses on the analysis of concepts and issues that form the foundation of the orientations and perspectives of nursing theories. This will, we hope, add to a comprehensive study of nursing's theoretical works.

Building on the foundation of the essays from the first edition, this edition contains several essays warranted by recent developments in the science and research of nursing. These chapters (11, 12, and 13) address the topics of pragmatism, biography, and evidence-based nursing. We believe the currency and relevance of ongoing debates about these topics in both the nursing scene and the broader epistemological and health care world make the presentations timely and critical in providing the bases for responsible discussions and development.

The chapters on systems (chapter 8) and transculturality (chapter 14) were written by new authors and address current thinking and innovative directions, and the chapters on interaction (chapter 5) and self-care (chapter 4) have been completely rewritten to incorporate current debates. The authors of the remaining chapters have edited their original work in order to assure the currency of the material. It has been rewarding to us as editors to revisit the work and help fine-tune it here and there.

Our first edition, with contributions by scholars from Germany, Norway, and the United States, has been well received since its publication. We have been told by many readers, especially colleagues in the U.S., that it had broadened their perspectives and exposed them to innovative thinking. We are delighted that our publisher presented us with the opportunity to elaborate on that work. We hope it will meet with approval similar to the earlier version and that it will kindle interests and point the reader toward new directions.

BACKGROUND TO THE FIRST EDITION

The idea for this book came about when Ingrid and I were together in Berlin in the summer of 1996. She had been talking with a German publisher who was interested in publishing a book in nursing theories. This led to our discussing the current situation in the discipline of nursing both in the U.S. and in Europe regarding theory development and theoretical discourse. We both felt there was a great need for a theory book that did not just elaborate on the contents of nursing theories, but that examined the conceptual and philosophical ideas behind nursing theories. Such a book, we thought, could assist advanced students in nursing to comprehend nursing's major theoretical ideas from foundational issues pertaining to theory development and relationship to nursing practice.

The idea in the beginning was to work on such a book to be published in German, with contributions by both American and German-speaking scholars in nursing. But as we got into the actual development of the outline and preparation of the manuscript, it became apparent that there would be great merit and excitement in publishing the book in German and English concurrently. Although it is quite true that European nurses and nursing scholars are exposed widely to theoretical work published in English, American readers have not had many opportunities to read analytical work regarding nursing theory written by German-speaking scholars, except for a limited number of journal articles published in English. In this age of globalism and multiculturalism, we find it exciting to present views and studies of nursing's theoretical issues by scholars not only with different philosophical orientations but also with different linguistic, cultural, and academic backgrounds. Thus we have contributions by four American authors, one Norwegian scholar whose advanced education is from the United States, and five German authors. The contributors have performed remarkable feats of pulling together sources of information and knowledge that undergird each theme, and at the same time remaining utterly critical and analytical in their expositions. We are sure all contributors would agree with us that the intent of the book is to raise critical questions fundamental to advancing nursing's theoretical work rather than to provide definitive answers about what is good or bad about nursing theories.

As with any edited book, it is quite amazing how one can achieve diversity in characteristics as we find in the chapters included in this book. Without the contributors' insights and knowledge, their diligence and perseverance, this book would not have materialized. We acknowledge the important contribution made by the translators who translated German manuscripts into English for the American publication, and those who translated English manuscripts into German for the German publication. We would not have a comprehensible work without their sensitivity and understanding regarding terms as used in nursing and philosophy. We are also grateful for the support of our American editor for two editions, Ruth Chasek at Springer, and our German editor for the first edition, Klaus Reinhardt at Huber.

Hesook Suzie Kim
Exeter, Rhode Island
Ingrid Kollak
Berlin, Germany

CHAPTER *1*

Introduction

Hesook Suzie Kim

Nursing's theoretical knowledge has a rich heritage in its development, dating back to the writings of Florence Nightingale and emanating from the work of many nursing scholars of the past three decades. Although there is a continuing debate about whether nursing theories, as they exist, are mature enough or rigorously developed, nursing theories, large and small, have become the cornerstone for understanding and guiding nursing practice in the current decade. However, there are many questions about nursing theories and their contents that trouble students of nursing, whether they are undergraduate or graduate students or practicing nurses.

One of the major difficulties voiced by many is related to the presence of numerous nursing theories, all of which claim to have answers to nursing questions and to provide guidance to nursing practice. Although nursing theories in general are presented with the supposition that they are oriented to describe and explain nursing's concern, each is based on assumptions, philosophies, values, perspectives, and scope that are unique. Different foundational ideas, both conceptual and philosophical, orient nursing theories to describe and explain the phenomena of concern to nursing in diverse ways. Though nursing theories in general are not presented with coherence among the theories' components, precision in conceptualization, and logic in structure, it is not too difficult to extract the theories' perspectives and assumptions that enlighten us about their orientations regarding how nursing phenomena are treated theoretically. A synopsis of nursing theories, mostly the so-called grand nursing theories, is given in Appendix A to orient readers to their foundations.

Many books written about nursing theories contain categorization of nursing theories into different sorts. For example, Meleis (1996) categorizes them as having systems, holistic, adaptation, and behavioral orientations, and puts them into theories on nursing clients, on human being-environment interactions, on interactions, and on nursing therapeutics. On the other hand, Parse (1987) treats five nursing theoretical models in terms of the totality and simultaneity paradigms. Obviously, different nursing theories have been developed with various conceptual and philosophical orientations, which usually lay foundations for the ways theorists view humans, human life, human relations, or practice. Theoretical assumptions that undergird theories stem from differing conceptual and philosophical orientations, and they have intimate connections to theories' substantive contents.

This approach to theory development depicts especially the grand theory development in nursing that occurred throughout the 1970s and 1980s. Thus, the so-called grand theories of nursing—such as Rogers' science of unitary human beings, Roy adaptation model, Orem's self-care model, Neuman's systems' framework, Parse's human-becoming theory, and Watson's theory of human care—are identifiable as having their foundational bases on specific ontological or philosophical orientations. Following this initial fervor of grand theorizing in nursing, however, nursing's theoretical work has focused on developing middle-range theories in the 1990s and the current decade (Liehr & Smith, 1999; Smith & Liehr, 2003). A list of middle-range theories in nursing is given in Appendix B, compiled from a review of the literature through 2004, in order to show the diverse subject matters addressed in these theories. Although some of the middle-range theories have been developed directly from specific grand theories such as those of Rogers and Roy (for example, the Rogerian theory of power by Barrett, 1992; and the urine control theory from the Roy model by Jirovex, Jenkins, Isenberg, & Baiardi, 1999), many have been developed independently, applying various theory development strategies such as the theory synthesis method of Walker and Avant (1995), as in the theory of unpleasant symptoms (Lenz & Pugh, 2003), and the grounded theory approach applied in many theories identified by Benoliel (1996). Thus, such middle-range theories are undergirded, though often not specified clearly, by various philosophical perspectives depending on their conceptual or methodological orientations and starting points. This means that there is a greater need at present to examine various conceptual and philosophical ideas that underpin nursing theories.

We offer in this book expositions that analyze selected nursing theories' conceptual and philosophical foundations so that nursing theories are not only understood in terms of their contents but also from their foundational ideas. This is based on the belief that users of nursing theories for research, practice, or education must have an understanding and enlightenment about theories regarding what the theories aim to describe and explain, and also from what ontological and epistemological perspectives such theoretical descriptions and explanations are developed. This, we believe, can be done only through in-depth analyses of the foundational ideas, examined within broad contexts from which different conceptual and philosophical orientations originate.

THEMES AS THE BASES FOR THEORETICAL UNDERSTANDING

In this edition, we have included thirteen themes as the basic orientations in nursing theories for examination in this book. These themes have become the major ideas that underline nursing's theoretical development, and have provided different starting points for theory development and contents. Six of them are thought to have conceptual foci as their starting points, while three are primarily oriented to the ontology of humans and one is specifically oriented to a philosophy of nursing. A chapter on pragmatism has been added in order to address the impact of this philosophy on nursing knowledge development and practice. The chapters on biography and evidence-based nursing address ideas relevant to practice and theory development.

A conceptual focus refers to a specific conceptualization of human aspects or nursing practice and provides an angle of vision regarding the phenomena with which a theory is concerned in offering understanding and explanation. In nursing theories, a conceptual focus often is a way of organizing our understanding of human phenomena. Conceptual themes have grounding in different domains of nursing, that is, in what Kim (1987, 2000) differentiated as the client domain, the client-nurse domain, the environment domain, and the practice domain.

Included in our analyses of nursing theories are the conceptual foci of *adaptation, human needs and needs, illness as risk,* and *self-care* grounded in the client domain, which are concerned specifically with the conceptualization of clients, client phenomena, and clients' nursing problems. These four themes are different conceptual orientations framing the phenomena in the client domain. Theories with their focus on these concepts view nursing clients primarily in terms of (a) how well they respond to forces that impinge on them (adaptation focus); (b) in what state they are in with respect to what they need or require in order to sustain or grow (human needs focus); (c) how attribution of illness as risk and the conceptualization of health and illness as a continuum determine and influence the ways clients experience illness and patienthood; and (d) how effective and efficient they are in handling obligations of living (self-care focus).

In addition, *human interaction* as a theme in the client-nurse domain offers the bases for examining nursing theories' orientations on client-nurse interaction. Nursing has traditionally been interested in studying interaction as client-nurse interaction. This is viewed as both the medium through which nursing care is processed and as the mode with which nursing produces its therapeutic effectiveness. We also include analysis of the concept of *transculturality* in relation to nursing theories. The concept of transculturality is considered to have reference to the environment domain, as culture is an environmental context in relation to human health. The concept of transculturality is viewed as grounding nursing clients and nursing practice contextually within cultural frames

The themes of *holism, systems,* and *existential phenomenology* provide the analyses of nursing theories from their ontological beginnings. These are themes adopted by nursing theories as three that provide specific ontological perspectives regarding humans, human entity, and human experiences. The theme of *caring and humanism* provides a framework for examining nursing theory from the philosophy of nursing perspective.

The philosophy of *pragmatism* is taken up because during the last two decades it has become one of the most debated and often controversial orientations regarding knowledge and human practice. Two new chapters on *biography and biographical work* and *evidence-based nursing* deal with recent themes that have emerged in the nursing scene as relevant concepts for nursing practice and theory development.

A FRAMEWORK FOR THEORETICAL UNDERSTANDING

Many books have been written about theories in nursing (for example, Barnum, 1994; Fawcett, 2005; Fitzpatrick & Whall, 1996; Meleis, 2005). Most of these are oriented to the analysis and critique of theories by adopting certain criteria for identifying theoretical assumptions, distinguishing contents, and evaluating the maturity, completeness, and logic of theory. In general, theories and theoretical frameworks are examined with respect to different components and aspects related to them. These are as follows:

1. Theoretical Perspectives—provides insights to the theory's worldviews and angle of vision regarding the phenomena of interest from the conceptual, ontological, and epistemological orientations
2. Basic Assumptions and Premises—further illuminates the theory's orientations regarding how one is to understand and explain nursing phenomena
3. Concepts and Their Definitions—specifies major concepts used in the theory and their conceptualizations
4. Theoretical Structure and Statements—specifies the form of theory and its structure and the nature of theoretical statements developed for the theory
5. Chronological Order of Progression—provides an understanding regarding the order with which a given theory has progressed over time
6. Theorist(s) and Major Proponents—provides insights into the theorist's scientific orientations that undergird the theory development

Comprehending nursing theories require multifaceted approaches, beginning with a descriptive understanding of theories, which comes from a thorough reading of original work. From this initial understanding, one can move toward a critical understanding based on analysis and evaluation of a given theory in terms of what it proposes as well as the foundation from which its proposals originate. It further involves a strategic understanding through which one can gain an appreciation of the processes of theory development and the background under which a given theory has emerged. This can be done by analysis of a given theory's evolutionary progression and through an in-depth understanding of the philosophical and theoretical commitments of the major proponents of a given theory. Table 1.1 shows how such multilevel approaches may focus on different aspects of understanding nursing theories.

This book does not attempt to analyze nursing theories from all of these analytical schemas, but is mainly oriented to the study of nursing theories from the analysis of foundational perspectives. The authors' aim is to provide a review and analysis of nursing theories that can add to the comprehension of theoretical work in nursing using an approach that is different from those adopted by major authors who focus on analyzing theories for content and logical structure. Our approach is to examine nursing theories from the analysis of conceptual and philosophical perspectives that undergird nursing theories. The themes identified as the major conceptual and philosophical orientations are examined for their meaning, ontological orientations, and epistemological implications. Theories relevant to each of the themes are then examined and contrasted in the context of the theme's definitional, ontological, and epistemological discussions. Hence, the reviews are oriented to identifying and examining the foundations on which the theories are developed. This level of studying theories will provide the reader with an appreciation of theories' perspectives and

TABLE 1.1   Multifaceted Approach to Theoretical Comprehension

Types of Analysis	Aspects of Theory Comprehension
Thorough Reading	Understanding the language and structure of theory
Analysis of Contents for Metaparadigm Orientation	Understanding the scope of theory
Analysis of Theory Structure	Understanding the theoretical precision and logic-in-use in terms of concepts and theoretical statements
Analysis of Coherence Among Components	Understanding the coherence and organization among theoretical components
Analysis of Foundational Perspectives	Understanding the conceptual and philosophical orientations regarding the images of humans and nursing, conceptualization of key phenomena, and theoretical explanation
Analysis of Theory Progression	Understanding the theory development process
Study of Theorist/Major Proponents	Understanding the theorist's perspectives and visions regarding theory development

philosophical issues pertinent to theory development in nursing. This orientation has guided the analyses offered in the following chapters.

The concept of human need is analyzed from a general analytic perspective in chapter 2, identifying some of the key need theories in nursing, while chapter 6 offers a discourse analysis of the current status of the concept of needs in nursing. In chapter 3, the concept of adaptation is analyzed in its meanings used in relation to populations and species and individuals. It furthermore addresses their implications for nursing's theoretical approaches regarding client phenomena.

The concept of self-care is examined in chapter 4 focusing on the meanings and social implications of upholding this as a valued concept. Issues of interaction and communication are analyzed in chapter 5 in relation to specific nursing theories dealing with client-nurse interaction.

In chapter 7, holism is investigated for its philosophical roots, identifying diverse orientations and multiple interpretations of this philosophy. It is then examined in relation to nursing theories, especially in terms of the theory of unitary human beings by Rogers, and implications of diverse holistic philosophies on nursing theory development. The concept of philosophy of system is examined in chapter 8, tracing it from the general systems orientation and new systems perspectives. Nursing theories with a systems focus are then examined in their specific orientations within the concept of system.

In chapter 9, the philosophy of existential phenomenology is described, tracing its philosophical roots in phenomenology and existentialism, and Parse's theory of human becoming is examined within the tenets of existential phenomenology. Chapter 10 offers an in-depth analysis of philosophies of humanism and caring and their implications for nursing theory development. The historical and philosophical origins of humanism and caring are traced and analyzed to depict and contrast how these philosophies are adopted in nursing theories. In chapter 11 an exposition on the philosophy of pragmatism is offered in relation to ontology, epistemology, and human conduct. It then examines implications of this philosophy on nursing practice and nursing knowledge development.

New developments relevant to nursing practice and knowledge development dealing with biography and evidence-based nursing are analyzed in chapters 12 and 13.

In chapter 14 an analysis of the concepts of culture and transculturality is offered in relation to its meanings for clients and nursing practice. This chapter uses the German situation as the background for discussing the perspectives of universalism versus culture-specificity in dealing with understanding people's lives and nursing practice. Multicultural context of living and nursing practice of the current scene in most countries raises questions regarding how our notions about differences by cultures and "otherness" need to be aligned with concepts of fairness and equality. Transculturality and multiculturalism are paradoxically associated with other philosophies and principles critical to our knowledge and practice.

Chapter 15 deals with the conceptualizations of health/illness as a continuum and illness as risk, and offers a postmodern critique that raises questions regarding the meaning of normality and abnormality and implications of illness concept as risk in developing theories about clients and health care in nursing.

In chapter 16 a postscript is offered with an examination of the culture of German nursing and nursing science.

REFERENCES

Barnum, B. J. S. (1994). *Nursing theory: Analysis, application, evaluation* (4th ed.). Philadelphia: Lippincott.

Barrett, E. A. M. (1992). Innovative imagery: A health-patterning modality for nursing practice. *Journal of Holistic Nursing, 10,* 154–166.

Benoliel, J. Q. (1996). Grounded theory and nursing knowledge. *Qualitative Health Research, 6,* 406–428.

Fawcett, J. (2005). *Contemporary nursing knowledge: Analysis and evaluation of nursing models and theories.* Philadelphia: Davis.

Fitzpatrick, J. J., & Whall, A. L. (1996). *Conceptual models of nursing: Analysis and application* (3rd ed.). Stamford, CT: Appleton & Lange.

Jirovex, M. M., Jenkins, J., Isenberg, M., & Baiardi, J. (1999). Urine control theory derived from Roy's conceptual framework. *Nursing Science Quarterly, 12,* 251–255.

Kim, H. S. (1987). Structuring the nursing knowledge system: A typology of four domains. *Scholarly Inquiry for Nursing Practice, 1,* 99–110.

Kim, H. S. (2000). *The nature of theoretical thinking in nursing* (2nd ed.). New York: Springer.

Lenz, E. R., & Pugh, L. C. (2003). The theory of unpleasant symptoms. In M. J. Smith & P. R. Liehr (Eds.), *Middle range theory for nursing* (pp. 69–90). New York: Springer.

Liehr, P., & Smith, M. J. (1999). Middle range theory: Spinning research and practice to create knowledge for the new millennium. *Advances in Nursing Science, 21,* 81–91.

Meleis, A. I. (2005). *Theoretical nursing: Development and progress* (Rev. 3rd ed.). Philadelphia: Lippincott Williams & Wilkins.

Parse, R. R. (1987). *Nursing science: Major paradigms, theories, and critiques* Philadelphia: Saunders.

Smith, M. J., & Liehr, P. R. (Eds.). (2003). *Middle range theory for nursing.* New York: Springer.

Walker, L. O., & Avant, K. C. (1995). *Strategies for theory construction in nursing* (3rd ed.). Norwalk, CT: Appleton & Lange.

CHAPTER 2

Human Needs and Nursing Theory

Jacqueline Fortin

The concept of *human needs*, as it relates to nursing practice and theory construction, does not lend itself to a clear and unambiguous definition. Rather, the literature reveals two major and often competing facets: that of a motivational drive that directs human behavior, and that of a force—politically driven and socially and culturally shaped. The two, however, are not necessarily independent. Holmes and Warelow (1997) have described them, in fact, as reflexive, because human needs defined as desires or wants shape the emergence of political and social policies. In turn, political ideologies and social and cultural forces shape the perceived needs of individuals or groups. Both facets, considered separately or together, play an important role in the conceptualization of needs as it relates to current nursing practice and nursing theory development.

From a scientific stance, the concept of human needs is of necessity an invented abstraction, ultimately defined within the parameters of the scientists' disciplinary alliance (e.g., biology, psychology, sociology, anthropology, nursing, or political science), theoretical orientation, and worldview. The concerns of those in the biological sciences evolve around physiological or somatic needs related to survival and health. Psychologists tend to expand the repertoire of needs to include higher-level needs, such as esteem, while social scientists place these and other social needs (e.g., affiliation) into the context of social interaction, culture, or international politics. Although each of these perspectives, to varying degrees, is important to nursing practice and theory development, nurse theorists traditionally have tended to draw mainly from needs theories that reflect objective, individualist accounts such as those of Abraham Maslow. Only recently has nursing begun to take note of the import of social and political forces within health care in general and nursing in particular (see for example, Holmes & Warelow, 1997; Yura & Walsh, 1988).

The broader conceptualization provides opportunity for exploring "images and details that are not readily apparent when viewed from one perspective" (Meleis, 1997, p. 183). For example, the broader conceptualization suggests a need for historical review and the need to distinguish human needs from socially constructed wants, desires, and satisfiers. At the same time, it raises cogent questions regarding the universality of needs, their contextual dependence, and their distinctly Western bias.

These issues are discussed in the first section of this chapter. Questions are raised rather than answered. The second section of the chapter presents an overview of nursing's needs theories with attention to how they are evolving.

CONCEPTUALIZATIONS OF HUMAN NEEDS

Marx (1964) was among the first modern theorists to link human needs to social and political forces. He proposed that the ideal society was one that recognized the needs of the people and fulfilled them. In contrast, Sites (1992) notes that Parsons and other sociologists took the position that biogenetic needs are transformed into need dispositions through the socialization process. Thus, "all explanation can be reduced to the social or cultural order under the assumption that humans are infinitely malleable" (Sites, p. 179). Malinowski attempted to define human nature by listing basic needs at various systems levels. He maintained that biological health was a necessity if social structural integrity and cultural unity were to be met (Turner, 1991b).

Since Marx and Malinowski, a host of scholars have attempted to tie social, cultural, and political forces to what is often characterized as the innate nature of man (Montagu, 1955), reflected either as a single human need—for adequacy (Combs, Richards, & Richards, 1976), or as a list of multiple needs that address those of the individual, family, community, and the nation (see for example, McHale & McHale, 1978).

The mid to late 1970s saw increased interest in human needs as they relate to the allocation of services and resources in both developed and developing nations. As human needs theories began to take on international significance, the tendency to reflect a Western bias became increasingly apparent (for a comprehensive discussion of this topic, see Galtung, 1980). As one example, Lederer (1980b), based on personal communication with Dr. Kinhide Mushakoji, notes that the Japanese language has no word comparable to "need." "[W]henever one tries to translate 'needs' into Japanese, something like wants, wishes, or desires will come out" (p. 8), making communication of needs difficult if not impossible. One can assume this would be problematic in other cultures as well. Analyzing Westernization from a different perspective, Holmes and Warelow (1997) chide Yura and Walsh for their "thinly disguised middle class liberal American ideology" (p. 461) in the development of their eclectic theory of human needs. Here, the problem is not communication, but rather the conceptualization of how needs are satisfied. Specifically, Yura and Walsh (1988) characterize the family as the "primary unit for human need fulfillment" (p. 96) although they recognize the role of the community, state, nation, and so on in facilitating need fulfillment.

Critics of Westernization challenge the underlying premise of the universality of basic human needs. They contend that such lists imply a model to be imitated by other cultures. Other questions revolve around the analytic stance toward epistemology that Westerners take. A list of needs and categories of needs can only be conceptualized as components or dimensions of a whole. Such conceptualizations can be problematic for scientists attempting to describe the holistic experiences (Galtung, 1980). As Galtung notes, however, the

> analytic versus holistic image is not a dichotomy of alternatives; it . . . can be seen as a both-and rather than an either-or. . . . The problem is not how to suppress analytic thinking in this field, but how to facilitate and promote holistic thinking. (p. 82)

Despite concerns of Western bias, most scholars agree that all humans possess certain organic or "basic needs" that must be satisfied for the sake of physical health (Mallmann & Marcus, 1980) and survival (Lederer, 1980a; Malinowski, 1944; Maslow, 1968, 1970; Montagu, 1955). However, McHale and McHale (1978) and others argue that people have desires and aspirations that go beyond physiologic or somatic needs and that the consequences when these needs are not met may be equally dire. Needs for social interaction, for example, are necessary for psychological well-being (Turner, 1987, 1991a, 1991b) and when not met may lead to feelings of loneliness and isolation (Linton, 1945), thereby threatening mental health. Less clear, perhaps, is the proposed interplay between the organic needs of individuals and their related satisfiers.

Personal, cultural, and societal values have a substantial influence on what is defined as a need and what mechanisms are considered appropriate for its satisfaction (McHale & McHale, 1978; Yura & Walsh, 1988). Montagu (1955) points out that while culture may play no role in the innate structure of a need, "[n]eeds function in a culture and culture modifies them" (p. 135). Others argue that it is not *needs* that are modified by social forces but their expressions as wants, wishes, desires, aspirations, and satisfiers. This stance raises the question of whether it is possible to distinguish needs from these related concepts.

ARE NEEDS OBJECTIVE AND UNIVERSAL?

The question of whether human needs are universal and objective is a poignant one and one that has engendered much scholarly debate. Some authors (see for example, McHale & McHale, 1978; Montagu, 1955, 1966) suggest that individual needs vary enormously in kind and in quality and particularly in relationship to the life cycle. Yet Linton (1945) and others (e.g., Watt, 1996) would argue it is not the need that varies, but rather the behaviors the need gives rise to. Thus, authors who favor the universal and objective conceptualization of needs contend it is not the notion of needs that is subjective, but rather the related desires and satisfiers that, according to Lederer (1980b), "differ in terms of space, time, and culture" (p. 5). Mallmann and Marcus (1980) suggest that the incorrect use of the term *need* is the basis for the terminological and conceptual confusion so prevalent in needs research.

Lederer (1980a) draws on the terminology used by Mallmann and Marcus (1980), who espouse to a universal and objective notion of needs. These authors characterize needs as "universal; and desires and satisfiers as spatially, temporally, and personally" determined (Mallmann & Marcus, 1980, p. 166). They contend, "[t]here is no one-to-one relation between needs and desires. Many desires are just distortions of needs" (p. 167). Mallmann and Marcus further maintain that individual attitudes are expressed by desires, whereas needs are an expression of universal human requirements—requirements people may not be aware of. Therefore, it is desires and satisfiers that theorists of the historical/subjective school are striving to understand and explain, for it is desires and satisfiers that are socially constructed and without objective content. The latter are linked with subjective feelings, and though individuals may not be conscious of their needs, they can readily articulate their correlated wants, desires, and satisfiers (Galtung, 1980). If we accept the distinction between needs and desires (satisfiers), we have a sound basis for the integration of the two needs approaches, the "universal/objective" and the "historical/subjective" (Lederer, 1980b, p. 8).

Holmes and Warelow (1997) take a different view. These authors suggest that if we accept the notion of reflexive interplay between needs and social context, then the search for universal need is futile. And this would surely be the case if we accepted the premise, put forth by Plant and colleagues, that needs are socially constructed and cannot be readily differentiated from wants (Plant, Lesser, & Taylor-Gooby, cited in Holmes & Warelow, 1980). It could be argued, however, that if we accept that the reflexive interplay is not between need and social context, but rather between the two facets of human need—one a motivational drive and the other a socially shaped force—then we could view them as two sides of the same coin. From this perspective, desires, wants, and satisfiers would be viewed as variables subject to manipulation. Motivational drives would be considered universal and designated as human needs. This does not mean a comprehensive list of all basic human needs is possible or even desirable, "but it does make sense to talk about certain classes of needs, such as 'security needs,' . . . 'identity needs'" (Galtung, 1980, p. 59), that will be experienced at some time by human beings everywhere, and to differentiate these from desires and satisfiers. Katrin Lederer (1980b) provides the following example:

> "I need a car," according to the above understanding would not be a needs statement. The person desires a car. The car is a satisfier. What the person might need is, for example, mobility, or status, or (speed) ecstasy. Under the person's personal set of living conditions, a car might be the adequate satisfier to meet any of the needs mentioned. (p. 5)

IS THERE A HIERARCHY OF NEEDS?

In theories of human need, the most pervasive assumption, whether implicit or explicit, is that of a needs hierarchy. The physiological needs linked to survival of the individual or group are usually addressed first with the connotation that they should be satisfied first, prior to higher-level mental or spiritual needs (Galtung, 1980; Maslow, 1970). For example, Montagu (1955, 1966) draws on the work of Malinowski to propose a two-structure hierarchy. The first level reflects "vital" basic human needs (e.g., for sleep, ingestion of food, activity, and escape from danger). Montagu (1966) maintains that these basic needs constitute the minimum biological conditions, which must be satisfied by any living group if its members are to survive. He further notes that the second level of the hierarchy addresses "non-vital" basic human needs, such as those related to security and social recognition, which must be satisfied in order to maintain an individual's mental health.

In a somewhat similar fashion, McHale and McHale (1978) propose that "sufficiency" and "growth" needs constitute a "second floor" in the needs hierarchy. Unlike basic universal needs, these second-floor needs are defined by each society for its members.

There is also a clear hierarchy in the human need system offered by Carlos Mallmann (1980) who classifies human needs according to four categories: Needs that are necessary for (a) existence (subsistence and security), (b) coexistence (belongingness and esteem), (c) growth (development and renewal), and (d) perfection (transcendence and maturity). Mallmann contends that satisfaction of each of the eight needs is a requirement if one is to avoid illness. Galtung (1980) also produced a hierarchical list of basic human needs he placed into four categories: security, welfare, identity, and freedom. Specific needs within each category bring the list to 28. Perhaps the author most often associated with a hierarchical structure of needs is Abraham Maslow.

Maslow

Unlike the social and political science scholars noted above, Maslow (1968, 1970) provides a set of objective "basic human needs" that reflect a different discipline, theoretical orientation, and worldview. For example, Maslow's (1954) seminal work on motivation and personality provided the contextual underpinnings from which his hierarchical model of human needs evolved. Educated as a psychologist, Maslow depicted the basic human needs as those necessary for survival or those needs that would produce frustration or psychopathology if not met.

Consistent with his interest in psychopathology, and as many other clinical psychologists have done, Maslow (1954) put aside the less understood cognitive and aesthetic needs, designating them as "prerequisites for the basic need satisfactions" (p. 92). Therefore, the cognitive desires to know and to understand and the overlapping aesthetic needs become part of the "gestalt" in Maslow's holistic dynamic view of personality.

Maslow's scientific philosophy or worldview (1954, 1968, 1970) emanates from organismic theory. His conception of man is of a "whole, functioning, adjusting individual" (1954, p. 25) who can best be understood from a holistic-analytic style. One essential characteristic of this form of analysis is its dependence on understanding the whole. However, to understand the dynamic whole, one must understand the role any given part plays within the gestalt of the whole. That is, the whole and its parts are mutually related; the whole is necessary to an understanding of the part and, in turn, the parts to an understanding of the whole. Based on organismic theory, Maslow proposed five basic human needs: physiological needs, safety needs, belongingness and love needs, esteem needs, and needs for self-actualization. According to Maslow, these needs constitute an inexact hierarchy beginning with the physiological needs and culminating in a drive for self-actualization.

Consistent with the physiological needs described by the authors cited above, Maslow's list includes the somatically based drives of hunger, thirst, sexual desire, and the need for rest, sleep, exercise and so on. Gratification of these physiological needs paves the way for satisfaction of the more socially oriented needs for safety and security. As physiological and safety needs are met, at least to some degree, needs for belongingness and love, self-esteem, and the desire for self-actualization emerge (Maslow, 1970). Leidy (1994) brings our attention to the fact that "[a]lthough Maslow's theory is frequently cited in the nursing literature and is commonly used as an underlying framework for clinical practice, it has been subjected to limited empirical scrutiny" (p. 277). This criticism has been echoed by Homes and Warelow (1997), and Minshull, Ross, and Turner (1986) as well.

Although there appears to be general agreement among the authors reviewed here, it is important to note there is currently no scientific basis for establishing a hierarchy of importance, particularly in higher-level needs. Intuitively most authors would agree it is more pressing for organic needs and safety needs to be met than higher-level needs, yet they do not maintain that people pursue maximum satisfaction of all of their organic needs before giving attention to those needs often characterized as higher level. Furthermore, the expression of human needs (wants, desires, satisfiers) and the gestalt of their interdependence will vary between individuals and groups over time and under varying conditions.

For example, McHale and McHale (1978) address the dimensions of international poverty and the dire social consequences when basic human needs are not met. Taking into account the interdependence of needs, these authors reflect on the vicious cycle that occurs in situations of social and economic deprivation. In relation to health, they note the following: "Poor nutrition lowers disease resistance. Hunger and ill-health impair productivity which, in turn, lessens the capacity to secure more food . . . and be more resistant to disease" (p. 31).

HUMAN NEEDS THEORIES IN NURSING

In 1991 and 1997, Meleis carried out a comprehensive analysis of nursing theories developed between 1950 and 1970. When their paradigmatic origins, time and period of development, and central questions and central concepts were taken into consideration, three distinct schools of thought emerged: needs, interaction, and outcome. The school of thought associated with needs "developed in response to the question 'What do nurses do?'" (1997, p. 185). Thus, Meleis identifies Henderson, Abdellah, and Orem as "needs theorists": Henderson's position emphasizes the nurse's role in complementing and supplementing individual's needs to maintain independence, while Abdellah specifies humans' need-related problems as the focus of nursing attention, and Orem conceptualizes her theory around the concept of self-care needs (1991, pp. 252–254; 1997, pp. 185–188). Theorists within this school, namely Henderson, Abdellah, and Orem, described the potential functions and roles of nurses in terms of patient needs, loosely based "on the fundamental needs of man" (Thorndike cited in Henderson, 1991, p. 16) or Maslow's hierarchy, respectively. Thus, needs theorists provided us with a "view of human beings that was slightly different but very close to the view provided by the biomedical model" (Meleis, 1997, p. 186).

The pioneering efforts of these theorists provide an excellent example of the reflexive nature of needs, namely, it reflects the interplay between the two facets of needs discussed above: one viewed as an internal motivational drive and another viewed as politically driven and socially and culturally shaped. In particular, the latter is clearly demonstrated in the works of Henderson (1991) and Abdellah (Abdellah &

Levine, 1986). The needs theories developed by these two theorists were shaped, in part, by the social and political forces that had come to bear on the profession as a result of "technological advancement and social change" (Dycus, Schmeiser, & Yancy, 1986, p. 94).

One driving social force undergirding the development of Henderson's and Abdellah's models was the recognition by the profession that changes in professional status could only be brought about by defining a scientific body of knowledge, a body of knowledge unique to nursing. A key objective, therefore, of these early efforts was to formulate models that were patient centered and that promoted independent nursing practice. The notion of need as a motivational drive that directs human behavior and that elicits consequences when the need is unmet provided a potential seedbed for such a model. Based on a conceptualization of the client in terms of human needs, and the nurse as one who could provide care when needs were unmet, these efforts were translated into Henderson's (1991) 14 conditions and Abdellah's typology of 21 nursing problems (Abdellah & Levine, 1986). The ultimate goal was to bring about radical change in nursing education and nursing practice.

Although Abdellah's writings are not specific as to theoretical statements, thoughtful analysis and critique of her works (e.g., Abdellah, 1957; Abdellah, Beland, Martin, & Metheney, 1960; Abdellah & Levine, 1986) by several nurse scholars (see for example, Dycus et al., 1986; Falco, 1995; Meleis, 1997; See, 1989) help this author to provide the context within which her typology of 21 problems was developed.

In response to the demand for problem-centered approaches in nursing education and nursing practice, Abdellah set out to develop a model that reflected scientific knowledge unique to nursing. She conducted descriptive investigations designed to explicate health care situations that are problematic to the patient or family and amenable to the professional functions of the nurse (See, 1989). The concepts, grounded in empirical data, formed categories that reflected needs, deficits, and problems that in turn provided the structure for the empirical listing of 21 groups of common nursing problems. Consistent with Maslow's (1954) theoretical orientation, the client is viewed as a whole made up of physiological, sociological, and psychological parts. This conceptualization of the client, along with types of interpersonal relationships between the nurse and patient and common elements of patient care, laid the groundwork for Abdellah's typology of 21 nursing problems listed below (Abdellah et al., 1960):

1. To maintain good hygiene and physical comfort
2. To promote optimal activity, exercise, rest, and sleep
3. To promote safety through prevention of accident, injury, or other trauma and through the prevention of the spread of infection
4. To maintain good body mechanics and prevent and correct deformities
5. To facilitate the maintenance of a supply of oxygen to all body cells
6. To facilitate the maintenance of nutrition of all body cells
7. To facilitate the maintenance of elimination
8. To facilitate the maintenance of fluid and electrolyte balance
9. To recognize the physiological responses of the body to disease conditions—pathological, physiological, and compensatory
10. To facilitate the maintenance of regulatory mechanisms and functions
11. To facilitate the maintenance of sensory function
12. To identify and accept positive and negative expressions, feelings, and reactions
13. To identify and accept the interrelatedness of emotions and organic illness
14. To facilitate the maintenance of effective verbal and nonverbal communication
15. To promote the development of productive interpersonal relationships
16. To facilitate progress toward achievements of personal spiritual goals
17. To create and/or maintain a therapeutic environment
18. To facilitate awareness of self as an individual with varying physical, emotional, and developmental needs
19. To accept the optimum possible goals in the light of limitations, physical and emotional
20. To use community resources as an aid in resolving problems arising from illness
21. To understand the role of social problems as influencing factors in the cause of illness (pp. 126–127)

Abdellah and Levine (1986) offer the list of 21 problems without defining the relationship of needs to problems. They do, however, characterize them as an "overt" or "covert" nursing problem or "a condition faced by the patient or family which the nurse can assist him or them to meet through the performance of her professional functions" (p. 54).

There is general agreement among nurse scholars that health, nursing problem, and problem solving are the three major concepts in Abdellah's writings (see, for example, Dycus et al., 1986; Falco, 1995; Meleis, 1997; See, 1989). Health is loosely defined by Abdellah as a reflection of "[s]elf-help ability developed and maintained at a level at which need satisfaction can take place without assistance" (Abdellah & Levine, 1986, p. 54). In earlier writings, Abdellah and colleagues (1960) linked health to need satisfaction; she did not, however, as See (1989) notes, "explicate in detail the distinction between satisfying health needs and nursing problems" (p. 128). Although there is no explicit mention of a hierarchy of needs, Abdellah indicated that "when for some reason any of these necessities—air, water, food, temperature, intactness of body tissue—departs from the optimum, a state of need can be said to exist" (Abdellah et al., 1960, p. 53). This would suggest that she considered some needs vital in contrast to those considered less vital, such as esteem needs.

The conceptualization of nursing problems is less clear and has generated dialogue about the primary thrust of the model. Abdellah and Levine (1986) define a nursing problem as "a condition faced by the patient or family which the nurse can assist him or them to meet through performance of professional functions" (p. 54). Falco (1995) argues that contrary to the client-centered orientation Abdellah professes, this definition "is more consistent with 'nursing functions' or 'nursing goals' than with client-centered problems" (p. 145). Consequently, the more nursing-centered orientation tends to magnify the concept of problem solving and the role of the nurse in the health care relationship. So, despite her stated shift from nursing problems to patient-client condition and outcomes (Abdellah & Levine, 1986), "scrutiny of the problem solving concept somewhat obscures the original intent of the model which was apparently to emphasize . . . the special patient condition which responds to nursing intervention" (See, 1989, p. 130). From the latter perspective, the clients' condition would be viewed as problems (needs) that act as a cue to guide nursing assessment and interventions.

Problem solving provides the final building block to Abdellah's writing. Defined as the process of identifying overt and covert problems, it is based on the assumption that correct identification of nursing problems, which may be emotional, sociological, or interpersonal in nature, is crucial to selecting the appropriate course of action (Falco, 1995).

Abdellah's model, in particular her list of 21 problems, is generally characterized as one based on Maslow's hierarchy of needs. Though the relationship between the conceptualizations of the two authors is sketchy, to her credit Abdellah does not overemphasize lower-level needs. In fact, many fall into the category of esteem needs and belonging and love (affiliation) needs.

There are notable similarities between Abdellah's 21 problems and Henderson's 14 components of basic nursing care (1991). There are also, however, distinct differences. Henderson's components are clearly client centered and considered in the context of four factors always present: (a) age; (b) temperament, emotional state, or passing mood; (c) social or cultural status; and (d) physical and intellectual capacity. In contrast, Abdellah's problems tend to be more nurse-centered, focused on nursing problems and nursing service. Henderson's 14 components of nursing care reflect her view of humans as biological, psychological, sociological, and spiritual beings. The basic needs of humans are reflected in the 14 components. However, congruent with the needs theorists, she notes that "these needs are satisfied by infinitely varied patterns of living, no two of which are alike" (Henderson, 1960, p. 3).

Henderson views health in the context of human functioning. According to Furukawa and Howe (1995), "[h]er definition of health is based on the individual's ability to function independently, as outlined in the 14 components" (p. 74). When the individual is unable to perform those activities independently, it is the nurse's duty to assist that individual (Henderson, 1991). To carry out this function, "[f]or Henderson the nurse must be knowledgeable, have some base for practicing individualized and humane care, and be a scientific problem solver" (Furukawa & Howe, 1995, p. 75).

The concept of needs is neither defined nor discussed in any depth by Henderson or Abdellah. However, it is important to remember that their focus was not on psychological theories of human behavior, but rather on client problems, nursing education, and nursing practice. Nonetheless, assumptions about the nature of humans and their needs influence implicitly and perhaps without awareness their theoretical thinking. As Abraham Maslow (cited in Wrightsman, 1992) wrote,

Every psychologist, however positivistic and antitheoretical he may claim to be has a full blown philosophy of human nature hidden away within him. It is as if he guided himself by a half-known map, which he disavows and denies, and which is therefore immune to intrusion or correction by newly acquired knowledge. (p. 38)

In any event, Abdellah and Henderson had a significant impact on nursing education and nursing practice. Their successes laid the groundwork for future generations.

CURRENT CONTEXTUAL FEATURES

From the 1970s to the 1990s a number of relevant changes were seen in nursing and the conceptualization of human needs. Nursing's earlier goals for defining a unique body of knowledge to guide practice and education had come to fruition and had become increasingly institutionalized in the nursing process. Scholarly debate turned to issues of philosophy, research methodology, holism, interpretivism and so on. At the same time, theories addressing human needs were maturing. The initial focus on the individual and innate motivational drives broadened to include the political and social issues raised by the notion of basic human needs. The debate has moved to issues such as universality, with some authors arguing that human needs are not universal, objective, or innate, but socially, culturally, and politically derived.

One major change in the perspective of conceptualizing needs in nursing has been in the contextualization of needs rather than focusing on "the basic human needs" conceptualizations, such as in "patients' needs" (Hupcey, 2000; Woo & Twinn, 2004), "health-care or nursing needs" (Betz, Redcay, & Tan, 2003; Hancock et al, 2003), "needs during hospitalization" (Hallstrom & Elander, 2001), or "needs of people in special circumstances" (Conner & Eller, 2004; Im & Choe, 2001; Keane, Brennan, & Pickett, 2000). In such approaches, the basic assumption seems to be that humans have different sets of needs arising out of specific contexts of life experiences such as being sick, being a patient in an intensive care unit or in a nursing home, or being a caregiver or a new immigrant. Such contextualizations of human needs also have stimulated advances in needs assessments within specific contexts, such as in the work of Davidson and colleagues (2004) for patients with heart failure. Although no specific theoretical perspective is taken up by these scholars in addressing human needs contextually, there certainly is a potential for advancement of middle-range theories from the perspective of contextualization of needs.

Drawing on the broader conceptualization of human needs theory and connecting it to nursing process, the work of Yura and Walsh (1978, 1988) remains within mainstream thinking in nursing. Suggesting that "the integrity of all of the human needs of the person(s) is the territory of nursing" (p. 70), these authors proposed an eclectic theory of human needs. Yura and Walsh identified 35 human needs of the client (person, family, and community) founded upon a number of international need theorists (e.g., Galtung, Mallmann, Maslow, McHale & McHale, Montagu) for theoretical substance. Unlike the Abdellah and Henderson theories, Yura and Walsh (1988) define need. Paraphrasing Montagu (1955) they note that

> Proponents of human need theory view the person as an integrated, organized whole who is motivated toward meeting human needs. A human need is viewed as an internal tension that results in an alteration in some state of the system. This tension expresses itself in goal-directed behavior. (Yura & Walsh, 1988, p. 70)

Working from this basic definition, these authors define their 35 problems in the context of the social and cultural insights wrought from their comprehensive literature review.

From a different perspective, Holmes and Warelow (1997) state that "needs . . . are always socially constructed" (p. 469). Therefore, they recommend making critical theory a force for change. They note there are two key tasks that critical theory must undertake: "first, the formulation of a theory of the good life and its relation to needs, commodities and consumption and, second, the clarification of the relationship between theory and practice" (p. 467). In addition, they recommend "praxis," a concept well known to nurses, as a method for "restructuring need interpretations" (p. 468).

The philosophical and theoretical differences between Holmes and Warelow (1997) and Yura and Walsh (1988) are provocative and highlight the two distinctly different approaches to human needs conceptualizations that are emerging. For Yura and Walsh, needs reside within the individual and those needs when unmet guide practice. In contrast, Holmes and Warelow view human needs as potent political and ethical issues that are socially constructed. No doubt more nurse scholars will enter the arena of needs theorizing as issues of access to care, treatment options, advanced technology, assisted suicide, and starvation move to the forefront of health care and nursing in this millennium. That, however, does not negate our need to continue to explore avenues to understanding the human needs of our clients (individuals, family, community) and how those needs best can be met, for that is not only the unique function of nursing, but it is also nursing's social mandate. The jury is still out on questions regarding the hierarchy of needs, interdependence of needs, importance of contextual features, and the term *need* as differentiated from wants, desires, or satisfiers, yet new pioneers in nursing are emerging.

REFERENCES

Abdellah, F. G. (1957). Methods of identifying covert aspects of nursing problems: A key to improved clinical teaching. *Nursing Research, 6*(11), 4–23.

Abdellah, F. G., Beland, I. L., Martin, A., & Metheney, R. V. (1960). *Patient centered approaches to nursing.* New York: Macmillan.

Abdellah, F. G., & Levine, E. (1986). *Better patient care through nursing research* (3rd ed.). New York: Macmillan.

Betz, C. L., Redcay, G., & Tan, S. (2003). Self-reported health care self-care needs of transition-age youth: A pilot study. *Issues in Comprehensive Pediatric Nursing, 26,* 159–181.

Combs, A. W., Richards, A. C., & Richards, F. (1976). *Perceptual psychology: A humanistic approach to the study of persons.* New York: Harper & Row.

Conner, N. E., & Eller, L. S. (2004). Spiritual perspectives, needs and nursing interventions of Christian African-Americans. *Journal of Advanced Nursing, 46,* 624–632.

Davidson, P., Cockburn, J., Daly, J., & Fisher, R. S. (2004). Patient-centered needs assessment: Rationale for a psychometric measure for assessing needs in heart failure. *Journal of Cardiovascular Nursing, 19,* 164–171.

Dycus, D. K., Schmeiser, D. N., & Yancy, R. (1986). Faye Glenn Abdellah. In A. Marriner (Ed.), *Nursing theorists and their work* (pp. 93–101). St. Louis, MO: Mosby.

Falco, S. M. (1995). Faye Glenn Abdellah. In J. B. George (Ed.), *Nursing theories: The base for professional nursing practice* (4th ed., pp. 143–158). Norwalk, CT: Appleton & Lange.

Furukawa, C. Y., & Howe, J. K. (1995). Virginia Henderson. In J. B. George (Ed.), *Nursing theories: The base for professional nursing practice* (4th ed., pp. 67–85). Norwalk, CT: Appleton & Lange.

Galtung, J. (1980). The basic needs approach. In K. Lederer (Ed.), *Human needs: A contribution to the current debate* (pp. 55–130). Cambridge, MA: Oelgeschlager, Gunn & Hain.

Hallstrom, I., & Elander, G. (2001). Needs during hospitalization: Definitions and descriptions made by patients. *Nursing Ethics, 8,* 409–418.

Hancock, K., Chang, E., Chenoweth, L., Clarke, M., Carroll, A., & Jeon, Y. (2003). Nursing needs of acutely ill older people. *Journal of Advanced Nursing, 44,* 507–516.

Henderson, V. A. (1991). *The nature of nursing: Reflections after 25 years.* New York: National League of Nursing Press.

Holmes, C. A., & Warelow, P. J. (1997). Culture, needs and nursing: A critical theory approach. *Journal of Advanced Nursing, 25,* 463–470.

Hupcey, J. E. (2000). Feeling safe: The psychosocial needs of ICU patients. *Journal of Nursing Scholarship, 32,* 361–367.

Im, E., & Choe, M. (2001). Physical activity of Korean immigrant women in the U.S.: Needs and attitudes. *International Journal of Nursing Studies, 38,* 567–577.

Keane, A., Brennan, A. M. W., & Pickett, M. (2000). A typology of residential fire survivors' multidimensional needs. *Western Journal of Nursing Research, 22,* 263–284.

Lederer, K. (Ed.). (1980a). Human needs: A contribution to the current debate. In K. Lederer (Ed.), *Human needs: A contribution to the current debate* (pp. 1–18). Cambridge, MA: Oelgeschlager, Gunn & Hain.

Lederer, K. (1980b). Needs methodology: The environmental case. In K. Lederer (Ed.), *Human needs: A contribution to the current debate* (pp. 259–278). Cambridge, MA: Oelgeschlager, Gunn & Hain.

Leidy, N. K. (1994). Operationalizing Maslow's theory: Developing and testing of the Basic Need Satisfaction Inventory. *Issues in Mental Health Nursing, 15,* 277–295.

Linton, R. (1945). *The cultural background of personality.* New York: Appleton-Century-Crofts.

Malinowski, B. (1944). *A scientific theory of culture and other essays.* Chapel Hill: University of North Carolina Press.

Mallmann, C. A. (1980). Society, needs, and rights: A systematic approach. In K. Lederer (Ed.), *Human needs: A contribution to the current debate* (pp. 37–54). Cambridge, MA. Oelgeschlager, Gunn & Hain.

Mallmann, C. A., & Marcus, S. (1980). Logical clarifications in the study of needs. In K. Lederer (Ed.), *Human needs: A contribution to the current debate* (pp. 163–185). Cambridge, MA: Oelgeschlager, Gunn & Hain.

Marx, K. (1964). *Economic and philosophical manuscripts of 1844* (M. Milligam, Trans.). New York: International.

Maslow, A. (1968). *Toward a psychology of being.* New York: Van Nostrand Reinhold.

Maslow, A. (1970). *Motivation and personality* (2nd ed.). New York: Harper & Row.

Maslow, A. H. (1954). *Motivation and personality.* New York: Harper & Brothers.

McHale, J., & McHale, M. C. (1978). *Basic human needs.* New Brunswick, NJ: Transaction Books.

Meleis, A. I. (1991). *Theoretical nursing: Development and progress* (2nd ed.). New York: Lippincott.

Meleis, A. I. (1997). *Theoretical nursing: Development and progress* (3rd ed.). Philadelphia: Lippincott.

Minshull, J., Ross, K., & Turner, J. (1986). The human needs model of nursing. *Journal of Advanced Nursing, 11,* 643–649.

Montagu, A. (1966). *On being human.* New York: Hawthorn Books.

Montagu, M. F. A. (1955). *The direction of human development: Biological and social bases.* New York: Harper & Brothers.

See, E. M. (1989). Abdellah's model of nursing: Twenty-one nursing problems. In J. J. Fitzpatrick & A. L. Whall (Eds.), *Conceptual models of nursing: Analysis and application* (2nd ed., pp. 123–136). Norwalk, CT: Appleton & Lange.

Sites, P. (1992). Human needs and control: A foundation for human science and critique. In R. H. Brown (Ed.), *Writing the social text: Poetics and politics in social science discourse* (pp. 177–197). New York: Aldine Gruyter.

Turner, J. H. (1987). Toward a sociological theory of motivation. *American Sociological Review, 52,* 15–27.

Turner, J. H. (1991a). Microtheorizing. In J. H. Turner (Ed.), *The structure of sociological theory* (5th ed., pp. 592–606). Belmont, CA: Wadsworth.

Turner, J. H. (1991b). The emergence of functionalism. In J. H. Turner (Ed.), *The structure of sociological theory* (5th ed., pp. 33–50). Belmont, CA: Wadsworth.

Watt, E. D. (1996). Human needs. In A. Kuper & J. Kuper (Eds.), *The social science encyclopedia* (2nd ed., pp. 383–384). New York: Routledge.

Woo, H., & Twinn, S. (2004). Health needs of Hong Kong Chinese pregnant adolescents. *Journal of Advanced Nursing, 45,* 595–602.

Wrightsman, L. S. (1992). *Assumptions about human nature: Implications for researchers and practitioners* (2nd ed.). Newbury Park, CA: Sage.

Yura, H., & Walsh, M. B. (Eds.). (1978). *Human needs and the nursing process.* New York: Appleton-Century-Crofts.

Yura, H., & Walsh, M. B. (1988). *The nursing process: Assessing, planning, implementing, evaluating* (5th ed.). Norwalk, CT: Appleton & Lange.

CHAPTER 3

Adaptation As a Basic Conceptual Focus in Nursing Theories

Donna Schwartz-Barcott

*A*daptation is a popular and long-standing term in nursing. It is used most frequently to capture a central concern of the discipline: an individual's adjustment to an illness, a disability, or health problem. It has been cited as a key term in the nursing literature since the mid 1950s, with the appearance of the first edition of the *Cumulative Index to Nursing and Allied Literature.* Since then, it has been used as a general subject heading to encompass the term in its most common dictionary meanings as (a) the act of process of adapting—as in adapting to a nursing home, or (b) the state of being adapted—as in being physically or psychologically well-adapted to diabetes. It also has been used as an adjective, referring to one's ability to adapt. Hall's (1991) article on adaptability as a personal resource influencing one's health uses the term in this manner.

Over the last 35 years, the primary emphasis in the nursing literature has been on adaptation as a process, one that can be conscious or unconscious; include physiological, psychological, or sociocultural mechanisms; or be seen as a success or failure. The focus on adaptation as an outcome has been secondary, although over the last 5 years it has gained almost equal attention in nursing, given the increased interest in developing and measuring patient outcomes.

Although the term has been used predominantly at the individual client level in nursing, it also has been employed at family and population levels and in the practice domain to address issues regarding the adaptability of nurses. For example, since the 1960s, there has been a small but continually increasing interest in how parents and families adjust when a member of the family, particularly a child, is acutely or chronically ill or disabled. The relatively rare citations at the population level deal mainly with how communities adapt to changing health needs or how a minority group attempts to deal with health problems associated with migration. In the practice domain, the predominant interest has been in the problems nurses face as students; as employees, in transition from being students to becoming professional nurses or from traditional roles into a new role (e.g., that of the nurse practitioner, operating room or home-care nurse, educator or administrator); or under new conditions (e.g., shift work) or difficult situations such as working with patients who are terminally ill.

As early as 1962, a small group of educators had begun to discuss and write about adaptation theory as a possible conceptual framework for nursing (Brown, 1963; Levine, 1966; Martin & Prange, 1962). They were looking for a conceptual framework that could be used to (a) develop more integrated curriculum, (b) serve as a theoretical basis for nursing practice, and (c) provide clues for improvement of patient care.

It was the broad conception of human phenomena—the unifying view of human biological, psychological, and social functioning underlying adaptation theory and its potential for integrating knowledge from diverse disciplines—that initially was so attractive and held such promise for nursing.

In the years that followed, nurses have drawn directly from the continuing development and refinement of various conceptualizations from both outside and within nursing. The conceptions underlying these efforts will be the focus of the remainder of this chapter.

BEGINNING CONCEPTUALIZATIONS OF ADAPTATION: POPULATIONS ADAPTING

In its most general form, *adaptation* has been used in a broad range of disciplines (including biology, physiology, genetics, anthropology, sociology, and psychology, as well as nursing) to refer to the mechanisms or processes that act to maintain a living entity in balance with its environment. That entity might be the human species, a society, a group, or an individual organism —a human being. However, the earliest scientific interest in the concept almost always is linked to biology and to Darwin's efforts at describing the mechanisms involved in long-term evolutionary change at the species or population level, first in plants, then in animals, and finally in the human species (Alland & McCay, 1973).

As a young naturalist, Darwin (1859) made a trip around the world on the now famous HMS Beagle. On the voyage, he accumulated a vast store of data and observed a wide range of species that seemed particularly well adapted to specific environmental niches. For example, on the Galapagos Islands, Darwin observed 13 species of finches that were apparently of common origin but had developed structural differences that suited them for a variety of niches. They differed in size and beak structure, depending on what they ate and whether they were ground or tree dwellers (Lerner, 1968). Retrospectively, Darwin tried to describe the process through which these changes in physical structure had occurred and how they were sustained across generations. Darwin went on to describe this process in terms of variability and natural selection. With the advent of population genetics in the 1930s, differential reproductive success provided the missing mechanism by which variability and natural selection resulted in transgenerational evolutionary change.

Thus, adaptation became closely aligned with the study of evolutionary change and survival. It was seen as a process by which a species interacted with and became fitted to its environment in order to obtain food, shelter, and protection from predation. Ultimately, this would ensure the biological survival of the species (*Encyclopedia of Sociology*, 1974). A basic assumption was that any living system exists within a given environment and it must adapt to that environment in order to survive. In this context, adaptation is not a conscious, goal-directed activity. It is the result of the differential reproductive success of populations, which is determined by the conditions of the moment, not by ultimate desirability or by the remote future (Washburn & Lancaster, 1968). In this context, it is worth noting the following here:

1. The process is based on a species or a population. It is the population, not an individual, that evolves. Individuals are part of the process but survival is at the population or species, not at the individual, level.

2. The response is to environmental conditions; the population either moves into a new environment or something changes in the population or species in response to the environment.
3. Analytically, one starts with a population that is already adapted to its environment.
4. Survival over a long time frame is the outcome of interest.

One major and enduring criticism of this theoretical work has been that the concept of adaptation is tautological, that is, whatever appears is considered adaptive. As Alland and McCay note (1973), this is illustrated in the supposedly "self evident" characteristic of biological adaptation whereby "organisms are surviving because they are adapted and they are adapted because they are surviving" (p. 144). The confusion is not helped when different forms of the term *adaptation* are used to label both the process and its outcome.

ADAPTATION AND THE EVOLUTION OF SOCIETIES

Parallel developments took place in anthropology and sociology in the mid nineteenth century among scholars interested in the evolution of societies. These early developments are associated with the writings of the English philosopher Herbert Spencer (Harris, 1968). By the 1900s, a major focus of those interested in societal evolution was on identifying the cultural and social mechanisms (e.g., technological, organizational, and ideational) that enhanced a society's adjustment to conditions of existence and thus increased its chances of survival (Carneiro, 1973; Service, 1968). In this context, the notion of environment was broadened to include not only the natural environment but also the social environment, although the unit of adaptation was still at the population level and the outcome was primarily on survival. The interest in societal adaptation and evolution has continued and currently can be seen in the works of scholars, including Carneiro (1973), Service (1968), Harris (1968), and McElroy and Townsend (1996) in anthropology; and Parsons (1964), Eisenstadt (1968), and Lenski, Lenski, and Nolan (1995) in sociology.

Although adaptation is most frequently linked with evolutionary change, it has also been studied throughout this time frame with regard to more short-term and nonevolutionary change. One would expect the type of adaptive mechanisms or processes involved with evolutionary change to be different from those dealing with short-term change. Based on a concern for identifying and distinguishing between these processes, Alland and McCay (1973) suggested that "adaptation" be considered as the physiological response of organisms (e.g., a homeostatic response to short-term variations in the environment, such as adaptations to temperature change) and that "transgenerational adaptation" be used as an outcome of the evolutionary process (p. 144).

ADAPTATION AT THE INDIVIDUAL LEVEL

René Dubos' 1965 book, *Man Adapting,* is continually cited as legitimizing and popularizing the image of the individual as a unit of adaptation—one in which health or disease is seen as a measure of the success or failure of an organism's efforts to respond to environmental challenges. Dubos was attempting to parallel Dobzhansky's (1962) work, *Mankind Evolving*—which dealt with the interplay between genetic endowment and environmental factors in humans—while at the same time shifting the focus from humankind as a whole to the individual human being: "*L'homme moyen environ,* trying as best he can to meet the emergencies of the day and to prepare for the uncertainties of the future" (Dobzhansky, p. xviii).

In the early 1960s, Dubos, already a renowned microbiologist for his work on antibiotics, was asked to give a series of presentations for the annual Sillman Foundation Lectures at Yale University, in conjunction with the 100th anniversary of the medical school. He used these lectures as a basis to explore broadly the issues related to the interplay between humans and their environment, while also addressing his growing concern about why bacteria, which at all times inhabit the human organism, only sometimes make people sick. His concern was based on his own research and on his wife's experience with tuberculosis during World War II, which Dubos described in a 1978 interview (Piel & Segerberg, 1990):

> Europe was at war. My first wife was French, born at Limoges. In 1939, at the beginning of the war, she came down with tuberculosis. I asked myself, "Why did she get tuberculosis, when we live as well as we do?" So I dug into her past and discovered that she'd had tuberculosis when she was about six or seven and had gotten well by herself, as most people do. Then why did she have a relapse? I theorized that the disasters in her family resulting from the war had caused her

very great anguish. I'm convinced that this anguish reactivated the tuberculosis that to all appearances had been cured. She died three years later. (p. 10)

Over time, Dubos became more and more aware that

prevalence and severity of microbial diseases were conditioned more by the ways of life of the persons afflicted than by the virulence and other properties of the etiological agents. Hence the need to learn more about man and his societies, in order to try to make sense of the pattern of his diseases. (Dubos, 1965, p. xxi)

In *Man Adapting,* Dubos (1965) weaves together examples from an amazing cross-disciplinary base of historical, physiological, and social science research related to human adaptation at the population and individual levels. He examines evolutionary and nonevolutionary changes. In the process, he creates an image of humans as individuals who adapt to their environment in ways that create distinctive disease patterns across diverse environments. This is the process of adaptation.

Dubos (1965) saw the individual human being as responding to the total environment—physicochemical, biological, and social. Kim (2000) summarizes well the fullness of this image in this way:

A person is thought to exercise adaptive abilities by selecting among alternatives to achieve a self-directed end, given the external conditions that are encountered at a given moment. Dubos' human, furthermore, is a product of the lasting and universal characteristics of human nature, inscribed in being, and yet is capable of establishing a personal history; thus, the person possesses both phylogenic and ontogenic adaptability. A person is seen as an organism responding to stimuli of environmental challenge in a manner that is based on rationality, i.e., that while some responses are based on the direct effects of the stimuli on the organism, most of a person's responses are usually determined not by such direct effects but by the symbolic interpretations he or she attaches to the stimuli.

Thus, Dubos' human treats and responds to actual environmental stimuli in a chained sequence of direct reactions, indirect reactions that occur as ripple effects of the direct reactions, and responses to personalized symbols that are generated by the impinging stimuli. This human trait, according to Dubos, makes the individual's responses to any environmental factors extremely personal (pp. 65–66).

The major explanatory thrust of Dubos' (1965) argument begins with the environment. He pays extensive attention to the factors—especially physical and chemical properties in our air, water, and food—that directly and indirectly give rise to disease. His primary concern is disease as the expression of the organism's failed efforts to respond adaptively to environmental challenges, although he acknowledges that survival and health are indicators of successful adaptation. In developing this argument, Dubos draws heavily on the physiological research and concepts of Cannon (1931) and Selye (1956). They contend that environmental factors give rise to physiological stress in organisms, which in turn makes them more vulnerable to disease. Thus, individuals' perceptions and symbolic interpretations of their environments often are seen as playing a major role in an individual's response and ultimately are linked to the success or failure of that response.

For Dubos (1965), intervention is aimed at helping "man function successfully in his environment—whether he is hunting the mammoth, toiling for his daily bread, or attempting to reach the moon" (p. xix).

ADAPTATION AND THEORY DEVELOPMENT IN NURSING

The most pervasive use of adaptation in the nursing literature is the image it creates of the individual patient attempting to adjust to the peculiarities of a specific disease or disability. Dubos' (1965) depiction of the human being as continuously adapting to environmental challenges is embedded in this image. Disease is just one of the many challenges one must contend with in a lifetime. For most writers in nursing, human adaptation is more of an assumption, a belief, that undergirds educational curriculum and practice than it is a scientific concept that can serve research and theory development.

For others, however, adaptation has presented a compelling theoretical framework, to be used initially as a guide for integrating educational curricula and later for underpinning nursing research. In the early 1960s, as noted previously, adaptation was one of the first theoretical frameworks to be considered for undergirding nursing curricula. Much of this early writing included summaries of the existing theoretical and research literature on adaptation from outside nursing. Nursing scholars began pulling out the basic assumptions and major theoretical concepts and relationships that seemed to have particular relevance to nursing. At times, some authors went on to consider adaptation as a conceptual base for integrating other theoretical schools of thought (e.g., socialization and individual psychodynamics).

In 1963, Pitel drew from the work of several well-established researchers, including Cannon (1932), Adolph (1956), and Selye (1956) to summarize the work being done on adaptation in physiology. She described the human being as a living organism, adapting to an ever-changing external environment via stimuli impinging upon the organism and its internal environment. Adaptation was defined as the adjustment of the organism to environmental change. The focus was on identifying normal physiological regulatory and control mechanisms and then explaining how these enabled the organism to maintain a constant internal environment, or homeostasis. Distinctions were made between environmental change of a short duration (such as daily fluctuations in outdoor temperatures); those that persist for an "appreciable period of time" (e.g., high or low environmental temperatures or altitudes); and those that are of a "very severe nature" (i.e., the physical stress of intense heat or cold, trauma, restraint, or mental stress). It was in regard to the latter that Seyle's stress syndrome was seen as playing a role. According to Pitel (1963),

> Any slight alteration of the internal environment (which may have originally arisen in the external environment) evokes regulatory responses to restore the internal environment to its original status. Cannon called this maintenance of a constant internal environment homeostasis. The adaptation is thus through internal regulation in the presence of environmental change. (p. 263)

Pitel did not mention specific nursing interventions from this work. She simply suggested that nurses who possess this broad perspective, especially knowledge of normal regulatory and control mechanisms, would be better able to detect physiological deviations from the norm (such as control mechanisms that are partially developed, impaired, or completely lacking) and create care plans that are more flexible. Ideally, these should take into account individual capabilities in adjusting to environmental change and helping individuals fit harmoniously with their environment. An example was given of the nurse who assists a patient in adjusting to life-supporting technology that takes the place of the patient's normal regulatory mechanisms.

In another article, Martin and Prange (1962) focused on the environmental changes that individuals normally encounter in their lives (i.e., birth, entering school, puberty, work and marriage, parenthood, involution, retirement and death). They linked successful and unsuccessful attempts at adapting to these changes with states of health or illness, respectively. Others, for example, Vassallo (1965) and Levine (1966), were inspired by the publication of Dubos' (1965) *Man Adapting* as a basis for summarizing current thought on adaptation. Levine focused more on the underlying theoretical explanation in Dubos' work and applied it to patient responses to a cerebral vascular accident and to how nursing care could be orchestrated across several phases of adaptation.

Some researchers began considering the possibility of integrating different theories within adaptation. Brown (1963) emphasized the "human organism's" capacity to learn and drew on theories of socialization from the writings of Talcott Parsons in sociology and George Herbert Mead in social psychology. She suggested that socialization could be seen as a major adaptive process that helps the individual become a social being and adapt to society by fulfilling roles and meeting the expectations of others, thereby maintaining integrity of personality. In a somewhat similar vein, but driven more by psychiatry than by sociology, Peplau (1963) focused on how individual behavior is molded over time and through an interpersonal field to gain a harmonious integration of behavior with that of others within the respective psychosocial field. From this angle, she suggested that "schizophrenia can be seen as massive adaptation or psychosocial behavior to overwhelmingly unfavorable conditions in an interpersonal field" (p. 274). This constitutes an example of the thinking that maladaptation leads to the occurrence of a disease state. Peplau extrapolated that by knowing the processes of adaptation underlying normal behavior, nurses would be better able to understand the origins of the abnormal.

A more systematic effort to develop a nursing theory with the conceptual focus on adaptation is seen in the Roy adaptation model. Initially proposed as a nursing framework by Callista Roy in 1970, this model and its subsequent refinements (Roy, 1976; Roy, 1984, Roy, 1997, Roy & Andrews, 1991, 1999; Roy & Roberts, 1981) are based on the assumptions inherent in Bertalanffy's general systems theory (1968) and Helson's adaptation level theory (1964). Roy views adaptation as a function of impinging stimuli and adaptation level that specifies where an individual is at a given moment in relation to all other preexisting stimuli and one's own internal resources. Hence, to Roy, individuals are adaptive systems that process stimuli through coping mechanisms that are teleologically present in human beings. Human beings are adaptive in the sense that "the human system has the capacity to adjust effectively to changes in the environment and, in turn, affects the environment" (Roy & Andrews, 1991, p. 7). In combining the assumptions of the general systems theory and human adaptation, Roy proposes in her adaptation model a view of human beings as systems that receive inputs as stimuli, process them through the systems' internal and feedback mechanisms, and produce outputs as behaviors that can either be adaptive or ineffective. More specifically, she believes in the goal-directedness and teleological features of humans, and views humans as systems that process "inputs," which are seen as a combined set of external stimuli and internal stimuli (equated with one's adaptation level at a given moment) through regulator and cognator mechanisms of coping.

To Roy, therefore, the essence of human adaptation is the interrelationship between the pooled effects of all stimuli of the environment (what she calls focal, contextual, and residual stimuli) and the individual's adaptation level, which is "the changing point that represents the person's ability to respond positively in a situation" (Roy & Andrews, 1991, p. 10). Behaviors as the outputs of coping are the responses of the adaptive system, and they reveal the nature of adapting by the human system to its environment. Behaviors as responses are either adaptive or ineffective in relation to whether they are promoting the person's integrity and the goals of adaptation. According to Roy, the human systems' goals of adaptation are survival, growth, reproduction, and mastery. To Roy, therefore, adaptation refers to immediate, short-term responses to ever-changing environment, and "adaptive" has a positive connotation in relation to the system's preestablished goals. In elaborating the model, Roy added to the basic tenets of the theory eight assumptions associated with humanism and veritivity (Roy & Andrews, 1991):

> In humanism, it is believed that the individual (a) shares in creative power, (b) behaves purposefully, not in a sequence of cause and effect, (c) possesses intrinsic holism, and (d) strives to maintain integrity and to realize the need for relationship. . . . In veritivity, it is believed that the individual in society is viewed in the context of the (a) purposefulness of human existence, (b) unity of purpose of humankind, (c) activity and creativity for the common good, and (d) value and meaning of life. (p. 6)

Hence, the notions of "creativity," communality of humans as social beings, and universal purpose of humankind are entrenched within the coping mechanisms of regulator and cognator. However, the manner in which such a juxtaposition influences the exact nature of adapting is unclear in the articulation of Roy's model. In addition, the Roy model does not specify how the universal goals of human systems and individual goals of adaptation play out in the process of adaptation for individuals in situations. The picture emerging from Roy's adaptation model is a view of humans who exhibit behaviors that are either adaptive or ineffective as judged by some external and objective criteria established in relation to the goals of adaptation. This makes the model circular in determining the nature of adaptation.

Besides those of Roy, other direct efforts at using adaptation for theory development and research in nursing began in the 1980s. In contrast to Dubos' (1965) focus on processes giving rise to a disease, nurse theorists and researchers turned their attention to how individuals adapt to the disease condition itself. The general question has been, How does any individual adjust to a specific disease, disability, or medical treatment (e.g., an implantable cardioverter defibrillator) that represents some degree of permanent change? These changes require some time (anywhere from a few days to 2 years) for the individual to reach his or her highest level of adjustment. Of these, the greatest attention by far has been on chronic or chronic-like disease (e.g., diabetes, epilepsy, or one of the many types of cancer).

Over the last 20 years, the more specific question has been, Why do some individuals do better than others? In order to address this, nurses have identified a number of indicators and outcome measures to separate the successes from the failures in individuals' levels of adjustment. Measures have been used to cover physical or physiological adjustment, such as comorbidity indexes, activity scales, and lab values such as glycosylated hemoglobin levels for those with diabetes; and psychosocial adjustment, for example, the psychosocial adjustment to illness scale and various measures of affect and depression (Craney, 1997; Peterson, 1996; Tsai, Tak, Moore, & Palencia, 2003; Wortell, 1995). A few have used a single measure, for example, Rosenberg's mastery scale or a quality of life questionnaire to capture an individual's overall adjustment (Crigger, 1993; Dales, 2001; Kessenich, 1997). Somewhat surprisingly, there has been very little debate in the literature about what it means to be "fit" or "adapted."

A few scholars have focused either on describing the overall process and identifying factors that influence it, for example, Taanila and colleagues (2002), Reed (1997) and Dwyer (1993); or on one aspect of the adaptation process (i.e., Wiklinski's phenomenological study [1993] of the use of humor among patients with cancer). Most,

however, have looked at the process from a quantitative and explanatory angle. Some have drawn on loose theoretical notions from Dubos' (1965) work, for example, Warner (1996), Peterson (1996), and
Wortell (1995), while most have used specific theories of coping and
adaptation (e.g., Lazarus & Folkman's theory of stress and coping
[1984], Taylor's theory of cognitive adaptation [1983], Roy's adaptation theory) on which to build their hypotheses. When using one of
the coping theories, researchers usually use the term *adaptation* to
refer to the outcome and *coping* to refer to the process.

The role of the environment is not easy to decipher in the above
research, although it is clear that the classic way of looking at environment and adaptation as influencing disease patterns is of little (if
any) interest to nursing scholars. "Environment" is rarely identified
as a central concept in explaining why some individuals adjust better
than others do. Instead, variables, such as social support, are considered potential resources within the environment that act as facilitators
in patients' efforts to adjust rather than the major element to which
the patient is adjusting.

REFERENCES

Adolph, E. F. (1956). General and specific characteristics of physiological
adaptations. *American Journal of Physiology, 184,* 18–28.

Alland, A., Jr., & McCay, B. (1973). The concept of adaptation in biological
and cultural evolution. In J. J. Honigmann (Ed.), *Handbook of social
and cultural anthropology* (pp. 143–178). Chicago: Rand McNally.

Bertalanffy, L. von. (1968). *General system theory: Foundations, development, applications.* New York: Braziller.

Brown, M. I. (1963, October-November). Socialization—A social theory of
adaptation. *Nursing Science,* 280–294.

Cannon, W. B. (1931). *The wisdom of the body.* New York: Norton.

Cannon, W. B. (1932). *The wisdom of the body.* New York: Norton.

Carneiro, R. L. (1973). The four faces of evolution. In J. J. Honigmann (Ed.),
Handbook of social and cultural anthropology (pp. 89–110). Chicago:
Rand McNally.

Craney, J. M. (1997). Implantable cardioverter defibrillators and their physical and psychosocial outcomes. (Doctoral dissertation, Boston College,
1996). *Dissertation Abstracts B, 57*(10), 6175.

Crigger, N. J. (1993). An adaptation model for women with multiple sclero-
sis. (Doctoral dissertation, University of Florida, 1992). *Dissertation
Abstracts B, 54*(5), 2437.

Dales, C. M. (2001). Adaptation to breast cancer following an autologous peripheral blood stem cell transplant: A prospective study. (Master's thesis, University of Windsor). *Dissertation Abstracts, MAI 40/03,* 678.

Darwin, C. (1859). *The origin of species by means of natural selection or the preservation of favored races in the struggle for life.* London: Murray.

Dobzhansky, T. (1962). *Mankind evolving.* New Haven, CT: Yale University Press.

Dubos, R. (1965). *Man adapting.* New Haven, CT: Yale University Press.

Dwyer, M. L. (1993). The oncology patient's experiences in making a treatment decision. (Doctoral dissertation, Catholic University of America, 1993). *Dissertation Abstracts B, 54*(3), 1330.

Eisenstadt, S. N. (1968). Social evolution. In *International encyclopedia of the social sciences* (Vol. 3, pp. 228–234). New York: Macmillan and Free Press.

Encyclopedia of sociology. (1974). Guilford, CT: Dushkin.

Hall, B. A. (1991). Adaptability: A personal resource of health. *Scholarly Inquiry in Nursing Practice, 5*(2), 95–112.

Harris, M. (1968). *The rise of anthropological theory: A history of theories of culture.* New York: Thomas Y. Crowell.

Helson, H. (1964). *Adaptation-level theory: An experimental and systematic approach to behavior.* New York: Harper & Row.

Kessenich, C. R. (1997). Quality of life of elderly women with spinal fractures secondary to osteoporosis. (Doctoral dissertation, University of Alabama at Birmingham, 1996). *Dissertation Abstracts B, 57*(8), 4976.

Kim, H. S. (2000). *The nature of theoretical thinking in nursing* (2nd ed.). New York: Springer.

Lazarus, R. S., & Folkman, S. (1984). *Stress, appraisal, and coping.* New York: Springer Publishing.

Lenski, G., Lenski, J., & Nolan, P. (1995). *Human societies: An introduction to macrosociology* (7th ed.). New York: McGraw-Hill.

Lerner, M. L. (1968). *Heredity, evolution and society.* San Francisco: Freeman.

Levine, M. E. (1966). Adaptation and assessment: A rationale for nursing intervention. *American Journal of Nursing, 66,* 2450–2453.

Martin, H. W., & Prange, A. J., Jr. (1962). Human adaptation: A conceptual approach to understanding patients. *The Canadian Nurse, 3*(58), 243–243.

McElroy, A., & Townsend, P. K. (1996). *Medical anthropology in ecological perspective.* Boulder, CO: Westview Press.

Parsons, T. (1964). Evolutionary universals in society. *American Sociological Review, 29,* 339–357.

Peplau, H. E. (1963). Interpersonal relations and the process of adaptation. *Nursing Science,* 272–279.

Peterson, J. Z. (1996). Changes in hope and coping in older adults during rehabilitation after hip fracture. (Doctoral dissertation, University of Florida, 1995). *Dissertation Abstracts B, 57*(2), 991.

Piel, G., & Segerberg, O., Jr. (1990). *The world of René Dubos: A collection from his writings.* New York: Henry Holt.

Pitel, M. (1963, October-November). Physiological adaptation in man. *Nursing Science,* 263–271.

Reed, D. B. (1997). Occupational rehabilitation of farmers with upper-extremity amputations. (Doctoral dissertation, University of Kentucky, 1996). *Dissertation Abstracts B, 57*(9), 5577.

Roy, C. (1976). *Introduction to nursing: An adaptation model.* Englewood Cliffs, NJ: Prentice-Hall.

Roy, C. (1984). *Introduction to nursing: An adaptation model* (2nd ed.). Englewood Cliffs, NJ: Prentice-Hall.

Roy, C. (1997). Future of the Roy model: Challenge to redefine adaptation. *Nursing Science Quarterly, 10,* 42–48.

Roy, C., & Andrews, H. A. (1991). *The Roy adaptation model: The definitive statement.* Norwalk, CT: Appleton & Lange.

Roy, C., & Andrews, H. A. (1999). *The Roy adaptation mode* (2nd ed.). Stamford, CT: Appleton & Lange.

Roy, C., & Roberts, S. L. (1981). *Theory construction in nursing: An adaptation model.* Englewood Cliffs, NJ: Prentice-Hall.

Selye, H. O. (1956). *The stress of life.* New York: McGraw-Hill.

Service, E. R. (1968). Cultural evolution. In *International encyclopedia of the social sciences* (Vol. 3, pp. 221–227). New York: Macmillan and Free Press.

Taanila, A., Syrjala, L., Kokkonen, J., & Jarvelin, M. (2002). Coping of parents with physically and/or intellectually disabled children. *Child: Care, Health and Development, 28,* 73–86.

Taylor, S. (1983). Adjustment to threatening events: A theory of cognitive adaptation. *American Psychologist, 38,* 1161-1173.

Tsai, P., Tak, S., Moore, C., & Palencia, I. (2003). Testing a theory of chronic pain. *Journal of Advanced Nursing, 43,* 158–169.

Vassallo, C. (1965, August). A concept of health. *Nursing Science,* 236–242.

Warner, L. S. (1996). The relationship of selected psychosocial and pathophysiological variables to depression in epilepsy patients. (Doctoral dissertation, Catholic University of America, 1996). *Dissertation Abstracts B, 57*(5), 3132.

Washburn, S. L., & Lancaster, J. B. (1968). Human evolution. In *International encyclopedia of the social sciences* (Vol. 3, pp. 215–221). New York: Macmillan and Free Press.

Wiklinski, B. A. C. (1993). Has humor a meaning for persons adapting to a cancer experience? A phenomenological question. (Doctoral dissertation,

Columbia University Teachers College, 1993). *Dissertation Abstracts B* *54*(12), 6137.

Wortell, T. H. (1995). The physiological and psychosocial adaptation of individuals with insulin-dependent diabetes and non-insulin dependent diabetes. (Doctoral dissertation, University of Miami, 1994). *Dissertation Abstracts B, 55*(7), 2651.

CHAPTER 4

The Concept of Self-Care*

Ingrid Kollak

The prefix *self* is frequently used in the current debate on the requirements and the provisions of the health system. Yet, the dynamics of this prefix—gathering momentum in the 1960s when self-help groups demanded alternatives to prevailing structures and in the 1970s when self-administered space was conquered for autonomous cultural work, new forms of living, women's projects, and so forth—now seems long spent. Thus, the question arises as to which meaning *self-care* has taken on in present discussions on the shaping of the health and social systems, both at the societal level as well as at the levels of organization and the individual. These are the questions inquired into in the following essay, which analyzes the meaning of the term "self-care" in different kinds of practice.

SELF-CARE AND SOCIETY

With Dorothea Orem's model of self-care, professional nursing possesses its own theoretical reflections on determining individual needs and the consequent organization of provision. On the basis of the definitions drawn up by the North American Nursing Diagnosis Association, self-care can be defined as the personal abilities and actions that enable individuals to plan, organize, and carry out everything

---

*Translated from German by Gerald Nixon.

that is necessary for their own care. Self-care covers day-to-day as well as specific activities of self-preservation (Kollak, 2003, p. 595).

The social discourse on self-care in the health and social systems is increasingly focusing on what the individual and what a society can or must provide. A society, it is argued, cannot pay the costs of all the services in the health and social care of the individual because this could trigger the collapse of the social system. Statutory insurances, such as the health insurance schemes found in many countries of Europe, are not all-embracing insurance policies but only give partial financial recognition for nursing at home that is provided, for example, by relatives or friends or by qualified nursing staff. Furthermore, it is said, individuals must be ready to make a greater contribution to their own health care scheme in the form of supplementary payments in order to do something for the preservation of their personal health and thus, ultimately, social health. What forms these personal endeavors might take—which are to generate health en masse—can be seen in countless guides to health, ranging from the right diet to the proper things to put in the medicine cabinet and from personalized fitness and wellness programs to the ABCs of miracle cures. Financial contributions to self-care flow into life insurance endowment policies and private pension plans, some of which are directly dependent on the development of share prices.

Apparently, however, there is no longer any universal faith in a system whose security lies in the hands of institutionalized structures. It is above all the young, the healthy, and the employed who assume that their statutory insurance contributions are financing others who do nothing to provide for their own care. Yet, the very notion of providing comprehensive cover for one's own self-care and one's own later life no longer has any solid foundation. Indeed, people's sense of security is declining, making them pessimistic and causing them to put money, if they can, into their savings accounts. This feeling of insecurity relates not only to concrete concerns about their job, their pension, and their health but also to a vague anxiety about how they will react, both physically and mentally, to the loss of one or other of these. This is not self-help as a form of emancipation from views imposed on us by others, a discussion we had during the 1960s; on the contrary, self-help appears as something menacing, as an existential and psychological burden. Moreover, the equally significant debate in those days about emancipation from all kinds of authority no longer plays any role in the present social discourse on self-help. This may be attributed to a general feeling that there is hardly any influence on politics and politicians and little power in social movements. The vacuum created seems to be filling with all kinds of other "authorities," which have attracted publicity through new ways and means of organizing self-care and providing for later life—not to mention the patients themselves, who have become their own experts.

An interest in one's own interpretation of life and an orientation towards one's own life circumstances has given way to a sometimes exaggerated notion of being personally responsible for all situations in life. This has triggered a self-denunciation that constantly puts people under pressure. The spectrum of models on offer ranges from the rich and beautiful and the eternally young to the sharp-witted elderly. One must look after oneself today in order to be fit and able tomorrow to fend off possible financial and social or physical and mental disasters. The attraction of this notion varies in degree, depending on people's physical and mental as well as financial resources.

The apparent necessity appears to be omnipresent for continuous self-interrogation as an expression of the all-pervading fear of individual and social derailment due to illness and loss or as a result of social hazards and catastrophes. In times of potential or real crisis (whether experienced individually through illness or socially in the form of a disaster) there is an increased longing for the preservation of a normal state of things. By means of this category of the "normal," it is apparently possible to arrive at a flexible classification of all imaginable states within the framework of what is above and below the mean value of normality. At the same time the notion is being fostered that, piece by piece, a gradual narrowing of differences is achievable, a progressive normalization. This notion of normalization applies both to the case of medicine being taken after blood tests have revealed irregularities and to that of interest rates being lowered in order to bolster the world economy.

In his book *Versuch über den Normalismus [An Essay on Normalism]* Jürgen Link (1997) examines the place that normalism occupies in modern cultures and asks how one can respond to the fear of an unnoticed individual or collective deviation from normality, which is possible at all times. He distinguishes two different strategies of normalization with which equilibrium can be restored to private and collective processes of life which have been thrown off balance: the *protonormalistic* strategy, which places emphasis on "'rigid' semantic and symbolic demarcations of boundaries" and the *flexible normalistic* strategy, aiming at "'adaptable' and 'loose' semantic and symbolic demarcations" (Link, 1997, p. 79).

In an age when apparently all offered therapies—ranging from heart transplant to faith healing—exist side by side, a regulating power is gaining significance that refers not only to an arbitrary body as a continually possible improvement of personal attributes and abilities but also to an arbitrary population as a continuous process of correction and reforms. This permanent regulation is taking hold in all areas of social practice by dividing them into the categories of "normal" and "pathological." Once this differentiation is accepted, a host of binary opposites come to mind: socially useful or useless, beneficial to the health or detrimental, shoring up an order or undermining it, authentic in communication or artificial, and so on.

THE NOTION OF SOCIALLY USEFUL SELF-CARE

The forms of self-care that are deemed useful in today's discussion of the health system are those that require a "normal effort" and demand "socially affordable services." The individual's own contribution in the form of supplementary charges or additional support work is taken for granted. This way of looking at things considers self-care to be an essential component of existing health and social care arrangements and something that may be fairly demanded of people. Such a comprehensive form of collective self-help with the support of relatives, friends, or neighbors is taken as the norm, the given, and is naturally factored in when calculations are made and the organization planned. Self-care understood in this way is one of the pillars of health and social care. Without it, the whole social system would collapse. The value of self-care is enhanced in the debate by being presented as a suitable means of decreasing excessive numbers of hospital beds, lengths of stay on the wards and, in a nutshell, reducing costs. And then, of course, as a component of the health and social systems, self-care is governed by existing bureaucratic legislation and regulation.

The service providers of this system are above all married or unmarried couples along with their sons and daughters: "In order to reduce the high costs of nursing in residential facilities, unqualified but dedicated helpers are 'rewarded' for nursing members of their family at home with a bit of pocket money" (Bartholomeyczik, 1997, p. 201). The right to incorporate or even demand the organized help of the family or neighbors in arranging care is justified by the (repeatedly publicized) pressures of economics and demography as well as those arising from the spectrum of diseases involved. Despite the fact that family and neighborhood structures are constantly changing, meeting these demands is seen as the only way forward and the nursing of sick family members is equated with housework. Having looked after her children, it is argued, every woman has the know-how to care for sick relatives, friends, or neighbors; men who nurse their old and sick wives grow with their task. Professional counseling, which is anchored in the measures to ensure quality in the statutory long-term care insurance scheme, is often not worthy of the name.

SELF-CARE AND ORGANIZATION

Nursing tends to orient itself towards holistic concepts, which regard the human being as a biopsychosocial unit. Treating the sick should involve the body in relation to awareness and in the context of the prevailing social organization of a society. And, what is more, trained and qualified staff should not only be able to nurse the sick but also to make a contribution towards promoting health among the population.[1]

In her theory of self-care Dorothea Orem puts forward a concept of professional care. The highly favorable reception given to Orem's much discussed self-care model by the nursing community can be attributed to its orientation towards resources. But it could also be asked from the opposite perspective: Why has self-care been made an issue at all when there is a basic assumption that all individuals have a personal interest in taking measures themselves to ensure that they lead a satisfactory life? Why is the ability to carry out self-care discussed at all if everyone possesses this ability and uses it either according to the general circumstances or depending on needs specifically related to their development or their disease? Based on these assumptions, self-care is the given; hence, what really needs to be at the center of the discussion is the form and the content of nursing and care. If the ability for self-care is overemphasized, one might conclude that the only thing that matters is to gain acceptance for greater personal contribution or, alternatively, for supplementary charges while letting external experts decide about the necessary personal contributions and the appropriate charges.

According to Orem's model, the necessary professional care is legitimized by the diagnosed deficit remaining when the possibilities of self-care are exhausted. This results in the necessity of organizing a system of care provision, ranging from instruction to support and even acting on behalf of the patient, called by Orem the "supportive-educative, partly compensatory and wholly compensatory nursing system" (1991). The model interprets these deficits in self-care as being temporarily or partially limiting and thus having to be compensated for by professional nursing.

It has become clear that the term "self-care" varies between a rather narrow and a broader definition of the necessary provision of care and its costs. The term is suited to legitimizing situations of both excessive and insufficient provision. It can be used to justify both insufficient care imposed from outside as well as the best possible care of one's own choice. The concept of self-care oscillates between the greatest amount of restriction and the greatest amount of freedom.

A narrow understanding of self-care gives priority to definitions of diseases and recovery targets drawn up by experts. Its focus is on self-care deficits, and its characteristic features are a tendency towards wholly compensatory nursing and a strict division of tasks, among the various professional groups as well as between qualified and unqualified nursing staff. In this narrow understanding of the term, an over-valuation of economic resources goes hand in hand with an undervaluation of the patients' personal resources. A broader understanding of self-care takes into consideration the degrees of illness and health of the persons concerned, regards self-care ability as being of great value, and puts a focus on supportive and consultative care provision. Personal resources are emphasized and the necessity of financial support is given justification. It appears at the moment that the former strategies of normalizing tasks in the field of social health prevail over the latter.

THE NOTION OF THE PROPER ORGANIZATION OF SELF-CARE

In the 1960s, opposition to the different forms of deciding diagnosis and treatment without the participation of the patient led to people getting together and forming self-help groups. They made a distinction between existing health and social care provided either by state-run institutions or by private, market-oriented organizations on the one hand and an alternative form of care provision based on free choice on the other. By forming self-help groups, they reacted not only to economic difficulties but also to such habits as the patronizing behavior of professionals and the belittling of existential crises.

Hence, the concerns of the critics of the strategy succinctly named "Help towards Self-help" were related, from its beginnings until well into the 1990s, above all to the unmet demands of the self-help movement for autonomy and free choice. So-called "staged self-help groups" thus attracted particular attention in that period. "Typical of such staged forms of organized self-help are therefore—apart from helping without charge—the spontaneity with which the groups are founded and the voluntary nature of the participation" (*Lexikon des Sozial- und Gesundheitswesen* [LSG], 1992).

Today one might say, cynically, that there are no limits to "helping without charge," but that would be to overlook the core of the statement relating to spontaneity and voluntary participation. It was precisely the absence of these two qualities that was the hallmark of the forms of organization considered to be "institutionalized." There was skepticism about what they could achieve:

> For one thing, in connection with the discussion on individualization and liberalization, a general skepticism has been gaining ground about social constellations such as the family, the neighborhood or a religion-based community. The obligation to help, which is anchored in such social constellations, is frequently perceived as a pressure which hinders the development of creativity, spontaneity and personal freedom. Furthermore, these social constellations entail wide-ranging obligations to help which impose on the members in many respects—in principle one could say in every respect—the duty to be there for each other. (*Lexikon des Sozial- und Gesundheitswesen* LSG, 1992)

Individualization and liberalization are still (or again) highly valued today, and for some reason or other, it is precisely the social constellations of family and neighborhood that seem to have been selected as suitable grounds for developing these qualities. Here, the public discourse is "liberal" enough to grant unmarried couples, same-sex partnerships, patchwork families, and others, free, self-financed and self-provided self-care.

And what has become of the organizations once labeled "staged"? In recent years these self-help groups have grown and now number many thousands. Under the heading "Berlin is the Capital of Self-help," the Berlin Self-help Contact and Information Office" (Selbsthilfe Kontakt-und Informationsstelle [SEKIS]) puts the present number of existing self-help groups at over 2,000 discussion groups as well as roughly 1,000 that have established themselves as clubs. Similar figures are also to be found in large cities of the United States.

Is self-help an outward expression of "organized helplessness" (Göpel, 1988, p. 154)? The Web site of the Berlin association named above provides only a very general description of the work of self-care groups: giving mutual support, gathering information and knowledge, developing alternative forms of coping with problems, reducing social isolation and anxiety, undertaking activities together, training self-assurance in dealing with professionals, developing perspectives and contents to fill life with, and encouraging each other to assert their rights (SEKIS, 2004). These offers are reminiscent of the flippant remark "Nice that we've been able to have a chat about it," although this observation refers solely to the outward presentation and is in no way meant to say anything about the actual work carried out by individual self-help groups.

The information provided by the SEKIS Web site on the political and theoretical foundations of the movement is also as general as one can possibly imagine, with the enumeration of the Ottawa Charter, the concept of empowerment, the tradition of the alternative movement as well as holism, autonomy, self-determination, and solidarity (SEKIS, 2004). The World Health Organization's (WHO) definition of health as a state of complete physical, mental, and social well-being was viewed by Fritz Simon as the "promise of salvation of a worldly-oriented sect" (Simon, 1996, p. 10). Oscillating between promised salvation and total inspection are also the possible meanings of the words listed above (empowerment, holism, etc.). As already stated, the concept of holism can be applied, on the one hand, to all areas of an arbitrary individual as a continuous improvement of abilities (e.g., dealing with professionals) and qualities (e.g., developing alternative forms of coping with problems). This interpretation recalls the historical roots of self-care in Germany, which dates back to 1929, the year of its entrenchment in the law. As conceptualized by the German Ministry of Labor, the aim of the law on "help towards self-help" was "to strengthen the will and vigor of the needy in such a way that they are able to maintain themselves through their own ability, effort and work" (Woeterbuch Soziale Arbeit, 1996, p. 490). The Ministry's formulation "maintain themselves through their own ability, effort and work" might be brought up-to-date with the term "empowerment."

SELF-CARE AND THE INDIVIDUAL

As we have already seen, the debate on the preservation of health through one's own personal effort leads to a continual self-interrogation. But this is not all; it also leads to comparing oneself to others. The wish to protect oneself against damage to one's health and against physical, mental, and social vulnerability seems to be concealed behind the practice of making comparisons with others. This is undoubtedly a part of the attraction of self-help groups. Yet, self-experience can also take on forms of personal self-examination in exceptional circumstances. These then find expression in peak performance, whether in sport, dieting, or in mental training. Profiting from these ascetic (though expensive) modes of self-castigation are the leisure, fitness, and "wellness" industries. What is of interest in these new forms of personal challenge is that through constant self-interrogation and persistent comparison with others, people are no less controlled from outside and no less determined by others than such dated therapies as sleeping cures or fattening diets, as propagated by Silas Weir Mitchell in his book *Fat and Blood and How to Make Them* (cited in Kollak, 1995, p. 165). Today this kind of book would be published by a famous model (or her ghostwriter) and called *How to Achieve Success and Beauty with the Light Diet. My Personal Tips and Tricks.*

THE NOTION OF THE RIGHT KIND OF CARE FOR THE SELF

The power of defining what is "normal" and what is "pathological," which is at the center of this debate, seems to have become a never-ending social and individual task. Should a legitimization be needed from the point of view of labor laws, then this is given by way of a medical diagnosis. Doctors are allotted the task of identifying health problems by inquiry and examination and of formulating the problems discovered in a diagnosis—no matter how vague these may appear. Patients, who reveal themselves to their doctor in the course of their conversation in order to obtain a diagnosis and therapy, do this because they require a legal justification or they hope to find a solution to their problem, or both.

In entrusting themselves to the hands of professionals, in believing the diagnoses, and in following advice on therapy, the patients act correctly. This relationship is of advantage to doctors because it increases their prestige as well as their income. In exchange, patients are certified sick and can stay away from work. They pay for the diagnosis, accept their dependence by doing so and, furthermore, they delegate responsibility to the doctor for the successful completion of all therapeutic measures.

This is comparable with the currently established procedures for certifying the need of long-term care in Germany. Even people in need of care require a legitimization from a doctor, and after submitting an application and undergoing an examination, they are put into a category of care corresponding to their state of health. Patients pay the care allowance they receive to a care provider or nursing home, for example.

"Expert in one's own case" is a phrase that has gained great prominence in this debate on the right kind of care for the individual. The impression is almost given that she or he could become the prized and treasured partner of every professional working in the health and social departments. What role does the patient play, as his or her "own expert" who has become the subject of social health empowerment? In my understanding of things, the meanings of these terms are too elusive. If we assume that individuals have an interest in independent self-care based on their needs, then, by analogy, they are experts in this matter, too. Declaring them experts just means that there are restrictions with regard to certain services or to the way these services are provided. This is the same level at which the debate on empowerment is taking place. Lay persons are trained by the professional either to accept subservience or to get the job done by themselves. The choice does not really seem attractive; there is a creeping sense of disempowerment.

Thus, the self-help movement in Germany, which is today organized in networks all over the country, deplores the fact that it is not accepted by professionals. On the SEKIS Web site, the lack of recognition is apparent when self-assurance in dealing with professionals is included in the list of the movement's aims or when members are urged to encourage each other to assert their rights (SEKIS, 2004). The difficulty of achieving equal rights in the work between patients and professionals seems to lie in the nature of the work itself: in cases of acute and chronic sickness, patients depend on immediate help or sustained support and need a medical legitimization of the state of their health, for example, in order to obtain money from insurance funds. Doctors, on the other hand, profit from this situation both financially and socially, in particular when they are highly specialized, for instance, as heart surgeons or even plastic surgeons.

A Tentative Summing Up
of the Discussion on Self-Care

In the current debate on social health, all conceivable meanings have been ascribed to the term "self-care." On the one hand, the aim of self-care is to help organize the normalization of social and individual life processes when the balance of these processes has been upset by hazards and disasters or by sickness, loss, and dependence. On the other hand, self-care is aimed at effectively sustaining individual and social normality in the long term. The resulting strategies that have been developed for the continuous improvement of personal abilities and qualities, as well as the constant reform of social conditions, are oriented towards either the greatest possible narrowing, fixing, and stabilizing of the "normality zone" or towards the greatest possible expansion and dynamics of the normality zone. Even if sometimes semantically "rigid" and sometimes semantically "loose" terms are brought into play, it must be taken into consideration "that we are talking about two polar types of strategy (constructed as ideal types) and not two [temporally] separate, discontinuous ones." Both strategies, in fact, operate in parallel and alternating fashion and are interwoven with each other on the field of normalism (Link, 1997, p. 81). In the end, the question remains whether, ultimately, the significance of the debate on self-care between the disintegration of existing systems of support and the development of emancipatory health promotion is to be judged in terms of the allocation of funds.

Note

1. This is in accordance with the new designation of the vocation of "health and sickness nurse" in Germany, protected by law since 2004.

References

Bartholomeyczik, S. (1997). Aufopferung oder Lohnarbeit? [Self-sacrifices or wage work?] In A. Mühlüm, S. Bartholomeyczik, & E. Göpel (Eds.), *Sozialarbeitswissenschaft, Pflegewissenschaft, Gesundheitswissenschaft* (pp. 199–202). Freiburg, Germany: Lambertus.
Göpel, E. (1988). Gesundheit ist mehr. Selbsthilfe im Gesundheitswesen. [Health care is more. Self-care in public health] In Selbsthilfezentrum

München [Self-help center of Munich] (Hrsg.), *Zurück in die Zukunft. Selbsthilfe und gesellschaftliche Entwicklung* (pp. 142–162). München, Germany: Profil.

Kollak, I. (1995). *Literatur und Hypnose. Der Mesmerismus und sein Einfluß auf die Literatur des 19. Jahrhunderts [Literature and hypnosis. Mesmerism and its influence on the literature of the 19th century].* Frankfurt, Germany: Campus.

Kollak, I. (2003). Selbstpflege [Self-care]. In *Pschyrembel Woerterbuch Pflege [Pschyrembel: Dictionary of nursing]* (pp. 595–596). Berlin: de Gruyter.

Lexikon des Sozial- und Gesundheitswesen [Dictionary of social and health sciences]. (1992). München, Germany: R. Oldenbourg.

Link, J. (1997). *Versuch über den Normalismus. Wie Normalität produziert wird [Attempt at normalism. How normality is produced].* Opladen, Germany: Westdeutscher.

Orem, D. E. (1991). *Nursing: Concepts of practice* (4th ed.). St. Louis, MO: Mosby.

Pschyrembel Wörterbuch Pflege [Pschyrembel: Dictionary of nursing]. (2003). Berlin: de Gruyter.

Selbsthilfe Kontakt- und Informationsstelle [Self-help contact and information center]. (2004). http://www.sekis-berlin.de

Simon, F. B. (1996). *Die andere Seite der Gesundheit. Ansätze einer systemischen Krankheits- und Therapietheorie [The other side of health. Starting points of a systemic illness and therapeutic theory].* Heidelberg, Germany: Carl-Auer.

Woeterbuch Soziale Arbeit [Dictionary of social work]. (1996). 4th ed. Weinhein, Germany: Beltz.

CHAPTER 5

The Concept of Interaction in Theory and Practice*

Susanne Wied

In the field of nursing and care, the term *interaction* is used in an exceedingly vague manner. There are three basic concepts to choose from, each of which will be examined in the theoretical section, in which no claim is made to any exhaustive treatment of the term's usage. The aim of this contribution, rather, is to look into and clarify aspects of the notion of interaction that are relevant to both the theory and practice of nursing.

Interaction has much to do with language. Today, it is scarcely possible to separate the term from the notion of communication, and also the written word constitutes a form of communication within the system of nursing and care.

In this contribution, the considerations are confined to interactions between people. It might be added, however, that should one wish to set aside the psychosocial conceptualization of the term, it is equally rewarding and important to examine interactions between fields or systems. But this means moving onto a different plane of the notion of interaction, leading to an abstract, epistemological discussion of the subject. Today there is greater acceptance of the theoretical side of nursing and such a discussion is now possible without

---

*Translated from German by Gerald Nixon.

producing what has been called "contemporary esoteric 'episto' babble." In addition to the now conventional use and application of fundamental psychological, humanistic, and sociological concepts in the context of nursing and care, we can identify newly specified concepts in, for example, kinesthetic, physical, or physiological contexts.

In the *Der Duden* (*[Duden Book of Loanwords]*, 1982) the term *interaction* is defined as "mutually related actions of two or more persons" and "reciprocal relationships between partners". The term is generally regarded as belonging to the fields of sociology and psychology. In Fuchs-Heinritz's *Dictionary of Sociology* (*[Lexikon der Soziologie]*, 1994) interaction is first defined in the basic sense of its Latin source as "reciprocal effect," before being divided into its manifold meanings; and among these a special place is given to "social interaction." According to the renowned sociologist, Talcott Parsons (1949), interaction denotes the social actions performed between two people (*ego* and *alter*). These actions are reciprocally oriented towards fulfilling the expectations of the other. Interaction is bound up with social roles and governed by common regulative norms. In the work of the social psychologist George Herbert Mead (1934), the focus is placed on the actions of partners performed through symbols that have the same meaning for both partners. Basing his assumptions on his ethnographic studies, Goffman (1967) distinguishes between centered and noncentered interaction. Here, the attention of the partners is directed towards common points of reference (e.g., social occasions); the partners cooperate in order to maintain these points of reference and if they are jeopardized, sanctions are imposed. Otherwise, in accumulating information, the interactants concentrate on their perception of each other. In their *Pragmatics of Human Communication* (1967) Watzlawick, Beaver, and Jackson consider interaction from the perspective of communication theory and defined systemically as the sending and receiving of messages between two or more persons. We will return to this theoretical approach at a later point.

In its colloquial usage, the term *interaction* is heard when topics take a psychosociological or sociopsychological turn—although, in effect, it is nebulously used in the basic sense of the mutual effects of whatever happens when two things come into contact with each other. In *Worterbuch der Psychiatrie und Medizinischen Psychologie* (*[Dictionary of Psychiatry and Medical Psychology]*, 1977), interaction is defined as "a kind of mutual relationship between the members of a group . . .", although it is not made clear whether it applies to the relationship between the individuals or between their messages. The interpretation is left to the reader. It is this very lack of clarity in the notion of relationship that causes the difficulty with, and the diffuse nature of the notion of interaction. When we talk about interaction, we are not writing, speaking, reading, or thinking about the same thing; as Mead would put it, we are not basing the linguistic symbol "interaction" on the same meaning.

INTERACTION AND NURSING THEORY

In order to illustrate the diffuse usage of the term, we should, in the following, consider in more detail the views of such nursing scholars as Meleis (1991), Fawcett (1993, 1995), Peplau (1962), King (1981), and Paterson and Zderad (1970/71, 1988), who categorize interaction as superordinate theoretical concept orders.

Meleis (1991) dates the rise of an "interactionist" school of thought in nursing to the 1950s and early 1960s. According to her, the theories of this school were centered on the development of a relationship between patient and nurse. They "focused their attention on the process of care and on the ongoing interaction between nurses and clients. Their theories were based on interactionism, phenomenology, and existentialist philosophy" (Meleis, 1991, p. 255). Accordingly, she categorizes the theories proposed by King, Paterson and Zderad, and Peplau as "interaction theories."

In defining the role of nursing, Meleis summarizes King's view as a "process of action, reaction, and interaction whereby nurse and client share information about their perceptions of the nursing situation and agree on goals" (Meleis, 1991, p. 256). She also summarizes the definition of interaction by Paterson and Zderad as a "human dialogue, intersubjective transaction, a shared situation, a transactional process, a presence of both patient and nurse" (1991, p. 256). Peplau's definition is summarized by Meleis as a "therapeutic interpersonal, serial, goal-oriented process; a health-focused human relationship" (1991, p. 256).

King puts the focus of nursing on "nurse-patient interactions that lead to goal attainment in a natural environment" (Meleis, 1991, p 256). Paterson and Zderad, on the other hand, see the focus of nursing in the assumption that the "patient is a unique being; the patient's perception of events; both patient and nurse are the focus" (Meleis, 1991, p. 256). For Peplau, the focus is on the "nurse-patient relationship and its phases: orientation, identification, exploitation, and resolution;

harnessing energy from anxiety and tension to positively defining, understanding, and meeting productively the problem at hand" (Meleis, 1991, p. 256).

According to King, the goals of nursing are to "help individuals maintain their health so they can function in their role" (Meleis, 1991, p. 257), while Paterson and Zderad consider them to be "to develop human potential, more well-being for both patient and nurse" (Meleis, 1991, p. 257). Peplau, on the other hand, sees nursing goals as "develop[ing] personality, making illness an eventful experience; forward movement of personality and other ongoing human processes in the direction of creative, constructive, productive personal and community living" (Meleis, 1991, p. 257).

Problems in nursing arise, according to King, "when nurse and patient do not perceive each other or the situation; they do not communicate information; transactions are not made; goals are not attained" (Meleis, 1991, p. 257). For Paterson and Zderad problems occur when "people with perceived needs [are] related to the health/illness quality of living" while, in Peplau's view, problems are the result of "unsuccessful or incomplete learning of life tasks; energy used in tensions and frustrations due to unmet needs" (Meleis, 1991, p. 257).

Thus, in Meleis' categorization of interaction theories we are presented with three different theoretical currents. King's approach has its source, first, in the publications of Peplau (and in other respects also in Martha Rogers) and, second, in the sociologically oriented studies of interaction carried out by authors like Parsons.

One aspect that does not stand out strongly enough in Meleis' categorization is the clear orientation towards systems theory expressed in King's writings. Indeed, in her further elaboration of interaction theories, Meleis defines interaction not from the point of view of communication theory but rather (if at all) from a humanistic standpoint in keeping with the approaches taken by Paterson and Zderad (see Meleis, 1991, pp. 258–260). We will return to these differences later.

Peplau's approach, on the other hand, is clearly derived from an analytically oriented psychiatry represented by Sullivan. Peplau has never claimed to have developed her own distinct theory. What she has done is to make the knowledge gained in a psychodynamically oriented psychiatry productive and fruitful for nursing, and this has given utmost clarity to her view of interaction. Here, we are dealing with individuals who have entered a relationship with each other that can be divided into clear phases and has clear objectives. Interaction is used as an instrument with which to release the potential for development in individuals and initiate processes of learning and maturing. In contrast to the systems approach, there is no separation between message, or information, and person; instead, one person is put in relation to another in the concept of transference and countertransference. With regard to nursing, we thus have a clear and unequivocal concept of action that can be very well applied to an analytical or psychodynamic setting.

When we move into a systems-oriented or family-oriented context of therapy, whether on the ward or elsewhere, we are drawn into problems of interface because we are mixing two notions of interaction: the relationship approach based on persons, and the systems approach based on information, on which a large part of King's theory (1981) is based. Here, however, it is necessary to separate—merely theoretically, of course—the person from the information, or message. The person as a "system" (which is vigorously disputed among sociologically oriented systems theorists), that is, an individual, exchanges information with another person, resulting in a system of its own that, detached from the individuals giving the information, constitutes interaction. The exchange of words and gestures in the system family (which King calls the interpersonal system), for example, results in a dynamic process that takes place independently of the participants or, as Watzlawick writes, "once structures of communication have been formed, they develop a life of their own which the individual participants are largely powerless to control" (Watzlawick, 1996, p. 48). These "self-organizing systems" are sometimes more "enduring" than the persons involved—a phenomenon that everyone knows who has enjoyed the peculiar fascination of family get-togethers. The same holds true for what King calls the "social systems" operating in hospitals. Here, patterns of communication continue to exist long after the roles originally allotted have changed. King does not consistently maintain the systems approach in her theory because she would otherwise demand from nurses a considerably greater ability to detach themselves. By regarding interaction as the exchange of information, we keep ourselves, as persons, as detached as we possibly can from what is taking place and instead analyze the "wholes" of the highly complex and labyrinthine process of communication in order to contribute to an explanation of, as well as a change in, the structures. Expressed in terms of the chaos theory, we destroy, in the therapeutic context, old attractors (patterns of order in chaotic vortices) only to establish new ones elsewhere. In the case of radical systems models, for example, that of Tschacher, we have no intention—contrary to humanistic or analytical approaches—of bringing ourselves to bear in our quality as individuals and human beings. That we nevertheless remain individuals and human beings constitutes the informal part of the relationship, not the professional. Here, Tschacher arrives at an important conclusion:

> It is quite possible that the new attractor leads to other problems as well as new sufferings. Who is to take responsibility in view of the complex causality of self-organized systems. The desire not to cause harm does not eliminate the risks involved in effective intervention. I fear that ethical notions of responsibility are—at least partially—irreconcilable with systems thinking since the latter can remain neither centered on the person nor linearly causal. (Tschacher, 1990, p. 162)

In her systems theory, King ultimately remains centered on the person—which, unfortunately with regard to interaction, waters down her otherwise sensible and logical approach. She thus defines interaction as a "process of perception and communication between person and person as well as person and environment, represented by verbal and non-verbal behaviors that are goal-directed" (Fawcett, 1995, p. 139). This definition remains unclear because of the notion of behavior that is introduced into it without being defined. And whether interaction is always goal-directed is a moot point. Furthermore, we must examine whether it is possible to describe an individual as a personal "system" without getting into difficulty with perhaps incompatible subsystems within the "system" of the human being. A satisfactory answer to this assumption has yet to be found. The counterhypothesis—put forward for example by Luhmann (1984) that we can equate individuals not with systems but with entities—is far more convincing from the point of view of a systems theory, but it is not possible to elaborate on this here. It must also be borne in mind that in her later writings Martha Rogers no longer speaks of the human being as an open system. However, with a mixed form of personal and informational interaction, which has no conceptual foundation, we are faced with a difficulty concerning the inner logic of King's theoretical edifice. Even though she calls her theory a general systems theory, her assumptions tend to be based on Parson's model of social roles within the "system" of society.

Paterson and Zderad's humanistic approach (O'Connor, 1993; Paterson & Zderad, 1970/71, 1988) presents people in dialogue with each other. It is based explicitly on Carl Rogers' humanistic psychology and on the philosophies of religion drawn up by Buber and

Marcel. These two authors chose phenomenology as their method. The key aspect of their notion of nursing is the ability to empathize, although they are at pains to stress that they are talking of "clinical empathy"—something that must be trained and does not lead to the merging of two persons and "being one" with each other but which, through the very ability to detach oneself, is able to create genuine therapeutic closeness (Zderad, 1969, pp. 655–657). What we find here is thus a humanistic rather than a systems or psychological approach: It is an approach in which interaction is understood as a deeply sincere and in no way "directive" encounter between people.

Humanistic and existentialist approaches to nursing enjoy great popularity among German-speaking students of nursing and also among conference participants who come into contact with nursing theory. However, one must not underestimate the dangers lurking in the admirably humane concepts of earlier thinkers. Without adequate training but with great moral goals, people who do not give sufficient reflection to how such methods are to be implemented quickly exhaust themselves. The profound existential and spiritual experience that can be gained in nursing urgently requires the ability to detach oneself. If not, it is possible that the basic concept of nursing is perverted and nurses cling to patients in order to fill their own empty existence. Unconsciously, they abuse their power in their dealings with the people entrusted to their care or, conversely, they allow themselves to be misused. The goal of "maturing" together with the patient demanded by humanistic theorists should be regarded with caution. In the writings of Carl Rogers and Martin Buber these goals are expressed with far greater modesty and with less pathos. It may be added that both men were quite aware that they were not true scientists or true philosophers. It is a fundamental, ethical disposition, which brings forth the desire to encounter people "without constraints" and "in a dialogue" rather than a scientific model drawn up from humanistic theories. Such a disposition is thus valuable for anyone working in a therapeutic context, especially in view of the ethical problems (e.g., systems thinking) discussed above. Nursing theorists, however, become involved in highly complicated communication structures (in systems terminology) when they present this disposition and this goal as a science in the presence of other scientists.

The question that remains is whether any purpose is served by categorizing such divergent currents of thought under the heading "interaction theories." The distinctions are clear enough when one reads Meleis' actual words, but they become greatly obscured in the pedestrian summaries of theory categorizations that have adorned nursing journals for years.

Fawcett's categorization is clearer (1995, p. 20). For her an "interactive approach" has a clear sociological foundation and is bound up with the notions of perception, communication, role, and self-image. She has no use for tabular categorizations of the supposed currents followed by different theorists, merely providing the reader with an overview of categorizations already undertaken by other authors.

Thus, for the context of nursing, no satisfactory definition of the term "interaction" has yet been found, even if the case studies described by Peplau (1962) and Friedemann (1996), for example, lead one to suspect that the authors have indeed drawn up a very clear concept of interaction for themselves.

INTERACTION AND HUMAN COMMUNICATION

Wittgenstein ends his *Tractatus Logico-Philosophicus* with the following words: "Whereof one cannot speak thereof one must be silent" (1963/1994, p. 115). Yet everyday we do the exact opposite and try to express in words and make understandable things that cannot be rendered understandable—the *ego* to the *alter*; or, as Canetti writes, "How much one must say in order to be heard when one is silent at last" (1976, p. 58).

It would be presumptuous to claim that one could explain such complex phenomena as interaction and communication in a complete and comprehensive manner. Our sense organs are by no means capable of recording all elements and although retrospective analysis (e.g., video replay) makes us all the wiser with the benefit of hindsight, we still have no chance of achieving this: After the event, in a two-dimensional perspective and with changes in sounds and colors, we have moved on to another plane, that is, that of communication technology. In spite of this, almost everyone believes they understand their fellows. There are a few who go insane in order not to have to carry on the business of believing they understand their fellows. And there are those, too, who, with the aid of such methods as hermeneutics or linguistic and systems analysis, try to pick up and follow the thread of wool through the labyrinth of human communication, thus spending their lives as philosophers, writers, or researchers in the field of communication and, of late, as nursing theorists.

A quite useful and practicable model for nursing, in the author's view, has been provided by the research studies undertaken by

Watzlawick and colleagues. Thus, the key axioms of this model will be presented briefly before turning to further concepts. Watzlawick's observation that "one cannot not communicate" has now apparently become an integral part of the repertoire of modern catchphrases such as "holistic nursing" or "maintaining standards." This observation, however, which forms his first pragmatic axiom (Watzlawick et al., 1967, p. 51), is the product of a research study carried out over many years on a solid systems theory basis. At the core of the research is the study of the pragmatics of human communication, the term "pragmatics" being taken from semiotics (in linguistics, the study of signs). The aim of the study was not to seek an explanation for the essence or nature of behavior but to describe the observable manifestations of human relationships. According to Watzlawick, the vehicle of such manifestations is communication (1967, p. 21).

Single acts of communication are called messages; a sequence of reciprocal messages between two or more persons is called interaction. These terms are thus intimately connected with each other.

The material for communication is understood to be every kind of sign, whether verbal or nonverbal, that is, all forms of behavior. As in semiotics, communication is divided into three fields: syntactics, semantics, and pragmatics. Syntactics deals purely with problems of sending and receiving information (codes, redundancy, etc.); semantics has to do with the meaning of message symbols; and pragmatics is concerned with the effects of communication on the behavior of those taking part in it. This division, of course, is purely theoretical and the three fields are closely interwoven in real-life communication. The study examined the basic features of communication as well as interference in it. Unlike King, Watzlawick does not go as far as to present the reader with an ideal model of communication; instead, especially through his analysis of its interference, he contributes to the possibility of developing more effective tools of understanding. A further observation by Watzlawick also deserves attention. Communication research has only natural language at its disposal, even if it is a question of meta-communication, that is, communication about communication. In contrast to what happens in mathematics, this leads to a lack of precision in formulating messages, a familiar phenomenon no doubt to anyone involved in nursing.

His first axiom, "One cannot not communicate" (Watzlawick et al., 1967, p. 51), is an axiom of meta-communication. His second axiom is "Every communication has a content and a relationship aspect such that the latter classifies the former and is therefore meta-communication." The content aspect simply transmits the message (or data) while the relationship aspect shows how the message is to be understood (Watzlawick et al., 1967, p. 54).

His third axiom is "The nature of a relationship is contingent upon the punctuation of the communicational sequences between the communicants" (Watzlawick et al., 1967, p. 59). It is not a question of whether this "punctuation" is good or bad but simply that it organizes behavioral events (Watzlawick et al., 1967, p. 56).

His fourth axiom states

> Human beings communicate both digitally and analogically. Digital language has a highly complex and powerful logical syntax but lacks inadequate semantics in the field of relationship, while analogue language possesses the semantics but has no adequate syntax for the unambiguous definition of the nature of relationships. (Watzlawick et al., 1967, p. 66–67).

Human beings alone have at their disposal both analogue and digital modes of communication, analogue language signifying more archaic forms such as gesturing or tone of speech; and digital language signifying, for example, abstractions in language, or as Bateson puts it, "There is nothing particularly five-like about the number five; there is nothing particularly table-like about the word 'table'" (Watzlawick et al., 1967, p. 62).

Watzlawick's fifth axiom is "All communicational interchanges are either symmetrical or complementary, depending on whether they are based on sameness or difference" (Watzlawick et al., 1967, p. 70). These axioms (which according to Watzlawick are only tentatively formulated) provide us with a well-structured instrument with which to observe interaction before becoming ensnared in interpretations, which make purpose-oriented interaction more difficult. Behavior, here, is not coupled as a stimulus/response pattern; nor is it related to Parson's notion of roles. In cases of interference in interaction it would be better to look at the communication structures drawn up by Watzlawick instead of resorting to the concept of stress, which King has built into her theory. It must be borne in mind that messages are not limited to the verbal (digital) plane and that most frequently it is nonverbal messages in particular that make up the more direct plane that determines a relationship.

We should now consider the reasons why in nursing it is preferable to choose an approach to interaction based on communication theory. The psychodynamic approach does not make full use of the knowledge secured by the neurosciences. Taking over a specific role (as mother, daughter, teacher, etc.) as a surface of projection or transference may have its attraction for the patient and has undoubtedly proved effective in psychotherapeutic practice (as suggested by Peplau, 1962, for example); however, in a context of bioscience-oriented psychiatry or somatics, clashes arise that draw nurses into interaction with neighboring professional groups in which there is a potential for conflict. Thus, they use up time and energy that would be better spent on interaction with the patient. This is not meant as a criticism of methods but as an appeal to examine whether theoretical approaches can be coupled with their respective practice. With regard to the humanistic approach, it has already been stated above that it may be used to form a personal inner attitude but not misused as a moral stick to be wielded every day in the theory and practice of nursing. The world has enough ills to recover from without adding nursing to them. It might be observed that, as far as our commitment and efficacy in the maturing and development of our fellow humans are concerned, we have just as little cause for immodesty as other professional groups. Thus, the more sober our view is of communication structures regarding patients, their relatives, our own and other professions as well as the conditions under which things are organized, the more realistic the prospects are of being able to work effectively with all the valuable approaches that have been formulated in recent years.

INTERACTION—A NURSING SCIENCE PERSPECTIVE

In the preceding sections we have been mainly concerned with sociologically and humanistically oriented concepts of interaction that have also been integrated by and large into classical nursing theories. However, further planes of interaction can be identified that are of significance in reflections on nursing science and nursing practice. These include processes of interaction at the physical, physiological, and kinesthetic levels, which will be elucidated by means of examples in the following.

The prime classical nursing theory, combining the knowledge of modern physics and systems theory in the context of nursing, is the *Science of the Unitary Human Being* (Rogers, 1970). This theory is based on the principle of "integrality," the name given to the reciprocal process, that is, "interaction," between the energy fields of human beings and their surroundings. It serves as a suitable theoretical framework when considering nursing from an integrative scientific perspective. The principles, formulated rather abstractly more than 30 years ago, sound like mere truisms in today's context of interdisciplinary research. Of epistemological significance, however, is the fact that some 10 years before other, now common names in nursing theory, Martha Rogers was a successful proponent of an integrative approach to knowledge that in other fields of science (as well as in large sections of the nursing scientific community) can still lead to serious difficulties today in conveying it to others. Her theory, now commonly available (albeit frequently in short definitions of the terminology), does not have to be presented in any detail here. Only a number of special features that concern our topic of interaction are to be outlined because, from a modern perspective, they need to be given more differentiated treatment in order to counteract misunderstandings and avoid erroneous interpretations in future. Rogers makes an often quoted statement (but one that is rarely discussed in nursing literature) with regard to the separation between life and nonlife. She postulates that this separation, deriving from the different ways in which the sciences of biology, chemistry, and physics developed, can no longer be maintained. By doing so, she touches upon a fundamental question of human ontology on which there is no unanimous judgment. This academic difference of opinion essentially dates back as far as antiquity and has continued until today in the debate on holism. Regarding oneself as a human being uncoupled from nonlife implies in itself an ontological separation from one's natural surroundings—without which interaction between separate entities would never exist. Moreover, this is a difficult issue with regard to the process of dying, which Rogers calls "transformation." If we introduce a plane of observation that defines us as an electromagnetic, or "energy," field in the physical sense (Rogers, 1970, p. 1990), we are able to understand energy fields—for example in the context of molecular and atomic or even subatomic quantum processes—without the classical separation of life and nonlife (Dürr & Popp, 2000, p. 211; Popp & Belussov, 2003, p. 7). These fields have a reciprocal effect on each other, which on the one hand allows us to speak of interaction, but on the other leads us to the next difficulty. Because of this, Martha Rogers apparently preferred to speak of "integrality," and rightly so. Depending on the elements related to each other in open systems one can, strictly speaking, no longer talk of interaction in a quantum mechanics sense because the physical processes may be studied in a temporary or permanent context—depending on the type of observation and experiment—but cannot be pinned down exactly. In these highly complex units of effect and being, it is no longer possible to undertake clear definitions without being hopelessly reductionist. There are not three dimensions of space; according to recent quantum models, our material composition consists of concatenations (Smolin, 2003).

On the other hand, mutual effects between biological systems are not proved to be wrong; they merely fail to describe the complete process. Thus, although it is postulated in integrated biophysics (Popp & Belussov, 2003, p. 67), for example—as in Rogers' theory—that the description of the individual elements does not represent the whole, for reasons of pragmatism the whole is divided into parts in order to be able to acquire any knowledge at all. For the logical consequence of a renunciation of all—basically reductionist—observation of system and field interactions ("nondifferentiation") is not only a renunciation of interactions of entities, however they are separated, but also a disintegration, a resolution into entities of ever greater complexity. In recent years this paradox has turned the development of scientific theories into a tightrope walk between the different systems of scientific and philosophical thinking on the one side and the banality of so-called esoterics on the other. Communicative interactions (theory development, interdisciplinary cooperation, media presentation) inevitably cause the break up of the fixed defining framework that was conventional in the past. This could lead in certain circumstances to the problem of a quasi-religious reliance on (scientific) systems of belief because the complexities are neither linearly logical nor completely ascertainable, even with all the technical resources at our disposal. The study of complementary therapy and nursing methods is therefore always bound up with methodological difficulties. This explains the apparent contradiction between the postulate of human beings and their environment belonging to a common system in the energy-field concept and the theory now being postulated by Popp and his colleagues, which clearly restricts the presence of biophotons with their corresponding mitogenetic radiation exclusively to "living systems" (Popp, 2004) in a currently valid context of quantum mechanics. If one accepts this supposed contradiction, the concept of integrated biophysics can be used as valuable basic research for further studies with regard to observable physiological and energy-based nursing phenomena, for example in the study of light and colors and their effects on human beings (Wied, 1998, 2001).

However, it must be realized, strictly speaking, that for example in therapeutic touch (TT), one can no longer speak of the interaction of two energy fields since the two entities (therapist and patient) are non-differentiated for a period of time within the greater organization of the meta-environment (in quantum physics, Eastern concepts, philosophies, and Martha Rogers, too, this system extends pan-dimensionally to the whole universe). This does not put regulatory systems out of force, such as our blood circulation and other hierarchically structured physiological systems; however, other processes that have not yet been sufficiently explained enable the body to trigger neuronal and mental blockades, for example, to reduce pain. Yoga, t'ai chi, chi gong, and so forth ultimately have the same foundations. Miracle cures, incidentally, cannot be expected. The physical systems of the living body are not immortal (they are irreversible and unidirectional) and remain so even in concepts of complementary therapy.

With a clear focus on the given cultural or temporal context of nursing, it is very helpful to make more use again of scientific knowledge in order to be better able to elucidate and develop systems of interaction such as those operating in kinesthetics, for example.

The concept of interaction in kinesthetics refers to the reciprocal effect of sensory systems (Buchholz, 2003, p. 370). The human being perceives differences in stimuli of touch and movement, and nursing activities are developed that are oriented towards implementing practicable patterns of movement for nurses and patients. The literature distinguishes between the one-sided communication of information; the step-by-step mutual communication of information; and the simultaneous, joint communication of information (direct exchange). The patterns of movement are formed according to how much each of the partners in this interaction contributes with regard to the components of time, place, and energy input. In this strategy the interaction plane is concrete and tangible as well as being simply organized as far as functions are concerned. Implemented with the right attitude on the part of nurses, it makes quite a considerable contribution to the potential well-being of clients and patients. Originally developed as part of modern dance (Maretta, 1976), this strategy requires further investigation by nursing scientists; for example, with regard to disorders that restrict movement patterns or are accompanied by spasticity. Psychomotor interaction between the partners takes place with different determinants than in the case of healthy children or mobile adults. At the same time the combination of touch and movement in intensive nursing in cases of coma, coma vigils, or in the nursing of those who are disabled is frequently just about the only form of inter-action available. In Watzlawick's terminology, this form of interaction is an element of the nonverbal, analogue system of communication. Movement and touch stimuli must be carried out professionally and be "goal-directed" in order to have the desired effect. Taking some-one fondly in one's arms or stroking his or her forehead is also done, of course—whether consciously or subconsciously—with the inten-tion of making one's situation easier to endure.

Fitting analogies are conceivable for other variables of interac-tion and are already put into practice in aromatherapy and music therapy. Color and light have already been mentioned. The sense of smell/aroma as well as sound/music/hearing are further fields of in-teraction that are worth researching in more depth with a view to ap-plying them to nursing situations. Phenomena that are still entirely in need of elucidation are transitions from interaction to coherence or resonance, that is, reverberations between two systems leading to the harmonization of elements within an emergent system—a process, in-cidentally, that by no means takes place harmoniously, because the one system is able to force its rhythm on the other through its pat-terns of interaction.

In summary, it can be said that in nursing theory and practice the concept of interaction has on the one hand uncoupled itself from its fixed usage in socio-psychological terminology; but, despite its justi-fied use in the abstract perspective of the systems-energy complex, it can be focused again on concrete areas of application.

REFERENCES

Buchholz, T. (2003). Kinästhetik [Kinesthetic]. In S. Wied & A. Warmbrunn (Eds.), *Pschyrembel Wörterbuch Pflege*. Berlin: de Gruyter.

Canetti, E. (1976). *Die Provinz des Menschen [The human province]*. Ham-burg, Germany: Fischer.

Der Duden. (1982). *Das Fremdwörterbuch [Book of Loanwords]*. Vol 6. Mannheim, Germany: Duden.

Dürr, H. P., & Popp, F. W. (2000). *Elemente des Lebens—Naturwis-senschaftliche Zugänge—Philosophische Positionen [Elements of life—Approaches of natural science—Philosophical viewpoint]*. Zug, Germany: Die Graue Ed. Kusterdingen.

Fawcett, J. (1993). *Analysis and evaluation of nursing theories*. Philadelphia: F. A. Davis.

Fawcett, J. (1995). *Analysis and evaluation of conceptual models of nursing* (3rd ed.). Philadelphia: F. A. Davis.

Friedemann, M. (1996). *Familien und umweltbezogene Pflege [Family and environmental nursing].* Bern, Switzerland: Huber.

Fuchs-Heinritz, W. (Ed.) (1994). *Lexikon der Soziologie [Dictionary of Sociology].* Opladen, Germany: Westdeutscher.

Goffman, I. (1967). *Interaction ritual: Essays in face-to-face behavior.* Chicago: Aldine.

King, I. M. (1981). *A theory for nursing: Systems, concepts, process.* Albany, NY: Delmar.

Luhmann, N. (1984). *Soziale Systeme [Social Systems].* Frankfurt, Germany: Suhrkamp.

Maretta, H. L. (1999). *Kinästhetik—Gesundheitsentwicklung und Menschliche Funktionen [Kinesthetic—Health development and human functioning].* Ullstein, Germany: Mosby.

Mead, G. H. (1934). *Mind, self, and society from the standpoint of a social behaviorist.* (Edited with introduction by C. W. Morris). Chicago: University of Chicago Press.

Meleis, A. (1991). *Theoretical nursing: Development and progress* (2nd ed.). Philadelphia: Lippincott.

O'Connor, N. (1993). *Paterson & Zderad: Humanistic nursing theory.* Newbury Park, CA: Sage.

Parsons, T. (1949).*The structure of social action.* Glencoe, IL: Free Press.

Paterson, J. G., & Zderad, L. T. (1970/71). All together through complementary syntheses. *Image: Journal of Nursing Scholarship, 4,* 13–16.

Paterson, J. G., & Zderad, L. T. (1988). *Humanistic nursing.* New York: National League for Nursing.

Peplau, H. E. (1962). *Interpersonal relations in nursing.* New York: Putnam.

Popp, F. A. (2004). *About the coherence of biophotons.* Retrieved December 5, 2004, from the International Institute of Biophysics Web site: www.lifescientists.de/ib0204e_1.htm

Popp, F. A., & Beloussov, L. (2003). *Integrative Biophysics—Biophotonics.* Dordrecht, Netherlands: Kluwer.

Rogers, M. (1970). *An introduction to the theoretical basis of nursing.* Philadelphia: F.A. Davis.

Smolin, L. (2003). Welcome to quantum gravity. Special selection. *Physics World, 16,* 702.

Tschacher, W. (1990). *Interaktion in selbstorganisierten Systemen [Interaction in the self-organized systems].* Heidelberg, Germany: Asanger.

Watzlawick, P., Beaver, J. H., & Jackson, D. D. (1967). *Pragmatics of human communication: A study of interactional patterns, pathologies, and paradoxes.* New York: Norton.

Watzlawick, P. (1996). *Menschliche Kommunikation. Formen, störungen, paradoxien [Pragmatics of human communication. Patterns, pathologies, paradoxes].* Bern, Switzerland: Huber. (Original work published in 1967)

Wied, S. (1998). Das Phänomen der Farbe und ihrer Wahrnehmung [The phenomenon of color and its perception]. Diploma dissertation, Humboldt University.

Wied, S. (2001). *Farbenräume* [Colorspace]. Bern, Switzerland: Huber.

Wittgenstein, L. (1963, 1994). *Tractatus Logico-Philosophicus.* Frankfurt, Germany: Suhrkamp.

Wörterbuch der Psychiatrie und medizinischen Psychologie [Dictionary of psychiatry and medical psychology]. (1977). München, Germany: Urban und Schwartzenberg.

Zderad, L. (1969). Empathic nursing. *Nursing Clinics of North America, 4,* 655–662.

CHAPTER 6

The Concept of Need in Nursing Theory

Penny Powers

This chapter picks up its central argument from the unanswered question in the previous chapter regarding the implication of conceptualizing human needs as universal versus socially and politically determined. A postmodern discourse analysis is offered here to examine nursing's conceptualization of human needs and nursing practice framed within such conceptualizations.

Most people could probably provide a definition of the word *need* in their native language. Nursing discourse, however, following psychology (Maslow, 1954, 1970), has used the word as concept, a technical and theoretical term that has played an important role in nursing theory and practice beginning with Peplau (1952). Nursing discourse concerning the concept of need is often referred to in the plural—needs—in an attempt to move away from the medical model of disease. A discipline-specific concept, however, possesses defining attributes, empirical referents, antecedents, and consequences (Walker & Avant, 1995). As a concept in nursing discourse, *need* functions as an abstract linguistic entity apart from patient situations in specific ways: (a) to organize discourse presented to nursing students about what it means to be a human being, (b) to provide a framework for organizing nursing interventions, and (c) to inform the way we think about nursing as a profession and its role in the social world.

The elevation of the word *need* to a technical term has proceeded without a formal definition, a concept analysis, or examination of the philosophical implications of using the word as a concept. Without these considerations, the concept of need has become taken for granted in nursing. The concept of need is found in many different contexts in nursing literature concerning practice, education, and theory, whereas its use in the discipline of psychology has decreased markedly.

It is the purpose of this chapter to provide one possible discourse analysis of the current status of the concept of need in nursing. Philosophical analysis provides important contributions to theoretical discourse in our discipline (Allen, 1986; Dzurec, 1989; Thompson, 1987). Smith, who has written a philosophical analysis of the concept of health (1981), states, "The method of testing ideas in philosophic inquiry is that of critical discussion . . . The major difference between philosophical inquiry and empirical science is that experiments are not performed in philosophic inquiry" (p.43). The concept of need is a good candidate for philosophical analysis in order to initiate discussion concerning its significance, relevance, and the consequences of its use (Thomson, 1987). This analysis does not presume there is some essential nature to the word or concept to be uncovered, discovered, invented, or proposed. Instead, it emphasizes that there is an important history to the concept of need that informs the manner in which it is currently used in nursing.

The claim of this analysis is that the use of the concept of need in nursing has philosophical implications that conflict with generally accepted goals of nursing. More specifically, this analysis claims that the way we as nurses use the concept (a) assumes that the standards or criteria used for judging the existence and relative weight of need statements are universally applicable to all people at all times (e.g., all prostatectomy patients need continuous urinary irrigation); (b) reflects a view of nursing's relationship to people that limits the autonomy and responsibility of both the nurse and the patient by severely limiting participation in the discourse to experts; (c) contributes to and reproduces an oppressive notion of the role of science and social agency in society; and (d) directs attention away from, or masks, important issues such as sexism, racism, power, knowledge, political action, and human emancipation.

The use of the concept of need without philosophical analysis results in unintended consequences such as the reproduction of social situations that contradict currently accepted ideals and aims of nursing. These contradictions can cause tension in the practice of a discipline (Giddens, 1979). The use of a Foucaultian perspective delineates the historical features of the concept and explains its use as an example of an oppressive discourse in Western society. Examining unintended consequences in this way provides a perspective for exposing discrepancies and explaining tensions within nursing discourse and practice.

THE WORD "NEED" AND NEED CLAIMS

The derivation, development, and refinement of the word *need* provides the starting point for this analysis (Powers, 1989). The root of the English word comes from old Teutonic and means violence, force, or constraint by or upon persons, as "I chopped the wood with need" (forcefully). Indeed, one old form of the word was "needforce," but this usage is now considered obsolete (*Oxford English Dictionary*, 1971). However, force is still detectable in modern synonym discussions where the emotional force implied by the word need is in contrast with the more formal word *necessity* (*Webster's New World Dictionary*, 1964). In the oldest use, the associated physical force was plainly visible between one person and another or between a person and an object. The most noticeable change in the evolution of the word for this analysis is that the location and direction of the force has been moved from outside a person to within a person. The only remaining vestige of compulsion is an emotional attachment to our opinion that we need something. We *feel* compelled instead of *being* compelled. For example the following sentence demonstrates the emotional attachment to the opinion, "I really need to get out there and pull those weeds out of my garden before they choke out my vegetable seedlings."

Need statements in modern English can be expressed on your own behalf, such as "I need a drink of water" or on behalf of someone else, such as "You need to lose 40 pounds" or for something else, such as "That house needs a fresh coat of paint." Need statements can also be implied by actions. For example, we assume that you change the baby's diapers because they need changing, without saying so unless you are asked. If you are asked for a reason, you often respond with a need statement.

The modern word no longer refers to externally applied force. It refers instead to an opinion about a compelling relationship to something. This opinion is identified by a socially proper linguistic expression, or implied in an action that is justified by a socially proper linguistic expression. "I need to stop and get some gas. The gauge is on 'E'."

It is important to emphasize that *the need is the statement,* not a physical condition, even when the statement is referring to something associated with a physical condition such as the empty gas tank. The gas tank has no physical condition that indicates need. The need is the statement by a person. The philosophical debate on this point continues, but the direction is clear (Michalos, 1988; Willard, 1987). All need statements are (explicitly or implicitly) *"in order to"* statements, that is, they are goal statements. Whenever a need statement is expressed, someone can always ask, *"Why* do you need that?" "I need some gas if we're going to make it to my sister's place." "I need a drink of water to quench my thirst." "You need to lose 40 pounds in order to get your diabetes under control." "You need two units of blood to stay alive." "That house needs a coat of paint to look attractive." "The baby's diapers needed changing in order to keep her bottom dry." Sometimes, the answers are self-evident, and the "in order to" justification is implied: "I need a drink of water because I'm thirsty. Why else would I say that?" Because need statements are assertions, there can be disagreement, even in the self-evident case: "I don't know, I thought maybe you needed some water to rinse your mouth, not because you were thirsty."

Fraser (1989) calls these self-evident cases *thin need statements.* They are not needs per se, but need statements, emphasizing the linguistic nature of our understanding of need. Need statements about food, water, and shelter are thin need statements that have self-evident, unexpressed "in order to" components. On the other hand, *thick need statements* are not self-evident cases and are normally accompanied by "in order to" justification clauses. New clothes, a nice house, good food are examples of thick need statements. "I need a new pair of shoes that have Velcro instead of laces because my arthritic fingers can't tie laces anymore without a lot of pain."

Need statements are in a form of argument. Need statements, or "in order to" statements, are examples of claim-grounds statements (Toulmin, Reike, & Janik, 1984). It is your claim that you need something, or that your patient needs something, or that the house needs something, and the "in order to" part of the statement constitutes the grounds (or reasons, or evidence) to support your claim. In the self-evident cases (the thin need statements) there probably won't be much disagreement, even though there can be. For example, I claim I need a drink of water and I give the grounds that I am thirsty. A listener may disagree with the claim that I need a drink of water, but cannot dispute my evidence that I am thirsty.

There is more often disagreement in thick need statements. Your claim can be disputed by challenging it with a counterclaim, complete with its own grounds, or by questioning whether your grounds actually do function to support your claim: "You may *feel* thirsty, but you do not *need* a drink of water because your body is overhydrated as it is." In the terms of informal logic, this latter challenge is about *warrants*. A warrant is the statement asserting the relevance of the grounds to the claim. A warrant is what shows that these grounds do support this claim. A warrant can be implicit or explicit, empirical or ethical, personal or social, depending on the type of claim. With the thin need claims, you usually don't provide a warrant unless you are specifically asked for it.

In the thin need statements, you don't usually supply grounds, much less a warrant, because the warrants as well as the grounds are implicit and usually self-evident. The sarcastic tone of the following sentence implies that the listener must be awfully dense to ask for justification for the claim that someone needs a drink of water: "I need a drink of water [claim] because I'm thirsty! [grounds] People do actually die from dehydration [warrant], you know!" Thus, a common warrant for thin need claims is that it is a good thing for person x to have y, or for x to have y now. Need claims are social/linguistic constructions based on assumptions about what human life consists of, including the social standards by which we judge goodness and rightness. Besides more often being asked for grounds, thick need statements also are asked more often for warrants: "I *need* new shoes with Velcro fasteners [claim] because my fingers hurt when I tie laces [grounds]. My fingers don't hurt when I use Velcro fasteners [warrant].

Need claims can be differentiated further from other types of claims people make. This differentiation is demonstrated by the fact that need is subject to different social criteria for evaluation than other kinds of claims, or arguments. Want statements, for example, are also claims, but the social/linguistic criteria for their evaluation are different from the social/linguistic criteria for the evaluation of need claims. When you say you want something, you always can be asked for your grounds in the same manner that a need statement is questioned. In other words, you can be asked, "Why do you want that?"

It is acceptable, however, in the case of a want claim, either to provide grounds or to refuse to provide grounds:

"I want some broccoli."

"Why?"

"I don't know, I just want broccoli, okay?"

This would not be an acceptable response to a need statement. A need statement requires the "in order to" justification and it is acceptable to ask the speaker for the grounds if it is not self-evident:

"I need broccoli."

"Why?"

"I just need broccoli, okay?"

"Come on, you have to have a *reason* to say you need broccoli."

"I need broccoli because I don't eat dairy products and so I get calcium from broccoli."

"Oh, okay. Now I understand why you *need* broccoli."

Want statements, therefore, cannot be disputed in the same way as need statements. You can ask for the grounds (the reasons) and you can question the speakers' judgment or their sanity, but you cannot argue the claim. If they want it, they want it. You can say why you wouldn't want it, or you can say why they shouldn't want it, but you can't say "You *don't* want that," unless you are (a) questioning their honesty (e.g., "You don't really want a drink of water, you're just trying to postpone going to bed."), or (b) teaching a child how to differentiate between want statements and need statements:

"I don't want a bath."

"Maybe not, but you sure do *need* a bath."

"I need a cookie."

"No, you *want* a cookie, but you sure don't *need* one."

Because our understanding of need is based on social/linguistic relationships (need claims), and these claims are not the same kind of thing as want claims, what kind of claims are they? Claims about need are examples of what Kuhn (1970) and Bernstein (1983) call judgmental statements. Bernstein distinguishes judgmental claims from subjective claims by saying that subjective claims cannot be disputed (i.e., "I really liked that movie") short of accusing someone of dishonesty or deceit. Judgmental claims, however, can be subject to dispute (e.g., "That movie was awful") and are judged by their support, that is, their grounds and warrants. Objective claims, on the other hand, (e.g., "That movie was filmed in Tanzania") are judged by appeal to objective criteria.

Need claims, therefore, belong in the judgmental category, and want claims are in the subjective category. Need claims always have supporting grounds and warrants, either explicit or implicit. This is to say, need claims are just as rational as objective claims. Such judgmental reasoning is often maligned as unscientific or subjective because of the acceptability of ethical warrants as support (Bernstein, 1983) and the possibility of counterclaims. Judgmental claims are judged more clearly by standards of social acceptability, not by so-called objective criteria, which in many views are also socially defined.

In summary, the following points have been supported: (a) In the evolution of the word *need*, the location of force has changed from an external visible compulsion to internal emotional force of compelling argument; (b) Need statements are claims, that is, a form of argument, subject to social/linguistic evaluation; (c) Need claims are subject to different social criteria with respect to their evaluation from other forms of argument, such as want claims, by virtue of the contrasting warrants that are socially/linguistically acceptable. These social standards undergo continuous evolution (Foucault, 1980) as do all social criteria.

THE CONCEPT OF NEED IN NURSING

The concept of need has been utilized widely in nursing theory and practice. Such an influential concept warrants scrutiny of its history, discourse, implications, and assumptions. The concept of need has a negative orientation among some nursing theorists because it reinforces a continued emphasis on human deficits (Meleis, 1997) that mirrors the biomedical deficit treatment model. Several early nursing theories have been characterized as need theories, but the concept itself was not defined by any of these authors (Meleis, 1997). In this category, Meleis includes Peplau, Henderson, and among more recent authors, Abdellah and Orem (Meleis, 1997). The work of psychologist Abraham Maslow (1954, 1970) is an important foundation for all of these theorists, especially for Peplau, who can be considered the main source of influence for Maslow's work in nursing (Peplau, 1952).

Nursing need theories were developed in answer to the functional question, What do nurses do? The answer for these theorists was that nurses meet or help patients to meet needs. The need theories focus on problems, and take a reductionist approach to human beings as a set of problems and nursing as a set of controlling functions (Meleis, 1997, p. 187). These early theories portray nurses as the decision-makers in the care process, and do not address the perception of the client, a view of the environment, or a process of interaction (Meleis, 1997, p. 187).

It is interesting to note that these theories are considered outdated foundational influences by some and yet these assumptions continue to inform nursing literature. There have been several more recent works that propose or apply an existing human-need model (Ellis & Nowlis, 1994; Minshull, Ross, & Turner 1986). Lilley (1987), for example, has developed the Human Needs Assessment scale based on Yura and Walsh (1983).

Interestingly, Maslow's work (1954, 1970) lacks a definition of need and also lacks any concept of a hierarchy of needs. However, Yura and Walsh (1983) have defined the concept of need more recently in nursing, as an objectively measurable internal tension resulting from an alteration in the individual. This definition reflects assumptions that have been discredited in philosophical literature. There is no adequate evidence for assuming the existence of a physically detectable internal tension based on a verbal statement of need (Michalos, 1988). Furthermore, this definition of need as an internal tension reifies a social/linguistic concept into a physical entity; locates the entity within individuals; and charges nurses to identify, name, and treat the condition. The goal of treatment is to eliminate the assumed alteration causing the tension. This process completely strips the social/linguistic, personal, and interactive nature of need identification in order to produce a science of needs. Nurses become the social agents of the resulting scientific body of knowledge that describes the alterations and the tensions, prescribes the treatments, and judges the outcomes by prescribed measurable criteria.

SOCIAL AGENTS OF NEED

The choice of a role for nurses of assessing and treating needs contains serious unexamined assumptions with regard to the notion of social agency (Allen, 1987). Nursing literature has not specifically addressed the philosophical notion of nurses as agents of social order. Social agents include such categories as teachers, police, bureaucrats, professionals, and other rule-enforcing authority figures that possess distinct bodies of knowledge about people and the social authority to do something about it. Social agents have always held higher status than occupations without such power or knowledge. According to Michel Foucault (1965, 1975, 1980), the notion of social agents (which he sometimes called disciplinary technologists in order to emphasize the technical role) has become an important consideration in modern discussions of power because of the great amount of knowledge and power and the large number of practices that have been developed in the social sciences. The training of social agents in each of the new areas of the human sciences has become widely institutionalized and acceptance of this category of person has become unquestioned.

The assumption of the acceptability of power and control over others for their own good is an explicit part of our education as nurses. For example, we are taught that science is a constantly evolving process toward truths that give social agents the tools to predict and control outcomes that facilitate the advancement of civilization, all of which is desirable. Academics produce the research that guides the practice that supports the research, which benefits society as a whole.

Nursing has a long-standing goal of increased power and influence in the social world, based on models from other professions. As another category of social agents, and as part of that role, nurses have the task of revealing and enforcing the normalized truths of their own brand of social science for the assumed order and benefit of all. Foucault presents compelling arguments to demonstrate that research in the social sciences is a powerful force for expanding the prediction and control of finer and finer details of people's lives (Foucault, 1980). The statistical average often becomes the enforced normal. Foucault claims that people in Western civilizations have generally come to accept the importance of the role of social agents (Foucault, 1979).

People have internalized the importance of being measured, examined, and compared to a standard, to the point that they compare themselves to published standards such as height/weight tables, normal blood pressure charts, or stages of grief. This large-scale social process results in social control of internal compulsions at all levels, from production to justification to expression (Dreyfus & Rabinow, 1983). This process is clearly reflected in the historical evolution of the word *need*. Need statements have been redefined as an internal tension and made subject to diagnosis and treatment by a social agent, using criteria that have been normalized from scientific averages. Patients are socialized to understand under what circumstances it is permissible for the claims of an individual to be overruled by a professional armed with a normal curve, scientific truth, and a nursing intervention.

The science of need gives members of society who are trained social agents the responsibility of enforcing dominant ideologies of the culture in which they have been carefully educated. One of the dominant ideologies in our Western society is male-centered, power-based empirical analytic science, which carries the assumptions of the value of efficiency, standardization, prediction, and control (Powers, 1992). If an individual does not conform to the influence of the dominant ideologies through social agents, the blame then falls on the individual, not on the science or the social agent. In this case, the problem lies with the person and her or his faulty socialization process or lack of compliance. Furthermore, people accept this blame when it is affixed by social agents who are supported by the vast power and knowledge of science, because science can be a very coercive model.

As nurses we readily accept the role of social agent based on social science without a philosophical analysis of the historical antecedents and present consequences of our position. This renders impossible a conscious decision about whether to acknowledge and participate in the process of extending the practices of prediction and control to newly defined subject areas in human life without acknowledging the social/linguistic nature of need claims made by embodied, situated speakers.

Nursing discourses include goals concerning patient advocacy, collaboration in decision making, patient teaching, patient perspective, environmental influences, cultural sensitivity, critical thinking, conflict resolution, and other so-called empowering strategies and perspectives. On the other hand, nursing actions based on the concept of need perpetuate the acceptability of oppression through scientific prediction and control (Meleis, 1985), using justifications phrased in terms of patient outcomes that are deceptive to both patients and nurses.

Nursing research on interventions is aimed at outcome measures such as compliance and normal responses (see Iowa Intervention Project, 1993). We use our discourse to construct the patient conditions we diagnose, the treatments we administer, and the units of measurement for the outcomes we seek, all in terms of normalized truth that has been standardized by research (see Carpenito, 1995). Patient education, for example, resembles oppression more than teaching, with the emphasis on outcomes instead of on understanding. This approach to the nurse-patient encounter assumes it is in the interests of society to produce outcomes, instead of fostering understanding from the patient perspective. We assume that the problems in patient compliance can be overcome with more science, more research, into more interventions that produce better outcomes.

ALTERNATIVE FUTURES FOR NURSING DISCOURSE ON NEED

Nursing literature has recently begun to address such topics as power and oppression. Allen and colleagues suggest that research about the conduct of research would be extremely useful in this regard (Allen, Allman, & Powers, 1991). Sawicki (1986) suggests a "politics of difference" for nursing literature, while Thompson (1987) suggests critical scholarship as an approach to the critique of domination in nursing. Hall, Stevens, and Meleis (1994) discuss the concept of marginalization, and Mason and colleagues (1994) address the empowering results of education for staff nurses. A critical social theory perspective of political agendas is examined by Dickerson and Campbell-Heider (1994). Though none of these discussions focus on the concept of need, there are some relevant writings in postmodern feminist theory.

Fraser, for example, suggests that emphasis be shifted to a discourse about need *identifications* instead of need *satisfactions* (1989). The importance of this distinction lies in the fact that restricting talk to need satisfactions assumes that the nature of the concept of needs is not problematic in the first place. Shifting talk away from need satisfaction to need identification is important because the former assumes that all needs are universal human qualities that are already identified and agreed upon, that is, they have assumed warrants for their expression in our social world.

Restricting dialogue to need satisfactions obscures the politically contestable nature of both thin and thick need statements. Thus, at first glance, it may seem obvious that people need housing, but less apparent is what kind of housing people need and what is an acceptable way of getting it, or being given it, or taking it. Talk about need identification, however, directs attention to the specifics of who decides what the need is, and what grounds and warrants are acceptable supports for the need claims. Talk about need identification amounts to letting people construct their own arguments for their need claims, to be communicatively achieved in an overtly political social world. This type of dialogue does not assume the existence of universal scientifically normalized needs whose satisfaction is assessed and prescribed by social agents. One effect of such a shift may be to emphasize understanding and negotiation instead of outcomes.

Fraser (1989) also notes that restricting talk about need to need satisfaction instead of need identification also serves to bypass discussion that the process of need identification in itself may be oppressive and favors dominant groups in the social world. Discourse in the social sciences concerning need satisfaction is thus restricted to norm-discovering, statistical, empirical analytic methodology, which has been described as necessarily resulting in oppression of subordinate groups (Foucault, 1979).

Fraser uses the concept of need specifically in this context to illustrate how a dominant ideology can co-opt a nondominant discourse, bypassing talk about the nature of need and instead talking about the distribution of need satisfactions. Foucault calls this process "the medicalization of social control" (O'Neill, 1986) because this kind of talk turns social/ethical discourse into a technical problem to be solved by social agents using normalized scientific truths. Medicalization of social control removes the inherently political nature of need identification from the discussion and creates new fields for social science and the education of new forms of social agents at the same time.

Talk about need and talk about rights have been described as characteristic of our form of late welfare capitalism (Fraser, 1989). From a Foucaultian perspective, this is to say that the only socially acceptable warrants for need claims in late welfare capitalist discourse are those that are constructed on the basis of social science, thus limiting participation in the discussion to those social agents educated to understand science. This process effectively eliminates talk about need identification by situated individuals who may or may not understand how science works. Instead, talk is limited to scientific discussion about the distribution of need satisfactions based on principles of welfare capitalism. Dreyfus and Rabinow (1983) say explicitly, "The administrative apparatus of the state posed welfare in terms of people's *needs* and happiness" (p. 139).

When people are acknowledged to have rights, there is an assumed definition of the good life, or what people have rights *to*. This definition provides the grounds and warrants for need goal statements, such as "I need *x* in order to get *y*," *y* being something to which you have a right. Oppressed groups are linguistically/scientifically acknowledged to have the same rights as everyone else, but can nevertheless experience discrimination. A group can be acknowledged to have a right to something, acknowledged to have a right to state the need to get it, but not acknowledged to have the right to access the means to get it. Similarly, other groups of people are simply not acknowledged socially to fit the definition of a "person" who has these rights, or are only acknowledged to have the right to a lesser quality of that something. Furthermore, subordinate groups tend to internalize these conditions as normal and unquestioned (Freire, 1972).

Two examples illustrate this form of oppression. First, consider that groups of citizens find it difficult to make a case to define their need for medical care in terms of care that does not discriminate against them on the basis of some social/linguistic category such as race. This difficulty arises because the need for medical care is already defined without reference to race by the hegemonic influence of medical discourse. The only case possible to make is one that refers to the distribution of medical care as it has already been defined. Even then, a redefinition of, say, illegal aliens as noncitizens effectively rules out their participation in the discourse. This move serves to retain the philosophical definition of needs to include their universal application to all humans, but removes illegal aliens from the category of human beings, thus denying them both the services and participation in the discussion.

Second, consider that discourse concerning the distribution of need satisfaction for scientifically normalized needs supports an illusion of choices. Thinking that we have rights to need satisfaction creates an illusion of autonomy. Instead, autonomous choices are severely limited because our needs are not self-defined. Instead, need has already been defined by the scientific research process instead of by the process of political discourse. Thus, autonomy is restricted to choices among methods of need satisfaction that may be wholly unsatisfactory or completely closed to that individual. Accordingly, as an immigrant you can assume you have a right to the good life, but find you have no right to the means to get it (Willard, 1987), and be completely at a loss to understand how to object to the manner in which this happened.

As nurses, we give patients illusions of choice that allow them to assume the right to have the choice implemented. At the same time, we sometimes deny the definition of "person" to someone, say, with a mental illness, or deny someone access to the means to get their need met because of the cost of advice about how to do it. This is part of the role of social agents because the general outcomes of research assume more importance than a single case.

Nurses are in a position to feel conflict between the assumptions of a trained social agent and the position of a member of an oppressed group. This is because nursing is traditionally a female occupation that simultaneously presents itself as being based on scientific research. The continually shifting dominant and subordinate relationships can cause tension within the practice of nursing. To patients we are dominant. To physicians and hospital administrators we are subordinate. To the lay public we are dominant. A nurse may be faced with trying to advocate *for* a patient *to* physicians, while at the same time trying to advocate *for* medical profession and its authority *to* the patient and uphold some degree of professionalism for herself or himself. This tension within nursing practice causes horizontal classism and racism within the discipline because of the self-deprecation that comes with oppressed group behavior (Freire, 1972; Roberts, 1983).

The goals of nursing, such as those found in the American Nursing Association's (ANA) Social Policy Statement, have received careful critique (Allen, 1987). One key goal of the discipline of nursing is professionalization, based partly on the criterion of the acquisition of a scientific body of knowledge and phrased in terms of people's needs, happiness, and health (Gamer, 1979). This goal reflects a desire among nurses for increased social power, prestige, and control. Based on the models from other professions, the goal requires an independent body of scientific knowledge that affords prediction and control of outcomes specific to the discipline. To this end, nursing has tried to ally with professional groups that achieved status on the basis of exclusion rather than empowerment (O'Neill , 1991).

Professionalism in these terms would mean the loss of perspectives from working-class nurses and nurses of color. In addition, nursing would remove itself from the strengths available from the discourses of unionism and feminism. The loss of these discourses would restrict the available subject positions from which nurses could speak in terms of need identification. Furthermore, professionalization in these terms would limit the possibility of discourses in nursing that are not based on traditional social science.

CONCLUSIONS

The concept of needs in nursing is a top-down, mechanistic, means-end, product-oriented list of technical functions for nurses in a role of social agency where the major goal is patient compliance with predetermined scientific categories. The process of assessing and treating need avoids revealing previously formed value decisions that were made without the mutual consent of individual patients and enforced without discussion. The warrants that provide the justification for this approach are efficiency, advancing scientific method, professionalization, and standardization.

The following recommendations for nursing arise from this discussion. Teaching nursing students the concept of need, in a list or a hierarchy, reinforces the assumption that needs are reified physical entities to be measured, diagnosed, and treated. Instead, we should emphasize talk about need statements as claims, made by embodied, situated speakers and supported by grounds and warrants that mean something in the context of the lives of speaker and listener. Nurses can encourage a person's ability to determine and support his or her own need claims, even if it contradicts our own. The concept of collaboration is lost when the underlying assumption of nurse as social agent gives so much weight to the ideal of compliance.

Students might well benefit from an appreciation of our position as patient advocates as well as a revised concept of social agency. These perspectives offer us opportunities apart from traditional professional goals.

Nurses can produce their own arguments, their own claims, grounds, and warrants in an arena of public discourse (Thompson, 1987). An argument can be made for nursing not as a science, but as a practical and moral way of being in the world (Yarling & McElmurry, 1986) that entails practical reasoning and informed judgment. New to academia, the discipline of nursing has the opportunity to demonstrate the operation of a practice discipline that is informed by many interrelated bodies of knowledge, including its own widely varying discourses in service to communicably achieved moral ideals through the efforts of situated human beings. It would be difficult to estimate the intended and untended consequences of the concept of needs on nursing at this point in its history. Although nursing practice has long been informed by this concept, further analysis of the discourse of needs seems warranted.

REFERENCES

Allen, D. (1986). Using philosophical and historical methodologies to understand the concept of health. In P. Chinn (Ed.), *Nursing research methodology* (pp. 157–168). Rockville, MD: Aspen.

Allen, D. (1987). The social policy statement: A reappraisal. *Advances in Nursing Science, 10,* 39–48.

Allen, D., Allman, K., & Powers, P. (1991). Feminist research without gender. *Advances in Nursing Science, 13,* 49.

Bernstein, R. (1983). *Beyond objectivism and relativism: Science, hermeneutics and praxis.* Philadelphia: University of Pennsylvania Press.

Carpenito, L. J. (1995). *Nursing diagnosis: Application to clinical practice* (6th ed.). Philadelphia: Lippincott.

Dickerson, S. S., & Campbell-Heider, N. (1994). Interpreting political agendas from a critical social theory perspective. *Nursing Outlook, 42,* 265–271.

Dreyfus, H., & Rabinow, P. (1983). *Michel Foucault, Beyond structuralism and hermeneutics.* Chicago: University of Chicago Press.

Dzurec, L. (1989). The necessity for and evolution of multiple paradigms for nursing research: A poststructuralist perspective. *Advances in Nursing Science, 11,* 69–77.

Ellis, J. R., & Nowlis, E. A. (1994). *Nursing: A human needs approach* (5th ed.). Hagerstown, MD: Lippincott.

Foucault, M. (1965). *Madness and civilization* (R. Howard, Trans.). New York: Vintage/Random House. (Original work published in 1961)

Foucault, M. (1975). *The birth of the clinic: An archeology of medical perception* (A. Sheridan Smith, Trans.). New York: Vintage/Random House. (Original work published in 1963)

Foucault, M. (1979). *Discipline and punish: The birth of the prison* (A. Sheridan, Trans.). New York: Vintage/Random House. (Original work published in 1975)

Foucault, M. (1980). *The history of sexuality* (Vols. 1–3). (R. Hurley, Trans.). New York: Random House. (Original work published in 1976)

Fraser, N. (1989). *Unruly practices: Power, discourse and gender in contemporary social theory.* Minneapolis: University of Minnesota Press.

Freire, P. (1972). *Pedagogy of the oppressed.* New York: Penguin Books. (Original work published in 1970)

Gamer, M. (1979). The ideology of professionalism. *Nursing Outlook, 27,* 108–111.

Giddens, A. (1979). *Central problems in social theory.* London: Macmillan.

Hall, J. M., Stevens, P. E., & Meleis, A. I. (1994). Marginalization: A guiding concept for valuing diversity in nursing knowledge. *Advances in Nursing Science, 16,* 23–41.

Iowa Intervention Project. (1993). *NIC Interventions linked to NANDA diagnoses.* Iowa City, IA: Iowa Intervention Project.

Kuhn, T. (1970). *The structure of scientific revolutions* (2nd ed.). Chicago: University of Chicago Press.

Lilley, L. (1987). Human need fulfillment alteration in the client with uterine cancer. *Cancer Nursing, 10,* 327–337.

Maslow, A. (1954). *Motivation and personality.* New York: Harper & Row.

Maslow, A. (1970). *Motivation and personality* (2nd ed.). New York: Harper & Row.

Mason, D. J., Costello-Nickitas, D. M., Scanlan, J. M., & Magnuson, B. A. (1994). Empowering nurses for politically astute change in the workplace. *Journal of Continuing Education in Nursing, 22,* 5–10.

Meleis, A. (1997). *Theoretical nursing: Development and progress* (3rd ed.). Philadelphia: Lippincott.

Michalos, A. (1988). Meeting current needs. *Dialogue, 27,* 507–515.

Minshull, J., Ross, K., & Turner, J. (1986). The human needs model of nursing. *Journal of Advanced Nursing, 11,* 643–649.

O'Neill, J. (1986). The medicalization of social control. *Canadian Review of Sociology and Anthropology, 23,* 350–364.

O'Neill, S. (1991, February). *The drive for professionalism in nursing: A reflection of classism and racism.* Paper presented at the conference "Critical Theory and Feminist Theory in Nursing," Medical College of Toledo, Ohio.

Oxford English Dictionary (Compact Ed.). (1971). London: Oxford University Press.

Peplau, H. (1952). *Interpersonal relations in nursing.* New York: Putnam.

Powers, P. (1989). *Needs—A concept analysis.* Unpublished manuscript.

Powers, P. (1992). *Needs in nursing.* Unpublished master's thesis, University of Washington, Seattle.

Roberts, S. (1983). Oppressed group behavior: Implications for nursing. *Advances in Nursing Science, 6,* 21–30.

Sawicki, J. (1986). Foucault and feminism: Toward a politics of difference. *Hypatia, 1,* 23–36.

Smith, J. (1981). The idea of health: A philosophical inquiry. *Advances in Nursing Science, 4,* 43–50.

Thompson, J. (1987). Critical scholarship: The critique of domination in nursing. *Advances in Nursing Science, 10,* 27–38.

Thompson, J. (1990). Hermeneutic inquiry. In L. Moody (Ed.), *Advancing nursing science through research* (Vol. 2). Newbury Park, CA: Sage.

Thomson, G. (1987). *Needs.* New York: Routledge and Kegan Paul.

Toulmin, S., Reike, R., & Janik, A. (1984) *An introduction to reasoning* (2nd ed.). New York: Macmillan.

Walker, L., & Avant, K. (1995). *Strategies for theory construction in nursing* (3rd ed.). Norwalk, CT: Appleton & Lange.

Webster's New World Dictionary. (1964). New York: World.

Willard, L. (1987). Needs and rights. *Dialogue, 26,* 43–53.

Yarling, R., & McElmurry, B. (1986). The moral foundation of nursing. *Advances in Nursing Science, 8,* 63–73.

Yura, H., & Walsh, M. B. (1983). *The nursing process: Assessment, planning, implementing, evaluating* (3rd ed.). New York: Appleton-Century-Crofts.

CHAPTER 7

The Concept of Holism

Hesook Suzie Kim

Throughout its modern development, nursing has been intrigued with the notions of wholeness, holistic, and holism both in practice and theory. However, the meaning of these terms in nursing varied from context to context and from one period to the next because these themes were introduced into nursing practice and nursing theory with different motivations and perspectives. The terms are used to depict health conceptualizations, approaches toward health, nursing philosophy, ontological orientations, and theoretical perspectives, which creates a great deal of confusion in the nursing discourse. There are at least three specific sources of discourse in nursing that created this scenario.

The first wave of discourse occurred in the context of nursing practice. Holistic advocacy in nursing has been traced to Nightingale by Shealy (1985), who found in the pioneer's work a promotion for holistic principles applied to the care of the whole patient. The whole-patient approach emphasizes the need to consider the patient in terms of body, mind, and spirit, and in the person's "wholistic" relations to environment. Although this orientation stayed within nursing as a foundational idea, it was not until after World War II that a more sustaining wave of holistic emphasis appeared in nursing. In the 1950s and 1960s, especially in the United States, the idea of holistic nursing philosophy was advocated by many nursing leaders as the way to differentiate nursing from medicine in the form of comprehensive nursing care. The holistic nursing philosophy encompassing comprehensive nursing care was a position developed to orient nursing to focus on all aspects of the patient (including physical, psychological, social, and spiritual) in providing nursing care. This was seen as a departure from the biomedical focus of medicine that was viewed as reductionistic and oriented to disease and pathology rather than being focused on patients as persons. This notion of holism has been integrated into the central ideology of nursing that is often used as a slogan for nursing practice and nursing conceptualizations. More recently, the notion of holistic nursing began to embrace spiritual and psychosocial care and aesthetics in nursing (see, for example, Gaydos, 2003, and Taylor, 2004, among many articles published in *Journal of Holistic Nursing* and other similar journals).

The second wave can be identified with the general holistic health movement, which arose during the late 1960s and 1970s with the counterculture and New Age cultures. Rethinking the ideas of health, illness, and healthy living led to terms such as holistic health, holistic care, holistic nursing, and holistic medicine, which gave different meaning to the term *holistic.* Within this holistic health movement, *holistic* meant alternative therapies and healing practices that are not based on the traditional biomedicine and natural sciences (Williams, 1998).

Holistic views in this sense are based on the philosophy that emphasizes the integration of body, mind, and spirit as the ground for healing, a multidimensional approach to health practice, and the rejection of authoritarian approach to health care (Barratt et al., 2003; Deliman & Smolowe, 1982; Goldstein, 2003; Lowenberg, 1989). In a generic sense, these terms used in this context align with the philosophy of holism that views humans as unified wholes composed of many dimensions that function interdependently. Yet because they are so often used in conjunction with alternative therapies such as meditation, homeopathy, spiritual healing, touch therapy, imagery, and art therapy, the terms have very specific meanings when used as adjectives in association with health, nursing, medicine, practice, and care.

The term *holism,* on the other hand, appeared in the nursing discourse in relation to nursing theory development that began in earnest in the 1970s. For example, Donaldson and Crowley (1978) suggested that nursing should uphold holism as the guiding principle for the discipline's substantive structure. Nearly all of the major nursing theorists of the time, such as Rogers, Orem, Roy, Newman, Parse, King, and Neuman, regardless of their theoretical perspectives, espoused the holistic philosophy when they were writing about their theories or implications of their theories for nursing practice. This caused much confusion in sorting out which theorists had holism as their theories' orientations. The confusion was addressed to some extent by Parse, who differentiated nursing theories into simultaneity and totality paradigms (Parse, 1987), bypassing a judgment on holism. Owen and Holmes (1993) include Rogers, Levine, Parse, Watson, and Newman as those who espoused holistic concepts in their theoretical work. There are other claims of holism in nursing theories such as the ones made by Hudson (1988), Sarter (1988), and Schultz (1987). However, the versions of holism or the tenets of different holisms these authors hold are so varied and unclear that it is difficult to say who among them are qualified to be holists. Parse, for example, has adopted several concepts from Rogerian holism, such as unitary being, multidimensionality, and evolutionary process. However, Parse's theory can be viewed as more centrally rooted within the existential phenomenological ontology. Newman, who began her theoretical work with the Rogerian framework, is moving toward existential phenomenology and spiritualism although maintaining some tenets of holism. Watson's theory also can be considered as not espousing the mainstream holism from the ontological point of view (Owen & Holmes, 1993). Of these theorists, Rogers' work is considered in this chapter in order to discuss and raise questions about how holism is integrated into a theory as an ontological and epistemological orientation.

HOLISM—DEFINITIONS, PHILOSOPHICAL ORIENTATIONS, AND VARIETIES

The term *holism* comes from *hol-* or *holo-*, meaning complete, entire, without division, or whole; and *ism,* suggesting an ideology of wholes. As a term, its first formal use is attributed to Jan C. Smuts, the South African politician and statesman, in 1926 (Smuts, 1926). It refers in its simplistic sense to a philosophy that the nature or the universe needs to be viewed in terms of wholes that are irreducible to parts and are more than the sum of their parts. Philosophically, however, the term conveys ideas that are much more complex, including not only the irreducibility of wholes to parts and the wholistic unity but also evolution and emergence as the basic features of wholes. Inherent in some holisms are specific ideas regarding the relations of wholes with their environment, and hierarchical relations among the wholes. Holism has been applied in the conceptualizations and studies of living organisms, including humans, but also of physical systems, social institutions including societies and cultures, nature, and even the universe as a unity. With such diverse philosophies underpinning holism—some interrelated and others providing distinct perspectives—a discussion of holism in the nursing context is problematic.

Holism, or holistic idea, is viewed by many to have a long history, with some scholars tracing its roots back to the classical Greek period, and continuing transformations through the eighteenth and nineteenth centuries and most intensely in the twentieth century. Holism, as it developed at the close of the nineteenth century and at the beginning of the twentieth century, was a response to the reductionism, mechanism, and atomism that were becoming the dominant scientific philosophies not only for the so-called natural, hard sciences such as physics, chemistry and biology, but also in psychology, sociology, anthropology, and political sciences. Hence, scientific holism was a development to challenge the adequacies of various scientific approaches such as mechanism, reductionism, atomism, and dualism. The movement against these scientific approaches responded with various alternative forms of holism to consider units (whether biological organisms, institutions, societies or political entities) as wholes and to study them as *whole qua whole.* In this sense, scientific holism has risen with a unified agenda but one developed into multiple types and forms.

There are various ways of differentiating types of holisms. Phillips (1976) traces the development of holism in terms of *holism 1, holism 2,* and *holism 3,* in relation to their oppositions to mechanistic (analytic) method, reductionism, and atomism. His arguments are directed to critiquing the epistemological bases of holisms rather than the holism's ontology. Phillips identifies holism 1 as organicism, representing a set of five interrelated ideas regarding organic wholes, which for Phillips are the starting points for discussing three types of holism:

1. The analytic approach as typified by the physico-chemical sciences proves inadequate when applied to certain cases, for example, to a biological organism, to society, or even to reality as a whole.
2. The whole is more than the sum of its parts.
3. The whole determines the nature of its parts.
4. The parts cannot be understood if considered in isolation from the whole.
5. The parts are dynamically related or interdependent. (Phillips, 1976, p. 6)

Phillips suggests that all of the characteristics of holism 1 are logically based on the Hegelian theory of internal relations set against the mechanistic (analytic) method of science (1976, pp. 6–20). Hence, Phillips' holism 1 was a development that connects the ontology of holism with the theory of internal relations as its basis of epistemology. Phillips acknowledges that holism 1 in its original form as biological organicism changed into a much more complex notion after about 1930 (1976, p. 29).

According to Phillips, holism 2 emerged with a specifically antireductionist agenda with the major thesis that "the properties of organic wholes or systems, *after* they have been found, cannot be explained in terms of the properties of the parts" (1976, p. 34). Holism 2 is seen as specifically opposed to the methodological individualism of Popper and other social scientists. On the other hand, holism 3 espouses that "it is necessary to have terms referring to whole and their properties" (Phillips, 1976, p. 37). This thesis finds support in the holism of general system theory of Bertalanffy (1969) and Koestler (1967). Through his analysis of various forms of holistic theories within the tradition of holism, which includes biological organicism, general system theory, functionalism, structuralism, and gestalt psychology, Phillips concludes that the following three holists' positions are in general indisputable: (a) the emphasis on the dynamic relation among the parts of an organic whole, (b) the idea that it is difficult to predict emerging properties through the study of parts, and (c) the notion that new concepts are necessary in order to study organic wholes scientifically. However, the holists are wrong to think that "there is anything here that is antithetical to the traditional analytic (or atomistic, or reductionistic) method" (Phillips, 1976, p. 123). He also concludes that holism is "an eminently unworkable doctrine" (p. 123). Hence, he disputes the validity of holism's epistemological foundation, and suggests that logically there is nothing that should deter holists from using the analytic or mechanistic method in the study of wholes.

From a different perspective, Harrington (1996) identifies several different origins of holism as a philosophy that sprang up against the growing "disenchantment" with the mechanistic scientific ethos of the early twentieth century. She saw this holistic science not as a movement based on a single perspective, but as "a family of approaches," the central tenet of which was "the need to do justice to organismic purposiveness or teleological functioning" (Harrington, 1996, p. xvii). Different holistic approaches were developed with varying commitments to the ideas that (a) organisms must be viewed

not as mere sums of their elementary parts and processes but as
wholes having distinct characteristics as wholes; (b) the ontological
categories of humans as body and mind (as in dualism) must be rejected, and humans must be considered as wholes and studied as
wholes; (c) organismic or systemic processes for any given system
must be viewed in the context of a larger system or the universe; and
(d) the mechanistic science ("the machine science") must be rejected
with the new science of "wholeness" in order for humanity to regain
its true dignity (Harrington, 1996, pp. xvii–xix). Harrington sees this
new holistic science of life and mind as being influential not only as a
"more authentic vision of life and mind" in which knowledge in biology, psychology, and sociology was developing in new directions, but
also as a "blueprint for visualizing" a more authentic future in the political arena (Harrington, 1995, 1996). Hence, unlike Phillips, Harrington offers a view of holism from its penetration into the collective,
cultural life in a historical context. Under the guise of holistic thinking, the twentieth century is entrenched in diverse and somewhat
paradoxical development of political and cultural ideologies such as
totalitarianism, political unitarianism, and cultural determinism as
well as a movement toward humanistic ideologies.

Several other ways of differentiating holism can point to the variety of terms used to describe differences in holisms. From the perspective of environmental ethics, Marietta (1995) proposes three
forms of holism: (a) biocentric holism, in which all living things are
considered to be wholes living with the natural environment, (b) ecocentric holism, or environmental holism, that views the natural system as a whole, and (c) holistic anthropocentrism that recognizes
humans as a part of nature but also as a distinct holistic entity. Kermode (2002), in a similar position, raises concerns regarding environmental decay in relation to health emanating from a strong holistic
interaction between humans and biosphere.

On a different note and from a sociological perspective, James
(1984) differentiates *holism of content* from *holism of form*. Holism of
content is advocated by social theorists who view the characteristics
of social wholes as qualitatively distinct from the characteristics of
their parts, insisting that social theories must incorporate the ontology of social wholes in their explanations. On the other hand, holism
of form is epistemologically oriented, and is a view that each term in
a theory "owes its meaning to its relations with the others" (James,
1984, p. 3). This means that all terms of theories are defined in relation to each other and within the given theories. Holism thus is

viewed separately, although it can be related in important ways, from either the ontological or the epistemological stance.

Again from a sociological perspective, Chattopadhyaya (1967) offers different versions of holism as biological organicism, idealistic organicism, psychological organicism, functionalism, and structural functionalism, all of which are seen to adhere to the notion that human actions must be explained in the appropriate social context as a whole. Täljedal (1997) offers yet another terminology to differentiate versions of holism in medicine and medical sociology: strong and weak holisms. According to him, strong holism is based on the "layer ontology" of viewing human beings as constituted by a set of distinct yet integrative levels of organization, whereas weak holism espouses conceptualizations of health in the context of individuals as wholes. These are similar to Kolcaba's differentiation of holism into systemic holism, organismic holism, and whole-person holism, all of which are based on the ways patients are conceptualized (Kolcaba, 1997). Viewing none of these versions satisfactory for nursing, he suggests "person-based" holism as a solution: to consolidate systemic and organismic holisms with the whole-person holism as an ecumenical way of handling knowledge development in nursing (Kolcaba, 1997). Cava (2000), on the other hand, insists that holism should be considered as a way to move away from nursing's preoccupation with "excessive proximity preference." To Cava, holism allows taking into account distance concerns that impinge on patients' illness experiences and concerns.

In all of this diversity in holism and holistic philosophy, there are four influential and sustaining themes from several eminent scientists and philosophers. The first is based on the tenets of organicism that evolved into viewing an organism as a whole that has functional relationships with its environment. Organicism also introduced the idea of teleology as the basis of the whole organism's survival, growth, and change.

The second theme comes from general system theory (GST) of Bertalanffy and Koestler's hierarchical conceptualization of systems. The major tenets of GST as a general science of wholeness include the concept of system as organized wholes, the elements of which are interdependent and in mutual interaction; and the principles of emergence, entropy and negentropy, equifinality, and so forth, applicable to systems regardless of the nature of parts and their relationships among the parts (Bertalanffy, 1969). Added to these notions of GST is Koestler's (1967) concept of open hierarchical systems for which he states that

[w]hat we find are intermediary structures on a series of levels in an ascending order of complexity: sub-wholes which display, according to the way you look at them, some of the characteristics commonly attributed to wholes and some of the characteristics commonly attributed to parts." (p. 48)

Inherent in this conceptualization of hierarchy is the idea that no entity is fundamentally a part or a whole except when the entities are considered in relation to one another. Entities therefore are

subordinated as *parts* to the higher centers in the hierarchy, but at the same time function as quasi-autonomous *wholes*. They are Janus-faced. The face turned upward, toward the higher levels, is that of a dependent part; the face turned downward, towards its own constituents, is that of a whole of remarkable self-sufficiency (Koestler, 1978, p. 27)

These systems-based ideas for holism thus do not require holists to use organismic metaphors in addressing wholes as units of analysis.

The third theme undergirding various holisms comes from the idea of evolution, drawing from Darwin's inspiring work that changed the way scientists looked at life, development, and change. In holism, Teilhard de Chardin's evolutionary ideas are cited often. Teilhard de Chardin (1959) espoused that humans and other entities are constantly evolving toward progressively higher, more complex and sophisticated, and more perfectly unified entities. Although the evolutionism of Teilhard de Chardin was oriented to the final point of evolution in the unity of humanity and nature with God, the idea of evolution as a holistic one undercuts many versions of holism.

The fourth theme is related to the thinking that unites all things, that is, all of reality as a whole. David Bohm's version of holism, which may be termed as universal holism, is based on the idea that the phenomena of the universe need to be expressed in terms of wholeness and movement (Bohm, 1980). In his conceptualization of universal holism, Bohm states that "each particle is only an abstraction of a relatively invariant form of movement in the whole field of the universe" and that "elementary particles are on-going movements that are mutually dependent because ultimately they merge and interpenetrate" (1980, p. 29). His version of holism thus relates the wholeness to the entire reality, uniting it with what he calls holomovement.

It is evident then that holisms (not as a single philosophy but as multiple, different philosophies), both from the ontological and epistemological contexts, are based on many ideas. None of the holisms espoused by philosophers or scientists endorse all tenets that are considered to be related to holism. The following are the major ideas that can undergird various holisms:

- An entity is considered a whole when it is composed of parts that are interdependent and in mutual interaction.
- Wholeness is inherent in reality and is the essential character of entities.
- The whole is more than the sum of its parts, and is distinct in its characteristics from its parts.
- The whole determines the nature of its parts, and the parts have ontological significance in the context of the whole.
- The whole is an emergent entity and follows evolutionary processes toward increasing complexity and diversity.
- An entity as a whole is in constant interaction with its environment.
- An entity as a whole is embedded in a larger whole inasmuch as all entities as wholes are organized in a hierarchical level of interaction and interdependence.
- There are distinct principles that govern the behaviors and characteristics of wholes, which are only applicable to wholes.

Although it is possible to categorize holism in many different versions, as seen in the preceding section, for the purpose of exposition in nursing we identify four types that endorse various combinations of the holistic ideas discussed above: entitative holism, anthropocentric holism, hierarchical systemic holism, and universal cosmic holism. The differences among these holisms are depicted in Figure 7.1.

Entitative holism considers living and nonliving entities of reality to be wholes. Each class of entity as a whole possesses unique characteristics that are different from its constituent parts and is governed by specific sets of holistic processes that define its behaviors as a whole unit. Within this holism, different holistic entities are viewed as being governed by explanatory principles of change and behaviors that may be unique. This form of holism aligns with the scientific holism that opposes reductionism and atomism, but not necessarily mechanism.

Anthropocentric holism focuses on humans as holistic units with characteristics and processes distinct from other animate and inanimate entities of the world. This version of holism highlights the interpenetrating, interdependent nature of body, mind, and spirit (soul) as a whole. It also views humans as having a distinct holistic character

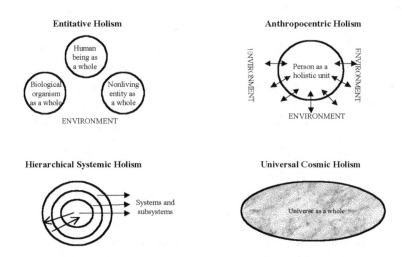

FIGURE 7.1 Representation of different types of holism.

that is different from other entities of the world and unique in itself. Humans as wholes are in interaction with the environment; however, the environment is not necessarily considered to be a whole itself or composed of other types of wholes. In this holism, human beings exist, experience, and behave as wholes through the processes that unite and integrate all aspects of human beings. Thus, illness is explained not in terms of an elevated blood sugar level or an enlarged cardiac valve, but in terms of the individual's state or experience that results from the integration of such phenomenon through holistic processes. Humans' relationships with their environment are viewed either as complementary and interdependent or as controlling and selective through human processes. This version of holism is often considered in conjunction with humanism, because the ontological center in both is the humans. Gestalt psychology is in line with this version of holism. Anthropocentric holism therefore is akin to organicism, with a distinction made between humans and all other living things on an ontological basis. In nursing, the holistic theories of Levine and Roy as well as the biopsychosocial model of clients align closely with this version of holism.

Hierarchical systemic holism refers to holism that identifies with many tenets of GST and the systems perspective. Epistemologically, this version of holism aligns quite well with pragmatism and constructivism, without a commitment to the ontology that wholeness is inherent in entities themselves. However, some adherents may subscribe to the hierarchical systemic characteristic as the inherent and true features of entities in a universal system of systems. Basically, this holism represents the idea that entities of the universe as wholes are systems that have sub- and supersystem relations among them, forming a hierarchy. Hierarchical relationships among systems are sometimes viewed as being organized through a control process such as cybernetics, while at other times they are considered to be in interdependent relationships. However, the notion of hierarchy suggests one part of a whole as a unit can be the point of attention at an analytic moment, while that same unit becomes part of a higher-level unit (or system) when the point of attention is shifted to that higher level. Hence, an entity as a system is a whole and not a whole, depending on how that entity is viewed or analyzed. Because of this, parts are referred to within this version of holism as subsystems, holding all characteristics of a system at their levels of analysis. Talcott Parsons' theory of social system (1951) aligns with this version in sociology. In nursing, the conceptual models of King, Roy, and Neuman partly align with this version.

Universal cosmic holism adheres to the notion that the universe in its totality is a whole, organized through processes that unite and integrate all elements contained within the universe to emerge and change as a whole. The universe is seen to possess a unitary pattern that permeates and is interpenetrating in all elements. The processes of the universe are often expressed in terms of multidimensionality, evolution and emergence toward increasing complexity and diversity, and unity. In this model, humans are integral parts of the universe, inseparable and connected within the universal character. Humans as well as all separate entities, living and nonliving, must be understood in terms of the universe, in the image of the total cosmos. In that sense, humans lose their unique features. Morowitz (1972) states in the same context that "[e]ach living thing is a dissipative structure, that is, it does not endure in and of itself but only as a result of the continual flow in the system" (p. 156). This points to the possibility that holism can lead to a different kind of reduction. Ecological holism, which is in line with this version, has been viewed as "totalitarian" (Kheel, 1985) and as projecting a "fascist understanding of the environment" (Regan, 1981). The picture of this universal cosmic holism is well depicted in Francis Thompson's poem that says "thou canst not stir a flower/Without troubling of a star." The major tenets of this holism are the interconnectedness of all elements of the universe and the interpenetration of the universal patterns in all elements, unifying them into one unitary movement, such as the concept of holomovement espoused by Bohm (1980). Martha Rogers' science of unitary human beings (1980) adopts some of the tenets of this version of holism.

What I have discussed so far points to the diversity in the philosophy of holism and the possible difficulty of judging a theory or conceptual model to be truly holistic. However, there are also other fundamental issues associated with the philosophy of holism as the foundation for science and scientific work from an epistemological stance. There are at least three issues that pose difficulties in developing science from the holistic philosophy: (a) developing explanations in terms of *whole qua whole*, (b) the issue of holistic reduction, and (c) problems of method in relation to conceptualization and measurement. First, although there are several theoretical principles in holism associated with the fundamental tenets identified earlier, theoreticians are finding it hard to develop explanations of behaviors or states of wholes through the explication of holistic processes. Theoretically, holistic processes are often identifiable only descriptively, without pointing to explanations of holistic behaviors or states. Second, on the other hand, holistic theories may lead to reduction of a kind that is different from the physical reductionism. Holistic reduction prevents views and understandings of human experiences from particular, distinct orientations, especially when humans are considered parts in ecocentric or universal holism (Gadow, 1992). Third, because one of the major tenets of holism is conceptualizing wholes as uniquely wholes and not in terms of parts, it is necessary to conceptualize holistic phenomena with new language (as specified in Phillips' holism 3). This means there is a need for a unified science—for example, for all sciences that deal with humans or living organisms (or even for all sciences)—united by a new set of scientific language and general theoretical principles. Holism, with its stance against analytic reductionism and decomposition, must come up with concepts that specify phenomena of wholes. For example, human phenomena in holism then would need to be conceptualized from a unified, holistic perspective, not from the biological, psychological, social, or nursing perspectives because such perspectives would only be addressing partial views. Holism points to a science without perspective, thus a new way of defining different scientific disciplines must be developed within holism. This is a challenge that cannot be taken lightly.

ROGERS' SCIENCE OF UNITARY HUMAN BEINGS

Rogers' science of unitary human beings as a theoretical framework was first proposed in 1970 and has gone through several stages of conceptual and theoretical revisions. The theory, as it was proposed in 1970 and labeled as "a science of unitary man" in 1980, had a strong alliance with the holism of general system theory, especially that of Bertalanffy, field theory, and the general evolutionary tenets (Rogers, 1970, 1980). From these, she adopted the notions of humans as open systems and complex energy fields. The concept of energy field refers to the entitative feature of humans and environment, meaning that humans and environment are "energy fields" rather than that humans and environment *have* energy. The pattern of energy field was depicted as "a mosaic of waves" in Rogers' earlier work, but is changed later to refer to a single wave. She also conceptualized a human as "a unified whole possessing his own integrity and manifesting characteristics that are more than and different from the sum of his parts" (1970, p. 47). By 1983, Rogers emphasized the irreducibility of human energy field, which concept she viewed as representative of her paradigm to be "unitary" rather than "holistic." In 1970, she embraced the notion that "man and environment are continuously exchanging matter and energy with one another" (1970, p. 54), but later dropped this "exchange assumption" completely, replacing it with the idea of mutual process and integration of the human and environment energy fields.

Rogers conceptualized human beings as continuously changing their life patterns (patterning) toward increasing complexity and negentropy. Life patterning is viewed in terms of the wholeness of the unitary human being, expressed as the human energy field. The patterns of life processes are seen as being manifested through the unitary human being's mutual, simultaneous integrating process with the environment through the principles of homeodynamics, specified as helicy, resonancy, synchrony, and reciprocity. The principles of synchrony and reciprocity were combined into the principle of complementarity, which later became the principle of integrality (Rogers, 1986, 1990a, 1990b).

Rogers also began her conceptualization of negentropic journey in a linear space-time notion, but later anchored it in multidimensional context. In doing so, she moved toward the universal, cosmic holism, stating, "the integrality of people and their environments coordinates with a pandimensional universe of open systems, points to a new paradigm" (Rogers, 1992, p. 28). By 1992 then, Rogers had moved to view her framework as rooted in a pandimensional view of people and their world, moving beyond the usual notions of multidimensionality of universal existence. As specified in her writings by 1992, Rogers' science of unitary human beings is based on the following assumptions and conceptualizations:

- A pandimensional worldview is a way of perceiving reality within a universe of open systems. Hence, all reality is pandimensional. Pandimensionality refers to "an infinite domain without limit" that is nonlinear and without spatial or temporal attributes. Pandimensionality "expresses the idea of a unitary whole." (Rogers, 1992, p. 31)
- Within this view, the fundamental units of both the living and the nonliving are energy fields that are infinite, pandimensional, and in continuous motion. An energy field is perceived as a single wave. The human energy field and the environmental energy field are identified as distinct fields. The human energy field can be conceptualized for a single human being or groups by which either an individual or a group is considered irreducible and indivisible, once they are conceptualized as a singular unit. Each human energy field (either as a singular individual or as a group) is integral with its own environmental field that is unique to it.
- Human beings and their respective environments both are unitary and irreducible wholes.
- The distinguishing characteristic of an energy field perceived as a single wave is patterning that eventuates from the mutual process of the human-environmental fields based on the principles of homeodynamics (of resonancy, helicy, and integrality). Field patterning is characterized by change that is continuous, relative, innovative, creative, increasingly diverse, and unpredictable.
- Field patterning is emergent and unpredictable. Causality is rejected.
- "The evolution of life and nonlife is a dynamic, irreducible, non-linear process characterized by increasing complexification of energy field patterning" (Rogers, 1992, p. 31). Hence, all entities in the universe follow this evolutionary process.
- Nursing based on a science of unitary human beings is "inseparable from the new world view and the process of change," and the phenomena of concern for nursing from this view are people and their world in a pandimensional universe.

What, then, is the essence of Rogers' epistemology and of her holism? Rogers' epistemological position for her science of unitary human beings is constructivism, in which the conceptualization and language of the science are viewed as constructions to make the subject matter unique to nursing. She stressed that the definitions, meanings, and principles of her science are only valid within the context of the science of unitary human beings. Rogers was also a perspectivist because she acknowledged the legitimacy of viewing humans and environments in other ways, especially from disciplinary perspectives other than the one she espoused, that is, the study of unitary, irreducible, indivisible human and environmental fields as the unique focus of nursing. Hence, to Rogers, humans possess many distinct characteristics that may be conceptualized differently according to specific disciplines' foci of attention. To her, nursing's phenomena of concern need to be people and their environments, conceptualized in a pandimensional worldview as unitary, irreducible, indivisible human and environmental fields. She did not say why this must be so. She insisted this is a unique way for nursing to conceptualize its subject matter.

Rogers' position on holism is a paradoxical one: She suggested that the term "holistic" not be used to indicate her notion of unitary human beings in her later writings, and yet she believed that her worldview was holistic. One of Rogers' important assertions is the negation of parts in wholes. The notion of parts is irrelevant within the concept of unitary wholes that are irreducible and indivisible. Hence, to Rogers, no parts are identifiable in wholes. This is a departure from the general positions of holism that acknowledge the existence or possibility of parts within wholes, but align with David Bohm's idea that fragmentation results from the way of seeing the universe and is not the essential character of the holistic universe. In addition, Rogers embraced various aspects of entitative, anthropocentric, and universal cosmic holism without reconciling the diverse orientations these three versions of holism support.

Rogers viewed unitary human beings and unitary environments as distinct fields within a universe of open systems, suggesting that a universe is constituted by fields considered to be wholes. Fields as wholes are viewed to be irreducible and indivisible. She also suggested that all living and nonliving entities change in an evolutionary sense in a dynamic, irreducible, and nonlinear process. These views align with the tenets of the entitative holism. However, Rogers' conceptualization of field as the fundamental holistic unit is arbitrary and fluid.

This means that her notion of field may refer to entities that have specific boundaries, such as human beings, as well as those that are defined as fields when analytic needs arise. Environments as fields are relative to the focused human fields. This means that an environmental field relative to one specific human field embraces other human fields in an irreducible, indivisible whole that is the respective environmental field. If each and every human field is unitary, is it possible for any human field, completely embedded into an environmental field of another human being, to lose its identity as a unitary being? If this is so, then how is it possible for one human field to retain its unitary wholeness, while it is also possible for it to be embraced into an irreducible, indivisible environmental field? In discussing the theory of accelerating evolution derived from Rogers' science of unitary human beings, Rogers seemed to suggest the environmental field as a nonhuman field. If this is the case, then Rogers' environmental field must be conceptualized as devoid of humans. Both conceptualizations of environmental field—one that embraces all other humans and the other excluding humans—present logical problems in relation to field patterning and mutual processing. Furthermore, Rogers suggested that unitary human beings as wholes that are conceptualized as irreducible and indivisible at one point may be subsumed within other wholes that are irreducible and indivisible at another point, for example, the conceptualization of family energy field or crowd as an energy field. This relative conceptualization of field and the specific identification of human energy field and environmental energy field point to various logical problems.

On the other hand, Rogers' focus is on human beings, whose energy fields are viewed as unique and in a continuous mutual process with their unique environmental fields. This notion is close to the anthropocentric holism in which the central focus is the humans and their relationships with environment. Rogers also views the human and environmental change and evolution to be interpenetrating, coordinated, and together in a single wave patterning. This view, reflecting David Bohm's holism, leans toward the universal cosmic holism. This orientation shifts the focus of study from humans to the universe, thus making it difficult to conceptualize the appropriate phenomena of concern for nursing.

Therefore, Rogers' holism is eclectic and contains several points, as raised earlier, that need to be reconciled. It is an abstract system that needs to be specified further in terms of language and conceptualization as well as through research. In addition, although Rogers indicates that "people's capacity to participate knowingly in the process of change" (1990) is inherent in this science, this idea is nowhere apparent in the conceptualization of field patterning expressed through the principles of homeodynamics. This vision of holism, then, highlights the integrality of humans and their environment rather than humans' proactive (both positive and negative) potential to influence the process of change.

CONCLUSIONS

The concept of holism as examined in this chapter is associated with complex and multiple sets of ideas used as ontological and epistemological bases for science. The term *holism* is used both casually and seriously in the literature, especially in the nursing literature. Nearly all of the nursing theorists used the term *holism* or *holistic* in describing their theories, often without specifying which assumptions of holism are incorporated into their theories. Besides Rogers, whose work was discussed in this chapter, Roy, Newman, Neuman, Parse, Orem, Levine, King, and Watson support one or two of the holistic tenets in their theories and theoretical models. Holism as nursing philosophy and as the basis for theory development in nursing has been with us for a long time. It is difficult to say what the future is for holism in nursing unless we are able to address why holism is necessary, desirable, essential, or important for nursing conceptualizations and nursing practice. If it is answered from an ontological perspective, then holism must be addressed from the way we conceptualize nursing clients as human beings. If it is answered from an epistemological perspective, then holism points to new ways of developing knowledge. In nursing, we must also address the question of how significantly holistic nursing theories accommodate essential and important issues of nursing practice. Phillips' despair that "holism is an eminently unworkable doctrine" must be overcome by various logical, empirical, and conceptual means, if nursing is to continue in its insistence to hold on to holism as its major orientation.

REFERENCES

Barratt, B., Marchand, L., Scheder, J., Plane, M. B., Maberry, R., Applebaum, D., Rakel, D., & Rabago, D. (2003). Themes of holism, empowerment, access, and legitimacy define complementary, alternative, and integrative medicine in relation to conventional biomedicine. *Journal of Alternative and Complementary Medicine, 9,* 937–947.

Bertalanffy, L. von (1969). *General system theory: Foundations, development, applications.* New York: Braziller.

Bohm, D. (1980). *Wholeness and the implicate order.* London: Routledge and Kegan Paul.

Cava, P. (2000). The error of excessive proximity preference—A modest proposal for understanding holism. *Nursing Philosophy, 1,* 20–25.

Chattopadhyaya, D. (1967). *Individuals and societies: A methodological inquiry.* New York: Allied.

Deliman, Y., & Smolowe, J. (1982). *Holistic medicine.* Reston, VA: Prentice-Hall.

Donaldson, S. K., & Crowley, D. M. (1978). The discipline of nursing. *Nursing Outlook, 26,* 113-120.

Fodor, J., & Lepore, E. (1992). *Holism: A shopper's guide.* Cambridge, MA: Blackwell.

Gadow, S. (1992). Existential ecology: The human/natural world. *Social Science and Medicine, 35,* 596–602.

Gaydos, H. L. B. (2003). The cocreative aesthetic process: A new model for aesthetics in nursing. *International Journal for Human Caring, 7,* 40–44.

Goldstein, M. S. (2003). Complementary and alternative medicine: Its emerging role in oncology. *Journal of Psychosocial Oncology, 21*(2), 1–21.

Harrington, A. (1995). Metaphoric connections: Holistic science in the shadow of the Third Reich. *Social Research, 62,* 357–386.

Harrington, A. (1996). *Reenchanted science: Holism in German culture from Wilhelm II to Hitler.* Princeton, NJ: Princeton University Press.

Hudson, R. (1988). Whole or parts: A theoretical perspective on person. *Australian Journal of Advanced Nursing, 6,* 12–20.

James, S. (1984). *The content of social explanation.* Cambridge, MA: Cambridge University Press.

Kermode, S. (2002). The natural holistic imperative. *Australian Journal of Holistic Nursing, 9*(2), 4–13.

Kheel, M. (1985). The liberation of nature: A circular affair. *Environmental Ethics, 7,* 135–149.

Koestler, A. (1967). *The ghost in the machine.* New York: Macmillan.

Koestler, A. (1978). *Janus: A summing up.* New York: Random House.

Kolcaba, R. (1997). The primary holisms in nursing. *Journal of Advanced Nursing, 25,* 290–296.

Lowenberg, J. S. (1989). *Caring and responsibility: The crossroads between holistic practice and traditional medicine.* Philadelphia: University of Pennsylvania Press.

Marietta, D., Jr. (1995). *For people and the planet: Holism and humanism in environmental ethics.* Philadelphia: Temple University Press.

Morowitz, H. J. (1972). Biology as a cosmological science. *Main Currents in Modern Thought, 28,* 156.

Owen, M. J., & Holmes, C. A. (1993). 'Holism' in the discourse of nursing. *Journal of Advanced Nursing, 18,* 1688–1695.

Parse, R. R (1987). *Nursing science: Major paradigms, theories, and critiques.* Philadelphia: Saunders.

Parsons, T. (1951). *The social system.* New York: Free Press.

Phillips, D. C. (1976). *Holistic thought in social science.* Stanford, CA: Stanford University Press.

Regan, T. (1981). The nature and possibility of an environmental ethic. *Environmental Ethics, 3,* 19–34.

Rogers, M. E. (1970). *An introduction to the theoretical basis of nursing.* Philadelphia: Davis.

Rogers, M. E. (1980). Nursing: A science of unitary man. In J. P. Riehl & C. Roy (Eds.), *Conceptual models for nursing practice* (2nd ed., pp. 329–337). New York: Appleton-Century-Crofts.

Rogers, M. E. (1986). Science of unitary human beings. In V. M. Malinski (Ed.), *Explorations on Martha Rogers' science of unitary human beings* (pp. 3–8). Norwalk, CT: Appleton-Century-Crofts.

Rogers, M. E. (1990a). Nursing: Science of unitary, irreducible, human beings: Update 1990. In E. A. M. Barrett (Ed.), *Visions of Rogers' science-based nursing* (pp. 5–11). New York: National League for Nursing.

Rogers, M. E. (1990b). Space-age paradigm for new frontiers in nursing. In M. E. Parker (Ed.), *Nursing theories in practice* (pp. 105–112). New York: National League for Nursing.

Rogers, M. E. (1992). Nursing science and the space age. *Nursing Science Quarterly, 5,* 27–34.

Sarter, B. (1988). Philosophical sources of nursing theory. *Nursing Science Quarterly, 1,* 52–59.

Schultz, P. R. (1987). Toward holistic inquiry in nursing. A proposal for synthesis of patterns and methods. *Scholarly Inquiry for Nursing Practice, 1,* 135–146.

Shealy, M. C. (1985). Florence Nightingale 1820–1910: An evolutionary mind in the context of holism. *Journal of Holistic Nursing Practice, 3*(1), 4–6.

Smuts, J. C. (1926). *Holism and evolution.* London: Oxford University Press.

Täljedal, I. (1997). Weak and strong holism. *Scandinavian Journal of Social Medicine, 25,* 67–69.

Taylor, B. (2004). Technical, practical, and emancipatory reflection for practicing holistically. *Journal of Holistic Nursing, 22,* 73–84.

Teilhard de Chardin, P. (1959). *The phenomenon of man. With an introduction by Sir Julian Huxley* (B. Wall, Trans.). New York: Harper & Row. (Originally published in 1955)

Williams, A. (1998). Therapeutic landscapes in holistic medicine. *Social Science and Medicine, 46,* 1193–1203.

CHAPTER *8*

Systems Theory and Nursing Theories*

Heiko Kleve

Following Niklas Luhmann (1995a, p. 15) we can still assume (perhaps even more so now than ever before) that "'systems theory' [is] today a collective term for very different meanings and very different levels of analysis." Consequently, the term "does not convey an unequivocal meaning" (Luhmann, 1995a, p.15). Because of this, the word *system* is likewise to be seen in a polyvalent light, depending on the particular theory within which it is defined or within which it is employed in order to provide descriptions and explanations. The classical definition of "system" is borrowed from Aristotle (cf. Ulfig, 1999, p. 137), namely, *as a whole which is composed of parts but which is more than or something different from merely the sum of its parts.* Because systems theory thinking is often associated with this definition of system, theories of systems are not infrequently viewed as being holistic (deriving from the Greek noun *holon*, meaning a whole). Such theories, it is commonly stated, are not interested so much in the scientific method of analysis, preferred since the days of Newton and Descartes, that dissects phenomena into their component parts; rather, systems theories are thought to favor a holistic view of things, that is, observation of the interactions between the parts that make the wholes what they are—something more than or

---

*Translated from German by Gerald Nixon.

something different from the sum of their individual parts (cf., among others, Capra, 1991).

Nursing theories, too, which also make use of the term "system" to describe and explain the phenomena of nursing, draw upon the concept of wholeness (see Neuman, 1997; Roy & Andrews, 1997) or holism (see King, 1997) in order to distinguish themselves from other theories. However, when we consider this use of the notion of holism in systems-based nursing theories, we see already that more recent concepts of systems have not yet received due attention in the theory of nursing. The truth is that the concept of holism no longer plays any significant role in current approaches of systems theory; on the contrary, it is either viewed rather critically or is even completely rejected. The critiques of holistic concepts, as to be found, for example, in postmodern philosophies and theories of science (see Lyotard, 1979/1994, p. 42ff; Welsch, 1987, p. 54ff.), have now also found their way into systems theory. More recent systems theories have thus taken a critical stance towards attempts wishing to observe the whole; they mark themselves off from the great systems philosophers, who along with Hegel deem the whole to be the ultimate truth and declare along with Adorno (1951), "The whole is not the ultimate truth" (p. 80). More recent systems theory thinking describes itself as *difference theory* thinking, that is, a way of thinking that reflects that both systems themselves as well as all systemic observations of the world are constituted by differences and constitute differences (cf. Clam, 2002). As a result, holism or holistic observation remains an unattainable ideal since the complexity of the world is observed through mechanisms of the (differential) reduction of this complexity but, as a result, the observation of the world cannot be holistic.

An extremely popular systems theory and one that has become increasingly important in recent years differs fundamentally, even paradigmatically, from systems theories that postulate holism. This is the sociological theory of self-referential systems put forward by the sociologist Niklas Luhmann (1927–1998). Especially with his books *Soziale Systeme. Grundriß einer allgemeinen Theorie* (Luhmann, 1984/1995a) and *Die Gesellschaft der Gesellschaft* (Luhmann, 1997), Luhmann has set standards for subsequent discourses on systems theory that should no longer be ignored when attempting to use systems theory in nursing science today. Luhmann's development of systems theory has now come to be regarded as a *general systems theory* (see Krieger, 1996), thus apparently superseding the classical general concept of systems developed as early as the 1950s and 1960s by the founder of interdisciplinary thinking on systems, Ludwig von Bertalanffy. It therefore seems appropriate to suggest that a nursing science interested in systems should devote its attention to the theory of self-referential systems.

As Jens Friebe (1999) has remarked, "applying his [Luhmann's] systems theory to nursing issues remains a problem to be solved" (p. 154). Resolving this problem is not easy though, because nursing needs theories to be oriented towards practical application while Luhmann "does not, however, develop applied science" (Friebe, 1999, p. 154). I hope to disprove this assessment in this chapter. For as soon as we look at the history of the reception of Luhmann's systems theory up to present (cf. de Berg & Schmidt, 2000), we are able to agree with Dirk Baecker's (1994) statement that "paradoxically the very abstractions that are involved here—lofty as they may be—turn out to be remarkably close to actual practice" (p. 13). It would exceed by far the bounds of this essay if I were even to begin to show the extent to which this systems theory has in the meantime been applied with considerable benefits in areas such as psychotherapy, family therapy, organizational development and consultancy, management, social work, and education (cf., among others, Gripp-Hagelstange, 2000). At all events it seems quite probable that for nursing, too, interesting benefits might be anticipated if nursing theorists were to examine more recent systems theory and make use of it as a basis for reflection.

However, before discussing any fundamental theorems of Luhmann's systems theory that might be profitably applied to nursing theory, the development of the paradigms of systems theory is first of all outlined in order, subsequently, to be able to place systems-based nursing theories (which came especially from the United States in the 1960s and 1970s) in their context and give a brief account of their core contents. The third step will be to outline a number of key theoretical elements of Luhmann's sociological systems theory, in the hope that they will provide an impetus for nursing to give increased consideration to this systems theory. In conclusion, a number of perspectives and questions are to be developed that are perhaps relevant in this context.

PARADIGM SHIFT IN SOCIOLOGICAL SYSTEMS THEORY

In the development of the sociological systems theory, one can distinguish at least three different paradigms (cf. Luhmann, 1984/1995a, p. 15ff.), whose postulates are structured by means of three operative distinctions: the part/whole distinction, the system/environment distinction and, finally, the identity/difference distinction (see also Kleve, 2000).

The First Paradigm of Systems Theory— The Part/Whole Distinction

The focus of this paradigm is on the wholeness or the unity of the system, in which the parts are conceived of as integrated system components that restrict each other's degree of freedom, thus bringing about something called "emergence" (cf. Willke, 1993, p. 278). Emergence refers to the properties of systems that only come into being when systems structure themselves as processes of mutually related parts. Emergent system properties are formed on account of the selective linking of system elements (in other words, on account of the relationships existing between the parts of the system) and can only be explained if the system is observed as a whole made up of interrelated elements rather than if the parts of the system are observed in isolation. One can imagine a family, for example, in which the members behave towards each other in a certain way, that is, according to certain rules and patterns of communication. These patterns and rules, inherent in the family system, first give rise to the members' individual behavior; therefore, if one wants to understand or explain their behavior, it is essential to try and identify the patterns and rules that structure the behavior of the individual family members. This explains why practitioners of systemic family therapy take a particular interest in the patterns and rules that—for the most part implicitly, latently—structure behavioral processes within families (cf. Simon, Clement, & Stierlin, 1999). Individual behavior patterns (e.g. children's symptoms such as bed-wetting and hyperactivity or illnesses such as anorexia) are thus regarded in systemic family therapy as functional contributions to the whole family system that serve to support the system's equilibrium, its homeostasis, and thus guarantee that the family structures are preserved.

However, it is precisely this systemic principle of the homeostatic preservation of structures that appears problematic because it amounts to nothing less than a latent conservatism of systems, to an affirmation of the system. Hence, systems theory is frequently criticized—on account of the very terminology that informs it as well as its key distinctions—for being primarily interested in system-maintaining processes that try, accordingly, to stabilize the holistic structures of the system. The transformation of systems, not to mention their breakdown, receives little attention, it is said. In the following it will become apparent why this criticism applies in particular to systems theories based on the part/whole distinction but by no means applies to those systems theories based on the next two paradigms elucidated below.

In sociology, the systems theory developed by Talcott Parsons is considered to be a classic theory based on the part/whole distinction. This theory has had a decisive influence on systems-based nursing theories (cf., Friebe, 1999) because these originated in the United States in the 1960s and 1970s at a time when the American sociologist was very popular (cf., Friebe, 1999, p. 148). (These theories are now becoming familiar in Germany, too, with the establishment of courses of study in nursing sciences.) From our vantage point today, these theories thus convey what one might call antiquated notions of systems that focus particularly on homeostatic system maintenance, and because this is their starting point, they are concerned with the goal of adapting individual behavior to the social or organizational structures of a society. Especially in the theory put forward by Sister Callista Roy and Heather A. Andrews (1997) the notion of adaptation already appears in the name these theoreticians give to their approach: adaptation model. But what is Parsons' concept of systems?

Parsons (1972) is interested above all in the question of how actions occur in social systems as emergent phenomena and maintain social systems. He answers this question with the so-called AGIL model. According to this model, social actions may arise when four functions are fulfilled: *a*daptation; *g*oal attainment; *i*ntegration; and *l*atent pattern maintenance. Each function is attributed to a different subsystem that is necessary in each case to enable an action to occur and thus an emergent action system to develop. *Adaptation* to changes in ecological conditions is made possible by the body, the biological behavioral system, so to speak. *Goal attainment,* that is, the intention and realization of the objectives and purposes of an action, is carried out by the personal system, that is to say the cognitive and emotional system of the psyche, the individual psychical personality. *Integration,* the embedding of actions into a network of relationships between bodies and personalities as well as the necessary coordination and attribution of actions, is dealt with by the social system involved (e.g., within the interaction of a family or an organization). The *latent pattern maintenance*—that is, the continuation (though perhaps dormant or in abeyance) of the action system with its routines, patterns, and rules—is made possible, finally, by the cultural system, or the social culture as such, that enables (so to speak) the upholding of standards, practices, patterns, and rules as well as of social roles, which can be invoked and brought into play at various times.

Parson's systems theory is also known as structural-functional theory, or as structural functionalism, because it assumes a predetermined structure and a systemic whole, in other words a structured system of social action, and asks—as a subordinated question to some extent—which functions must be fulfilled by which subsystems in order that the whole may constitute and maintain itself as a system. Structural functionalism as a holistic, sociological version of systems theory (cf., among others, Morel, Bauer, Meleghy, Miedenzu, Preglau, & Staubmann, 1997, p. 300) may be regarded as an unquestioned main focus of many classic concepts of systems (in nursing, too). The key factor, here, is that the subsystems—that is, the body (the biological system), the personality (the conscious, or the psychic system), the social aspect (the social system, e.g., a family, a group or an organization) and the cultural aspect (the cultural system of values, norms, roles, etc.)—are set in relation to each other in such a way as to enable their respective functions (adaptation, goal attainment, integration, and latent pattern maintenance) to "emerge." For, according to Parsons, "Action is system!" (Luhmann, 2002a, p. 19).

In several versions of systems theories that are closely or loosely oriented to Parsons' approach, the individual systems are sometimes imagined as Russian dolls, each contained within another like the layers of an onion, so to speak, and relating to each other in such a way that the larger system always contains the next smaller system (see, for example, King, 1997, p. 185). The only question is whether it is (still) helpful to describe systems with this or any other kind of spatial metaphor. Peter Fuchs (2001), at any rate, considers spatial metaphors an unsuitable means of arriving at descriptions of systems that are adequate for such a highly differentiated and complex society. He attempts to get the better of reifying descriptions, still predominant in systemic theories, too, by calling a system a *metaphor* intended to symbolize something that, strictly speaking, eludes definition. This metaphorical conceptualization of a system, however, only completely comes into its own in the third paradigm of systems theory. But in the late 1960s and early 1970s already, classic systems-theory orientation, with its adherence to the part/whole distinction, was gradually giving way to a second paradigm of systems theory.

The Second Paradigm of Systems Theory— The System/Environment Distinction

By the end of the 1960s, Luhmann (1970b) had already left structural functionalism, or structural-functional theory, behind. For him the phenomena primarily in need of explication were no longer systemic structures and their maintenance but the social function to be fulfilled in order, and then (on a secondary plane to some extent) to form systemic structures that first led to the emergence of systems. Hence, even in his early years, Luhmann no longer applied the term structural functionalism to his theory, speaking instead of a *functional-structural* theory. Thus, Luhmann begins by switching the priorities: His starting point is not the structure but the function.

Whereas in the structural-functional theory one presupposes certain system structures and subsequently inquires into the functional tasks (the AGIL model) that must be fulfilled in order for the systems to be maintained as part/whole relationships, the functional-structural theory is more versatile in its analytical possibilities. This is because the concept of structure is subordinated to the creation of distinctions with the result that, although distinctions (e.g., the primary system/environment distinction) must be presupposed in the differentiation of a system, already integrated structures need not be. A system is defined, accordingly, as an entity that marks itself off from its environment; as long as it can preserve its distinction from its environment, the system is maintained (as a body, psyche, or social system, say).

The principal question posed by the functional-structural theory is in this respect not addressed to the maintenance of systems but to the functions and tasks that the respective systems with their structures fulfill for their environments (e.g., for society or for other systems). Considered from the point of view of evolution theory, systems go into decline when other systems are able, in a functionally equivalent way, to solve a problem more adequately, thus asserting themselves in their environment, or when the problem for which a system attempts to find a solution by forming structures is eventually solved. Because of this functional-structural orientation, which can equally describe and explain system transformation and decline, this theory is also known as *equivalence functionalism* because the *particular* fulfillment of functions by systems can always be *compared* with other, *equally possible* (i.e., contingent) variants of function fulfillment. The question that can then be posed is whether functional systemic equivalents (alternatives) can be found that are able to fulfill to an even greater degree of satisfaction the functions that a given system more or less satisfactorily fulfills. Luhmann calls this comparative method the *functional method,* or *functional analysis* (cf. Luhmann, 1970a). Functional analysis continues to be a key method of systems theory (cf. Luhmann 1984/1995a, p. 83ff.) that enables us to compare different things, for example, different systemic structures, with each other based on the (perhaps identical) functions they fulfill. "Functional analysis uses relations to comprehend what is present as contingent and what is different as comparable" (Luhmann, 1984/1995a, p. 83).

In order to illustrate this method, one could again imagine a family in which a symptom occurs that requires therapy, for example, anorexia. If one assumes that, as a particular systemic action structure, the anorexia performs a function within the system of family relations, one can (for example, in family therapy) ask at least two questions: first, as to which function this might be; and second, which alternative (contingent) systemic structures are imaginable and ultimately achievable that are not accompanied by symptoms such as anorexia, but nevertheless serve the function to be fulfilled within the family.

As is made clear by this last example, finally, functional-structural theory is interested in system change, or system transformation; and in the form of equivalence functionalism or functional analysis, it provides at the same time a means of being able to analyze, describe, and explain this change as well as possibly also to initiate it in practice. Systems theory has experienced a further advance towards developing a sensitivity to transformation and dynamics by means of the third, current paradigm.

The Third Paradigm of Systems Theory— The Identity/Difference Distinction

Luhmann's book *Social Systems* (Luhmann, 1984/1995a) has further radicalized the focus placed by functional-structural theory on difference theory. With its third paradigm, systems theory has now (if it hadn't before) turned into a poststructuralist, or perhaps one could even say a postmodern theory, a theory that is primarily concerned with differences and the creation of differences and only subsequently (i.e., based on differences and the creation of differences) with the creation of structures and structure-creating processes (cf. Clam, 2002). The development of systems is regarded as a complex process of differentiation: A system is able to develop that marks itself off from an environment of operations, events, or distinctions that neither belong to it nor are associated with it only when recursive operations, events, or distinctions (in other words differences) are linked to each other in such a way that they are distinguishable from other operations, events, or distinctions. Thus, at the start of any system development there is a distinction between what belongs to the system (in the form of operations, events, or distinctions) and what is set apart from it systemically, namely its environment. In other words, the system only constitutes itself as a systemic identity when recursive operations of the same type set themselves apart from unassociated operations of a different type.

It is precisely this aspect that is referred to when one speaks of the identity/difference distinction in this paradigm of systems theory. For a system's identity is formed in its being different from its environment. A system is no longer regarded as a unity, no longer as a holistic structure; it is not, as Jean Clam (2000) puts it, "a thing that is present in the world, possesses an inner structure or organization and maintains a relationship to the world which operates via the 'interface' of its spatial borders" (p. 308). On the contrary, a system consists "solely of operations. . . . Beyond its operative actions, occurring successively from moment to moment, it is nothing. At the very moment the system discards its constitutive distinction between itself and its environment, it vanishes" (Clam, 2000, p. 308). When one tries to express this notion in more concrete (reifying, ontologizing) language, recourse is necessarily made to the kind of paradoxical formulation that gives a difference (the system, that is to say) the connotation of unity and equates it with identity. But the system is the difference (between system and environment).

Yet, strictly speaking, this notion of system eludes any attempt at definition. It is for this reason that Fuchs (2001), the systems theorist who has probably developed Luhmann's theory more intensively and more radically than anyone else, refuses to regard systems as (spatially determinable) objects or even as subjects. Instead, he calls them "unjects" and would like to have the concept of system understood purely as a metaphor:

> Construing the system as difference rules out the system as a thing, as subject/object, as a phenomenon. It is not the ONE, which can be elucidated, scanned and analysed through and through. System is (against the backdrop of classical logic) the paradoxical expression for an *operative difference*. It is also the expression for throwing the

scheme of being into disarray, for a destructive *neither/nor* with regard to the question of being. If one wants to have the system as an object, one must reify the difference of the system, i.e. one must make a systematic error, which need not inevitably cause any harm but will be fatal when it involves a theory of difference which then, quite unawares, turns into a theory of system. Systems theory is, upon close scrutiny, a theory of the *barrier* in the system/environment distinction and as such it is also a *barriered* theory. (Fuchs, 2001, p. 242).

Although, strictly speaking, the system is the difference, the distinction, the barrier between system and environment (cf., also Luhmann 2002a, p. 66ff.), systems *imagine* themselves to be unities. The way in which this happens is explained by the theory of self-referential systems. The concept of self-reference in particular points to the construction of systemic unity:

The theory of self-referential systems maintains that systems can differentiate only by self-reference, which is to say, only insofar as systems refer to themselves (be this to elements of the same system, to operations of the same system, or to the unity of the same system) in constituting their elements and their elemental operations. To make this possible, systems must create and employ a description of themselves; they must at least be able to use the difference between system and environment within themselves, for orientation and as a principle for creating information. Therefore self-referential closure is possible only in an environment, only under ecological conditions. (Luhmann 1984/1995a, p. 25).

Luhmann assumes that three types of self-referential systems in particular can be described and explained using the theory of difference, namely biological, psychical, and social systems. *Biological systems,* that is, living organisms, are created by the permanent and continuous recurrence of physical life processes (e.g., metabolism, the activity of the organs, and cell formation) and their distinction from an environment of, among other things, psychical and social systems. *Psychical systems* are produced by the permanent and continuous recurrence of consciously formed operations, that is, thoughts or the mind's focused attention, and their distinction from an environment of, among other things, biological and social systems. And *social systems,* that is, interactions or organizations, for instance, are constituted by the permanent and continuous recurrence of communicative operations and their distinction from an environment of, among other things, biological and psychical systems.

With regard to all three categories of system mentioned, the theoretical figure of self-reference denotes a property attributed exclusively to human subjects in early European philosophy: the (self-)identification of one's own, of one's own unity (e.g., the "I" of the psyche) through the distinction made in respect of otherness (e.g., the social "you"). The primary task of any system, whether it be of a biological, psychical, or social nature, is to refer to itself in such a way that it achieves stability as an operable unity and draws a boundary (puts up a barrier) between itself and its environment, which it can distinguish from itself. This is not only accomplished by the psyche but also, for example, by the bodily system and its subsystems, such as the stomach. If the stomach of a mammal were not able in this respect to differentiate, distinguish, and mark itself off from an external systemic environment (for example, from the food to be digested), it would digest itself. In order that systems do not sink into chaos, into entropy, they must—it might be summed up here—not only be able to distinguish themselves from their environment but also be able to keep up this distinction permanently. Thus, the forming of systemic structures always presupposes the forming of difference, which is reconfirmed with every operation carried out by the system, otherwise the system would disintegrate and be absorbed by its environment.

In order to stress this once more: According to this theory, systems distinguish themselves from their environment, and this distinction constitutes the system. It is in this respect that the theory of self-referential systems differs from so-called analytical systems theories; these theories likewise take into account the system/environment distinction but presuppose that an external observer (e.g., a scientist) must always establish this difference. Depending on his interests, he will regard one thing and then another as a system and will distinguish it from its particular environment. Luhmann's systems theory takes up this analytical conception of systems but radicalizes it by establishing that the system itself is also an observer (e.g., of itself). The system is itself thought of as an observer with regard to the differences it establishes in order to observe itself or others, for example, with regard to the question as to what others' observations of its self-observations may look like; that is, how others observe its observations.

> Here too one comes to a "sublation" [*Aufhebung*] of the older basic difference into a more complex theory, which now enables one to speak about the introduction of self-descriptions, self-observations, and self-simplifications within systems. One can now distinguish the system/environment difference as seen from the perspective of the

observer (e.g. that of a scientist) from the system/environment difference as it used in the system itself, the observer, in turn, being
conceivable himself only as a self-referential system. (Luhmann,
1984/1995a, p. 25).

Linked to the thesis of self-referential systems are extensive revolutionary transformations of the theory, two key ones of which I
would like, finally, to outline here.

First, self-reference means not only that systems refer to themselves through the recurrence of certain related operations, thus
marking themselves off from an environment, but also that differ-
ence-creating processes that have successfully been constituted as systems can acquire contact to their environment or to other systems
solely by means of self-contact, or self-reference. Each biological,
psychical, or social system can thus connect with its respective environment solely by means of reference to its own operations, that is,
indirectly. Accordingly, the biological system can only react to relevant processes occurring in the corresponding psyche or in relevant
social systems by means of its own bodily processes. And these psychical and social processes can only be distinguished by means of its
own bodily sensors. By analogy, the same can be said, of course, in respect of the psychical and social systems.

The psyche, for example, can only consciously perceive bodily
states to the degree permitted by the respective consciousness together with its thought operations. Further, the psyche can only
process communications by means of its own psychical faculties of
thought. The interfaces among body, psyche, and social system are
consequently boundaries at which various areas of complexity meet;
these areas provide each other with stimuli in order to form differences but do not overlap. In this way, communication, say, cannot
connect directly with what is happening in the psyche in terms of
thought but only in the form of conveyed information (with the help
of the biological system). But as soon as thoughts are conveyed, the
message along with what was conveyed (the information) are no
longer *thought* operations but occurrences within communication
that are no longer measured according to psychical but according to
social standards. The theory of self-referential systems makes a clear
distinction between the classes of system named above, thus enabling
the relations between the individual systems, the reciprocal relationships of observation, to be described with great precision.

Second, this does not mean, of course, that biological, psychical,
and social systems could exist without each other; on the contrary,

each of these systems presupposes itself as a relevant environment. They are thus interdependent, none of them being able to operate without the others. Luhmann (1984/1995a, p. 286ff.) speaks in this context of *interpenetration* and later of *structural coupling* (cf., Luhmann, 2002a, p. 118ff.). Fuchs (2001), moreover, uses the term *conditioned co-production* in order to highlight this fundamental interdependence, the reliance of system and environment on each other: "The system is not to be lifted out of its environment; it cannot be isolated. It is this *co*, this *concurrence*, this twoness that cannot be bisected to form two ones" (Fuchs, 2001, p. 15). Consequently, as can perhaps be readily understood, the social aspect cannot be differentiated into systems without the psychical and biological aspects coacting as conditions of this differentiation. However, what is interesting, especially for nursing, is above all the thesis that the biological, physical aspect cannot come into being without the social and psychical aspects being present as conditions of biological differentiation.

THE PART/WHOLE DISTINCTION AS THE STARTING POINT OF SYSTEMS-BASED NURSING THEORIES

The last two paradigms of systems theory described have yet to be taken up by nursing theory. In the discourse of health care studies in general, there is scarcely a more appropriate comment than that of Jost Bauch (2000), who sums it up as follows:

> In the perception which medicine and healthcare have of themselves and the world there is no visible history of consideration given to the ideas of systems theory of the kind put forward by Niklas Luhmann. Sociological systems theory has so far left not the slightest imprint in the description which healthcare has given of itself. (p. 387)

Bauch sees two reasons for this: First, with few exceptions (see, for example, Luhmann, 1990a, and to some extent Luhmann, 1975) Luhmann himself has given hardly any attention to the health system. By contrast, he has been published substantial systems-theory-based analyses in separate monographs on the economic system (Luhmann, 1988), the system of science (Luhmann, 1990a, 1994a), the system of law (Luhmann, 1993a), the system of art (Luhmann, 1995b), the political system (Luhmann, 2000a), the system of religion (Luhmann, 2000b), and the education system (Luhmann, 2002b).

Second, according to Bauch (2000, pp. 387–388), this conspicuous abstinence of Luhmann's with regard to the health system has to do with the fact that this system scarcely possesses any distinct reflective theories that provide a comprehensive sociological analysis of its position in society or of its particular functions and the work it does. Thus, a sociology of the health system may be able to offer sociological descriptions from outside; however, these remain unobservable by the health system itself because "there is no theoretical apparatus within this social system that might be able to take up and process such external theoretical descriptions" (Bauch, 2000, p. 388). For this reason there was evidently no inducement for Luhmann to concern himself to any great extent with the health system. He attempted, nonetheless, to ascertain the causes of this particular reflective deficit in sociology. One of the causes, he concluded, was that the health system fulfilled a social function (namely, the treatment of the sick) that apparently required no further justification and reflection as it was taken for granted (cf. Bauch, 2000, p. 388).

Furthermore, according to Luhmann (cf. Bauch, 2000, p. 389), this treatment seems to get along with a minimum of (reflective) communication—at least from the point of view of classical biomedicine and in comparison with other social systems. Whereas politics, law, or education relate to their psychical and social environments, to people or social institutions, through a variety of communication media, medicine—and nursing, too—relate more or less directly to the biological system, the body. That this (old, classical) point of view is becoming increasingly problematic, however, and that especially the health system now presents itself much more clearly as a system that also places an extremely strong emphasis on communication has been demonstrated in recent years in particular by the growing establishment of health care studies (cf. Bauch, 2000, p. 401ff.), including nursing studies (cf. also Mühlum, Bartholomeyczik, & Göpel, 1997). This can be explained by systems theory; I will come back to this later.

That American nursing theories have not yet taken up the last two paradigms of systems theory is partly due to the fact that they were developed in the 1960s and 1970s, a time when those concepts of systems theory were especially popular that were based on then modern approaches of general systems theory put forward by Ludwig von Bertalanffy or on the sociological systems theory of Talcott Parsons. Both approaches—that of Bertalanffy as well as that of Parsons—can be subsumed under the first paradigm of systems theory, postulating the part/whole distinction. Drawing upon Jens Friebe (1999, p. 148ff.),

I would like to give a brief outline of three such approaches of systems-oriented nursing theory, namely, those of Dorothy E. Johnson (1980), Imogene M. King (1995, 1997), and Betty Neuman (1997).

Dorothy E. Johnson (cf., Friebe 1999, pp. 148–149) regards nursing as a regulating force that becomes necessary when structural disorders of the system or a subsystem occur. Accordingly, the aim of nursing is to perform the function of encouraging or bringing about effective and useful behavior in patients in order to prevent disease, alleviate illness, and hasten recovery. This model is thus based above all on behavioural systems that react to environmental influences and whose aim is to prevent stress and process it functionally. If the human behavioral system does not succeed in preventing or functionally processing stress, nursing may become necessary. Nursing would then have to perform the required system regulation with the aim of protecting, stimulating, and supporting the stress-affected individual. As Friebe (1999, p. 149) makes clear, this concept is based on linear stress communication, on a stimulus/response model of behavioral psychology. What this model does not make visible, however, is that stress is by no means sufficiently observable through a reportedly stress-causing input from the environment; it is only observable when it is taken into consideration that individuals all have their own way of processing inputs from the environment cognitively as well as emotionally. As we will see below, this very perspective is a keystone of the theory of self-referential systems.

Imogene M. King (cf., Friebe, 1999, pp, 149–150) develops a broad system-oriented framework for nursing which, besides containing a theory of goal attainment, aims to provide a link to other theoretical approaches that are especially concerned with personal, interpersonal, and social systems. With this framework she attempts to create a holistic context for nursing theory that is oriented to Ludwig von Bertalanffy's ideas on a general systems theory. Of special significance for King is the formulation of a systems-based theory of interaction that foregrounds the reciprocal relationship between systems and their environments. This would appear to correspond to the second paradigm of systems theory, whose starting point is the system/environment distinction. According to this paradigm, of course, the system is not only influenced by the environment but also vice versa; permanent (cybernetic) feedback processes take place that go far beyond the confines of any one-sided notions of causality. With the help of the term "transaction," King develops a concept with which she tries to formulate goal-oriented nursing interaction. Nevertheless, this theory of interaction is insufficient, according to Friebe (1999, p. 149), because it is unable to accommodate both the dynamic developments and the differing symmetries of relationships in nursing.

A more comprehensive system model than that of either Johnson or King has been designed by Betty Neuman (cf., Friebe 1999, p. 151ff.), whose concept is also based on the systems of individual, group, and society and who observes the interactions of the systems and their respective environments in terms of the management of, defense against, and resistance to, stress. These processes of reacting to stress through management, defense, and resistance lead to an increasing relevance of various dimensions, especially those of a physiological, psychological, development-specific, sociocultural, and spiritual nature. If these dimensions are adequately functional, the personality remains intact and there is a stable equilibrium between the mind, the psyche, and the body. In the event of a disintegration of the personality, or an imbalance between the mental, psychological, and physiological dimensions, nursing becomes necessary (among other things). Nursing is entrusted with an extensive range of tasks "from limiting the possibilities of a confrontation with stress to a readjustment and re-orientation with a view to restoring basic resources" (Friebe, 1999, p. 152). For Neuman, too, it is a matter of stabilizing the system through nursing because stability is equated with well-being. After all, she is working towards a practice-oriented theory as a guide to nursing practice.

In summary, it can be concluded that the classical nursing theories, with their holistic intentions and classical system models, are focused on the maintenance of systems. There is no question that maintaining an individual's biological and psychical systems is an undeniable task of nursing; but it is quite a different matter whether the social systems in which people participate are likewise to be judged worthy of continued maintenance. Social systems in particular are capable of disrupting psychical and biological processes to such a degree that these are in danger of no longer being able to maintain themselves. We must, therefore, concur with Friebe (1999) with reference to the systems-based approaches described above when he states that these might well be able, on the one hand, to provide the basis for models of practice but, on the other, that they

> mostly suffer from the fact that they are invariably oriented to the individual's adjustment to social conditions and are not capable of integrating the asymmetries of interactions, internal psychical processes and changes in relationships. At the same time they frequently encour-

age the illusion that there is an unlimited ability to control social processes. (p. 154)

None of these criticisms, however, can be leveled at the theory of self-referential systems.

SYSTEMS THEORY AS THE THEORY OF SELF-REFERENTIAL SYSTEMS

In the following, the third paradigm of systems theory is taken up once more before, as a final step, a number of possible issues and perspectives are outlined for developing a nursing theory oriented towards current systems theory. Although the basic assumptions and features of this paradigm have already been presented, at least a brief account of further components of the theory ought to be given now, because if they are not understood, the theory of self-referential systems cannot be discussed in, or taken up by, nursing theory.

Let us begin with system formation, which comes about through self-referential processes in the biological, psychical, and social fields. In order for a system to be able to stabilize the system/environment distinction by which it is constituted, operations of the same type must connect with each other and refer to each other (Luhmann, 1990c). It is this process that first leads to the formation of a system, that is, to the formation of difference. Luhmann (1995a) proposes that this self-referential constitution of systems be named autopoeisis, a term taken from biology. The concept of autopoeisis (from the Greek *auto,* meaning "self," and *poein,* "to make") was put forward by the biological systems theorists Humberto Maturana and Francisco Varela (1987), who developed it originally in order to describe and explain the self-organisation of organisms. Luhmann applies the basic idea of autopoeisis, referring to biological systems, to psychical and social systems; all such systems are accordingly autopoietic—in other words self-referential, closed systems. Systems of this kind are organized in such a way that they "reproduce all the elementary components out of which they arise by means of a network of these elements themselves and in this way distinguish themselves from an environment—whether this takes the form of life, consciousness or (in the case of social systems) communication" (Luhmann 1995a, p. 266). At least three consequences ensue from the concept of autopoeisis for the further description of biological, psychical, and social systems.

First, operational closure and autonomy. Autopoietic systems are not directly influenced by the environment at the level of their operations. Consequently, occurrences in the environment cannot intervene when autopoietic systems are constituted; should this happen, autopoeisis—and thus the maintenance of the system—is endangered. For autopoeisis assumes that the self-reproduction of systems takes place exclusively through the system's own operations that can connect with each other because they are of the same type. Thus, according to this theory, so-called interventions are merely stimuli, irritations, or perturbations (Maturana & Varela, 1987) from the environment; whether and, if so, how the system reacts to these depends on its own operations. This theory manifestly goes beyond classical behaviorist stimulus/response models and, moreover, conventional intervention and control theories (cf., among others, Bardmann, Kersting, Vogel, & Woltmann, 1991) because to a certain extent, environmental stimuli as well as intervention and control operations offer the system opportunities to change. However, whether or how these opportunities are taken up by the system depends on the system's own autopoietic dynamics. In other words, every system interprets what is happening in its environment and reacts on the basis of these interpretations. Hence, a system's reactions are always determined by the system and not by the environment.

It is precisely this understanding of intervention and control that has been applauded in the professions in which new systems-theory thinking has exerted great influence (for example, in psychotherapy, family therapy, organization consultancy, education, and social work) because it provides an explanation for the practical experience among many professionals that the ability to plan interventions is extremely restricted (cf. Woltmann, 1991). Systems react in a certain way, and this can be influenced only to a very limited degree from outside. Nevertheless, it is possible that stimuli from the environment induce a system to undergo change.

The thesis that planned intervention is improbable but that stimulation of systems to undergo change is possible enables us to reconstruct, on the basis of systems theory (i.e., scientifically), the popular ethic of "supporting self-support" postulated by the caring professions.

Second, obtaining information as construction. Closely linked to the understanding of intervention as described above is the answer to the question of how autopoietic (i.e., self-referential, closed) systems obtain information. If the concept of autopoeisis is taken seriously, systems have no direct access to their environments in order to obtain information. *The environment is inaccessible to autopoietic systems with regard to operations and information.* The classical concept of information conveyance as the transmission of a message from a sender to a receiver cannot be integrated into this theory. An alternative and more suitable concept (and one upon which Luhmann [1995a, p. 68] bases his ideas) is provided by Gregory Bateson (1982), who asserts that information is "any difference that makes a difference" (p. 274). Accordingly, conveying information is not the transmission of identities (e.g., messages) but of differences. In order for a system to be able to generate information, it must be capable of observing changes of state, that is, differences, in its environment that likewise trigger changes of state, that is, differences, in its own internal operations. However, whether or how an autopoietic system observes environmental differences and processes these to form differences of its own depends first and foremost on its own operational structure and only to a lesser degree on the environment.

If we use this concept to describe and explain cognition, or psychical perception and the focusing of attention, we arrive ultimately in the domain of *constructivist* views (cf., Kleve, 1996), for instance, those of Immanuel Kant's *Critique of Pure Reason.* According to Kant (1787/1916), objective reality, the so-called "things themselves," is not attainable through cognition. Rather, cognition produces "things for us," realities that appear as they appear because our organs of perception "gauge" them as best they can, according to their capabilities. Systems theory radicalizes this classical constructivism through its theory of observation (cf., Luhmann, 1990a), which postulates that not only psychical systems and human subjects observe, but also biological and social systems—that is to say, that observation is thought of as a systemic process of difference forming, independent of the subject.

Once the primary system/environment distinction has become stabilized, a system can distinguish itself from its environment and describe itself as an identity; in doing so, it undertakes a process of self-observation by means of a reentry of the system/environment distinction into the one side of the distinction, namely into the system. The system can observe not only *that* it differs from its environment but also *how* it differs from its environment and thus identifies itself as something different from its environment. Self-observations are called *second-order observations* because they observe their (own past) observation. Second-order observations also occur when systems observe other systems while these themselves are observing. It is here that systems theory demonstrates its epistemological capacity. Understanding reality is viewed as observation based on distinctions and labels and these must be actively established. This perspective was opened up by the English logician George Spencer-Brown (1997), who couples the development of every form of reality with distinguishing and labeling. If one wishes to know why realities are what they are and appear to be what they appear to be, one should shift one's perspective from the appearance of reality to observations, which construct realities on the basis of certain distinctions and labels. The epistemological core is that—based on Spencer-Brown's logics of distinction and Heinz von Foerster's second-order cybernetics (Foerster, 1993)—every question as to the contents, attributes, or identities of reality is related to observers. Thus, the (classical epistemological) question as to "what," that is, the contents of observations, leads to the question of "how," that is, the genesis of observations.

Third, the operational division of biological, psychical, and social systems. Luhmann's theory describes biological, psychical, and social systems as autopoeitic systems and makes clear distinctions between them. Autopoeisis means, moreover, that systems permanently reproduce themselves with their own operations and elements. The question then arises, What are these operations and elements? In the case of biological and psychical systems the answer seems to present itself relatively quickly: organisms, as biological systems, reproduce themselves autopoietically through life processes (metabolism, cell division, etc.) while psychical systems are generated through permanent operations of thinking, of cognition. And, it must be added, biological and psychical systems are structurally coupled in such a way that not only do they presuppose each other but they are also capable of irritating each other to such an extent that changes occur in each of them. This would be a subject for a systems theory of psychosomatics (cf. Simon, 1993). But what about social systems? What are their elements?

For Luhmann (1995a, p. 191ff.), the operation that constitutes social systems is the communicative operation and thus the elements that differentiate social systems are communications. Accordingly, social systems are made up of communications. Human beings, as units of biological and psychical systems, belong to the environment of social systems. In this theory, therefore, human beings are not unimportant for the constitution of the social system; indeed, as units of biological and psychical systems, they are its prerequisite. Yet the dynamics of social systems cannot be explained by the observation of the individuals taking part in the system; this requires separate socio-logical, communicative analyses based on the understanding that the generation of social system's own emergent complexities cannot be at-tributed to anything biological or psychical. Social systems, that is, communications, also observe in their own separate way.

For Luhmann, the basis of (psychical and social) observations as well as the structural coupling of psychical and social systems is the category of *sense* (Luhmann, 1995a, p. 92ff.). Consciousness and the social system both operate on the basis of sense. Thoughts (as ele-ments of the psychical system) and communications (as elements of the social system) distinguish and label, that is, observe current hap-penings also in a context of other possibilities, or in a context of po-tentiality. This relationship between what is currently being thought or communicated on the one hand and potentially possible thoughts and communications on the other represents the category of sense. Sense, furthermore, is thought of as a medium in which thoughts and communications inscribe themselves as certain forms; what is impor-tant, however, is that this inscribing in the sense medium happens dif-ferently, according to whether it is done psychically through thoughts or socially through communications. And between consciousness and the social system there is an operational boundary separating con-sciousness and communication in such a way that thoughts and com-munications cannot be translated directly from one to the other. Indeed, although consciousness and communication may be linked to each other *structurally* via the sense medium, they nevertheless remain separated from each other *operationally*. Thus, no thought can be communicated directly while no communication can directly enter the consciousness (a detailed account of this is given in Luhmann (1995a, p. 191ff.) and Fuchs (1993).

Should a systems-oriented nursing theory wish to take up the ideas of systems theory based on the third paradigm, that is to say Luhmann's paradigm, it must at least set out from the components of theory hitherto described. If so, which questions and perspectives might arise for a systems-oriented nursing theory? A detailed an-swer—or indeed a conclusion—cannot be given in this contribution, of course. However, a number of speculative observations are to be hazarded nevertheless.

PERSPECTIVES AND QUESTIONS OF A THEORY OF SELF-REFERENTIAL SYSTEMS IN NURSING

Nursing is a practice that clearly has to do with all three autopoeitic classes of system—biological, psychical, and social—in equal measure. For this reason, nursing (like social work, incidentally; cf. Kleve, 1999, p. 56ff.) has a special affinity with holistic notions; by using them it aims to embed the unitary human being in the social system because it tries precisely to relate to this unity. As Bauch (2000) asserts, this holistic relationship with human beings can be observed in the entire health systems—at least it can if we describe the unity of the human body in terms of systems theory as a unity of the difference of two autopoeitic systems, namely those of the psyche and the body. From a sociological perspective of the theory of self-referential systems, the health service (and thus nursing, too, with its special tasks) has the primary function of treating the sick "and accordingly is concerned with the relationship between body and consciousness" (Bauch, 2000, p. 390) and, it might be added, in a social system (e.g., in a certain organization such as a hospital).

Bauch (2000) follows on directly from Luhmann's systems theory when he writes that "body and psyche . . . are two structurally coupled but at the same time autopoietic systems," (p. 390) whose relationship, however, is characterized by structural indifference and psychical inattention to bodily functions. Yet as soon as pain is felt, at the very least, an (acute or chronic) disease leads to the interruption of the psychical system's inattention to changes of state in the biological system. Pain is an emergent psychical occurrence stimulated by the body; it is thus information that comes into being when certain differences in the biological system lead to certain differences in the psychical system. As Fritz B. Simon (1995) writes from a systems theory perspective, the processes that

> we call "diseases of the body" are structurally determined reactions of the body to internal changes in the network of interactions of the components (structural and functional changes) or to perturbing interactions with the environment, e.g., with bacteria, too cold drinks or too hot bath water, or with colleagues at work or the loved ones at home. (p. 66)

Should such "structurally determined reactions of the body" occur, the perception of pain in the psychical system is a possible result.

In such circumstances it is the task of the health system to restore the state of structural indifference of body and psyche—to silence the body, as it were, by fighting the ailment, and hand in hand with this, by alleviating or taking away the pain. The precondition for the health system's coming into play is, of course, that changes in the state of the body become significant not only at the psychical level through (perceptible) pain but also at the social level, that is, they are communicated with the result that doctors, nurses, and others go into action. Hence, Simon (1995) places emphasis on the fact that psychically perceived changes in the state of the body only become symptoms when communication takes place. "Experiencing pain, sensing a disturbance in one's well-being or feeling ill require validation through communication in order to be recognized as a symptom, as a distinguishing feature of illness" (Simon, 1995, p. 66). From this point of view diseases, too, are systemic constructions that point to (psychical and social) observers whose observation takes place in a context of certain social, factual, and temporal conventions, and is thus relative and contingent. "Bodily, psychical and social occurrences or states first become symptoms when they are identified and labeled as 'symptoms' by observers communicating about them" (p. 66).

A systems-theory-oriented description of the reciprocal irritations of biological, psychical, and social systems thus presupposes first of all the strict *operational* decoupling of the three systems. Only now, as a second step, may it be asked how these systems can relate to each other in such a way that they become relevant for each other at the structural level and trigger changes in their states. A systems-based nursing theory could observe the relationship between nursing actions and these systems from precisely this perspective. Nursing would then be describable as a social practice relating to all the named systems without being able to establish, however, whether or how each of these systems changes. As long as nursing is not able to intervene directly in the biological system, all its actions can be considered communications within a social system. Consequently, nursing, too, is no more and no less than a stimulus offered in the social environment of biological, psychical, and social systems requiring nursing—with the aim, of course, of irritating these systems (in a positive way) such that their relationship to each other works towards controlling or curing disease or promoting health.

The theory of self-referential systems enables us to describe and explain social systems in a highly differentiated way. Besides the operation of social systems, communication, which has been discussed above, this description refers, for example, to the different types of social system (cf. Luhmann, 1997). Hence, we can distinguish at least three different social system types that might also be scrutinized more closely with regard to nursing: namely, interaction, organization, and society.

Interaction refers to social systems in which people are physically present (*face-to-face* contexts). These are generated when people observe each other and observe that this is precisely what happens: not only do they observe others but their observing is also observed by others. For interactive social systems of this kind, the axioms that apply are the classical axioms of pragmatic communication theory as postulated by Paul Watzlawick (1969). A systems-based nursing theory could take a close look at these axioms for nursing practice and inquire into the specific nature of nursing interaction and the effect this has on the psychical and biological systems of both the person being nursed as well as the person nursing. Jens Friebe (1999) has especially criticized the too narrowly viewed notions of interaction of classical systems-based nursing theories, which are not able to distinguish different (e.g., symmetric) forms of relationship. With the systems-oriented theory of interaction (see also Kieserling, 1999) recommended here, it would be possible to describe the various interactive dimensions of nursing and explain their dynamics.

Organizations are social systems that are formally organized, that is to say, they are bureaucratized and structured by legal precepts. They are characterized by a specific form of communication, by which they are held together, namely by decisions (cf. Luhmann, 2001). Organizations are based on membership and continue to exist even if interaction were to fall apart, that is, if communication among persons physically present were no longer to take place. As a rule, membership of organizations is connected with a certain role (cf. Nassehi & Nollmann, 1997), namely a *performing role* (for example, that assumed by a professional nurse), while patients take on the so-called *publication role*. By means of these roles it is determined whether and how individuals can participate in those systems, which in modern society perform such tasks as are necessary for human psychical and physical reproduction (autopoeisis), that is, in organizations (e.g., firms, schools, institutions of social welfare and health care, etc.). The question then arises as to how (through which mechanisms) a person's inclusion or exclusion is determined in organizations. Under which conditions do people have access to organizations, or when is this access barred to them? What organizational dynamics are set in motion in the case of inclusion (e.g., in a hospital), and what happens to people who are or continue to be excluded? These and other questions could be posed by a systems-based nursing theory that tries to analyze, for instance, the organizational contexts of nursing practice (e.g., in hospitals and certain nursing institutions or also in day care and nursing in the home).

Society is the name Luhmann (1997) gives to the overall social system that includes all (interactive and organizational) communication and that today, on the one hand, is only conceivable as a global society, and on the other, is divided into various functional systems. Because of this, sociological systems theory is above all concerned with describing and explaining the dynamics of autopoeitic functional systems, for example, those of the health service. With few exceptions Luhmann himself never published any comprehensive studies of the health system (see, for example, Luhmann, 1990b), to which nursing can, of course, be considered to belong. However, Simon (1995) and Bauch (2000) have undertaken studies of this social subsystem from a systems theory standpoint. Simon's aim is above all to demonstrate that health is one side of the illness/health distinction, which leads the observation, and that this side is generally only relevant in communication through its negation, that is, only through being what it isn't, namely illness. As we have seen above, the indifference between body and psyche—that is to say, the state of the psyche's inattention to the biological system—ceases at the point when the body makes itself noticed, at first in the psychical and then in the social system, as a result of pain and subsequently illness. It is precisely this situation that led Luhmann (1990b) to infer that the health system is a system of treating illness that observes society on the basis of the ill/well distinction and goes into action whenever it can diagnose bodies and label them as ill. Setting the system in motion goes hand in hand with the presupposition that it will identify illness; if this is successful, that is, communicatively endorsed (e.g., legally), money will flow. And money is, so to speak, the (economic) energy without which autopoeisis cannot be maintained in most functional systems.

If, however, the identifying of illness leads to the autopoeitic differentiation and the resulting dynamics of the health system, we can assume, along with Simon (1995), that

> the better the health system functions, the more people there are in a society who are ill. This is a fundamental paradox that results from

the logic of living systems. A large number of patients who have been successfully treated are not well after treatment but continue to be ill. (p. 194)

For it is through the identifying of illnesses and not through unimpaired health that this system secures its autopoeisis. Similar dynamics, incidentally, can be found in the system of social work (cf. Kleve, 2003) because both the health system and the social work system are social functional systems that are only set in motion after (biological, psychical, or social) deficits have been labeled; this labeling guarantees the continuation of autopoeisis. The problems that become clear in this connection with regard to the efficiency (economy) and effectiveness (attainment of goals) of the health system—and that also affect nursing—could be further elucidated with the help of a systems-based social theory.

Bauch (2000) attempts just such an elucidation when he observes that the health system is trying to develop a new systemic code and thus a new distinction to lead the observation: namely the difference between *health promoting* and *health impairing.* Hence, the health system is now going beyond the classical code "ill/well" due to its enormous social scope, which is also reflected in its differentiation into new sciences, for example, the health care and nursing sciences. The system of treating illnesses is only now becoming the health system, although the former continues of course to be a subsystem of the latter.

> The health system's area of responsibility is growing because the system is no longer related to the fact of illness alone. Society as a whole is becoming the reference and examination point of a sanitary project since all social behaviour patterns must be tested in a scheme of large-scale prevention for possible latent or manifest long-term pathological states." (Bauch, 2000, p. 400).

The goal of extending this system to cover the whole of society "in a scheme of large-scale prevention" is presumably health, although there are as yet no implementable and verifiable criteria for answering the question of what health is (cf. Simon, 1995). Even the World Health Organization, according to Simon (1995), provides "only a very dubious definition of this (in advertising very effective) term . . . when they want it to be understood as 'the state of complete physical, mental and social well-being'" (p. 10). This definition, he says, sounds more "like the promise of salvation given by a thoroughly worldly sect" (p. 10).

At best, this definition connotes a positive ideal which lives, however—like most ideals—because of the impossibility of attaining it. Nevertheless, a social system that is oriented to this ideal is potentially capable of labeling each and every person as ill in some physical, mental, or social respect. That this poses a problem, that it can lead to an explosion of costs and other difficulties (not only economic), is something quite obvious; but it also brings into focus a success story—that of the system's whole new areas of tasks: "prevention, promoting health, public health policy, wellness schemes, specific preventive measures (e.g. health and safety at work), infrastructural measures on environmental protection, furthering professionalisation in nursing practice, rehabilitation, etc." (Bauch, 2000, p. 400).

Summing up, one can say in conclusion that systems theory (and Luhmann's systems theory in particular) is able to describe and explain the social dynamics not only of the health system just described but also of nursing as well. With the help of the theory of self-referential systems, practice-oriented nursing is also able to observe especially the biological, psychical, and social dimensions of its tasks. This gives rise to numerous and possibly unwonted questions, only a small number of which I could touch upon here. It is now a matter of further narrowing down these questions in order to discover perhaps new and forward-pointing answers that are helpful and constructive for the perspectives of nursing and nursing science in a modern society.

REFERENCES

Adorno, T. W. (1951). *Minima Moralia. Reflexionen aus dem beschädigten Leben* [Minimal morality. Reflections from damaged life]. Frankfurt, Germany: Suhrkamp.

Baecker, D. (1994). *Postheroisches Management. Ein Vademecum* [Postheroic management. A handbook]. Berlin, Germany: Merve.

Bateson, G. (1982). *Geist und Natur. Eine notwendige Einheit* [Mind and nature. A necessary unit]. Frankfurt,Germany: Suhrkamp.

Bardmann, T. M., Kersting, H. J., Vogel, H. C., & Woltmann, B. (1991). *Irritation als Plan. Konstruktivistische Einredungen* [Irritation as plan. Constructivist perspective]. Aachen, Germany: Kersting.

Bauch, J. (2000). Selbst- und Fremdbeschreibung des Gesundheitswesens. Anmerkungen zu einem absonderlichen Sozialsystem [Internal and external descriptions of the health system. Notes on a peculiar social system]. In H. de Berg & J. Schmidt (Eds.), *Rezeption und Reflexion. Zur*

Resonanz der Systemtheorie Niklas Luhmanns außerhalb der Soziologie (pp. 387–410). Frankfurt, Germany: Suhrkamp.

Capra, F. (1991). *Wendezeit. Bausteine für ein neues Weltbild* [The turning point: Science, society, and the rising culture]. München, Germany: dtv.

Clam, J. (2000). Unbegegnete Theorie. Zur Luhmann-Rezeption in der Philosophie [The non-confined theory. Luhmann-reception in philosophy]. In H. de Berg, & J. Schmidt (Eds.), *Rezeption und Reflexion. Zur Resonanz der Systemtheorie Niklas Luhmanns außerhalb der Soziologie* (pp. 296–321). Frankfurt, Germany: Suhrkamp.

Clam, J. (2002). *Was heißt es, sich an Differenz statt an Identität zu orientieren? Zur De-ontologisierung in Philosophie und Sozialwissenschaften* [What does it mean to orient along differences instead of identity? On de-ontologization in philosophy and social sciences]. Konstanz, Germany: UVK.

de Berg, H., & Schmidt, J. (Eds.). (2000). *Rezeption und Reflexion. Zur Resonanz der Systemtheorie Niklas Luhmanns außerhalb der Soziologie* [Reception and reflection. On the perception of Niklas Luhmann's systems theory beyond sociology]. Frankfurt, Germany: Suhrkamp.

Foerster, H. von (1993). *Wissen und Gewissen. Versuch eine Brücke* [Knowledge and consciousness. Attempt of bridging]. Frankfurt, Germany: Suhrkamp.

Friebe, J. (1999). Applying social science concepts to nursing: Systems theory and beyond. In I. Kollak, & H. S. Kim (Eds.), *Pflegetheoretische Grundbegriffe* [Nursing theories: Conceptual and philosophical foundations] (pp. 145–161). Bern, Switzerland: Huber.

Fuchs, P. (1993). *Moderne Kommunikation. Zur Theorie des operativen Displacements* [Modern communication. On the theory of operative displacements]. Frankfurt, Germany: Suhrkamp.

Fuchs, P. (2001). *Die Metapher des Systems. Studien zur allgemein leitenden Frage, wie sich der Tänzer vom Tanz unterscheiden lasse* [The metaphor of systems. Studies on the overall leading question, how the dancer can be differentiated from the dance]. Weilerwist, Germany: Velbrück.

Gripp-Hagelstange, H. (Ed.). (2000). *Niklas Luhmanns Denken. Interdisziplinäre Einflüsse und Wirkungen* [The thinking of Niklas Luhmann. Interdisciplinary influences and effects]. Konstanz, Germany: UVK.

Johnson, D. E. (1980). The behavioral bystem model for nursing. In J. P. Riehl & C. Roy (Eds.), *Conceptual models for nursing practice* (pp. 207–216). New York: Appleton-Century-Crofts.

Kant, I. (1916). *Critique of pure reason* (J. M. D. Meiklejohn, Trans.). London: G. Bell. (Original work published in 1787)

Kieserling, A. (1999). *Kommunikation unter Anwesenden. Studien über Interaktionssysteme* [Communication among participants. Studies on interaction system]. Frankfurt, Germany: Suhrkamp.

King, I. M. (1995). A systems framework for nursing: The theory of goal attainment. In M. A. Frey & C, L, Sieloff (Eds.), *Advancing King's framework and theory of nursing*. Thousand Oaks, CA: Sage.

King, I. M. (1997). Ein systemischer Bezugsrahmen für die Pflege [A systems framework for nursing]. In D. Schaeffer, M. Moers, H. Steppe, & A. Meleis (Eds.), *Pflegetheorien. Beispiele aus den USA* [Nursing theories. Examples from the US] (pp. 181–196). Bern, Switzerland: Huber.

Kleve, H. (1996). *Konstruktivismus und Soziale Arbeit. Die konstruktivistische Wirklichkeitsauffassung und ihre Bedeutung für Sozialarbeit/Sozialpädagogik und Supervision* [Constructivism and social work. The constructivistic reality perception and its meaning for social work, social pedagogy and supervision]. Aachen, Germany: Kersting.

Kleve, H. (1999). *Postmoderne Sozialarbeit. Ein systemtheoretisch-konstruktivistischer Beitrag zur Sozialarbeitswissenschaft* [Postmodern social work. A system theoretical-constructivistic contribution to social work science]. Aachen, Germany: Kersting.

Kleve, H. (2000). Paradigmawechsel in der Systemtheorie und postmoderne Sozialarbeit [Changing the paradigm in system theory and postmodern social work]. In R. Merten (Ed.), *Systemtheorie Sozialer Arbeit. Neue Ansätze und veränderte Perspektiven* (pp. 47–66). Opladen, Germany: Leske & Budrich.

Kleve, H. (2003). Zwei Logiken des Helfens. Ambivalenz- und systemtheoretische Betrachtungen [Two logics of helping. Ambivalence and system theoretical consideration]. *Soziale Arbeit, Heft, 6,* 220–227.

Krieger, D. J. (1996). *Einführung in die allgemeine Systemtheorie* [Introduction into systems theory]. München, Germany: Fink/UTB.

Luhmann, N. (1970a). *Soziologie als Theorie sozialer Systeme. In: ders. Soziologische Aufklärung 1. Aufsätze zur Theorie sozialer Systeme* [Sociology as a theory of social systems. Sociological enlightenment 1. Essays on the theory of social systems] (pp. 113–136). Opladen, Germany: Westdeutscher.

Luhmann, N. (1970b). *Funktionale Methode und Systemtheorie. In: ders. Soziologische Aufklärung 1. Aufsätze zur Theorie sozialer Systeme* [Functional method and systems theory. Sociological enlightenment 1. Essays on the theory of social systems] (pp. 31–53). Opladen, Germany: Westdeutscher.

Luhmann, N. (1975). *Formen des Helfens im Wandel gesellschaftlicher Bedingungen. In: ders. Soziologische Aufklärung II. Aufsätze zur Theorie der Gesellschaft* [Models of helping in the changing social conditions. Sociological enlightenment 2. Essays on the theory of society] (pp. 134–149). Opladen, Germany: Westdeutscher.

Luhmann, N. (1988). *Die Wirtschaft der Gesellschaft* [Economy as a social system]. Frankfurt, Germany: Suhrkamp.

Luhmann, N. (1990a). *Die Wissenschaft der Gesellschaft* [Science as a social system]. Frankfurt, Germany: Suhrkamp.
Luhmann, N. (1990b). Der medizinische Code [The medical code]. In *ders: Soziologische Aufklärung 5. Konstruktivistische Perspektiven* [Sociological enlightenment 5. Constructivistic perspective] (pp. 183–195). Opladen, Germany: Westdeutscher.
Luhmann, N. (1990c). *Essays on self-reference.* New York: Columbia University Press.
Luhmann, N. (1993a). *Das Recht der Gesellschaft* [Law as a social system]. Frankfurt, Germany: Suhrkamp.
Luhmann, N. (1994a). The modernity of science (K. Behnke, Trans.). *New German Critique, 61,* 9–23.
Luhmann, N. (1995a). *Social systems* (J. Bednarz, Jr. & D. Baecker, Trans.). Stanford, CA: Stanford University Press. (Original work published in 1984)
Luhmann, N. (1995b). *Die Kunst der Gesellschaft* [Art as a social system]. Frankfurt, Germany: Suhrkamp.
Luhmann, N. (1997). *Die Gesellschaft der Gesellschaft* [The society as a social system] (2 Bände). Frankfurt, Germany: Suhrkamp.
Luhmann, N. (2000a). *Die Politik der Gesellschaft* [Politics as a social system]. Frankfurt, Germany: Suhrkamp.
Luhmann, N. (2000b). *Die Religion der Gesellschaft* [Religion as a social system]. Frankfurt, Germany: Suhrkamp.
Luhmann, N. (2000c). *The reality of the mass media* (K. Cross, Trans.). Stanford, CA: Stanford University Press.
Luhmann, N. (2001). *Organisation und Entscheidung* [Organization and decision]. Opladen, Germany: Westdeutscher.
Luhmann, N. (2002a). *Einführung in die Systemtheorie* [Introduction into systems theory]. Heidelberg, Germany: Carl-Auer-Systeme.
Luhmann, N. (2002b). *Das Erziehungssystem der Gesellschaft* [Education as a social system]. Frankfurt, Germany: Suhrkamp.
Lyotard, J. F. (1994). *Das postmoderne Wissen. Ein Bericht* [The postmodern knowledge. A report]. Wien, Austria: Passagen. (Original work published in 1979)
Maturana, H. R., & Varela, F. J. (1987). *Der Baum der Erkenntnis. Die biologischen Wurzeln des menschlichen Erkennens* [The tree of knowledge. The biological roots of human understanding]. München, Germany: Scherz/Goldmann.
Morel, J., Bauer, E., Meleghy, T., Miedenzu, H., Preglau, M., & Staubmann, H. (1997). *Soziologische Theorie. Abriß der Ansätze ihrer Hauptvertrerer* [Sociological theories. Summary of approaches and their main representations]. München, Germany: Oldenbourg
Mühlum, A., Bartholomeyczik, S., & Göpel, E. (1997). *Sozialarbeitswis-*

senschaft. Pflegewissenschaft. Gesundheitswissenschaft [Social work science, nursing science, health science]. Freiburg, Germany: Lambertus.

Nassehi, A., & Nollmann, G. (1997). Inklusionen. Organisationssoziologische Ergänzungen der Inklusions-Exklusionstheorie [Inclusions. Completions to inclusional and exclusional theories of the social science of organizations]. Soziale Systeme, 2, 393–411.

Neuman, B. (1997). Pflege und die Systemperspektive [Nursing and systems perspective]. In D. Schaeffer, M. Moers, H. Steppe, & A. Meleis, (Eds.), Pflegetheorien. Beispiele aus den USA (pp. 197–227). Bern, Switzerland: Huber.

Parsons, T. (1972). Das System moderner Gesellschaften [The system of modern societies]. Weinheim/München, Germany: Juventa.

Roy, C., & Andrews, H. A. (1997). Das Adaptionsmodell [The adaptation model]. In D. Schaeffer, M. Moers, H. Steppe, & A. Meleis, (Eds.), Pflegetheorien. Beispiele aus den USA (pp. 227–250). Bern, Switzerland: Huber.

Simon, F. B. (1993). Unterschiede, die Unterschiede machen. Klinische Epistemologie: Grundlage einer systemischen Psychiatrie und Psychosomatik [Differences that made differences. Clinical epistemology: Foundations of a systemic psychiatry and psychosomatics]. Frankfurt, Germany: Suhrkamp.

Simon, F. B. (1995). Die andere Seite der Gesundheit. Ansätze einer systemischen Krankheits- und Therapietheorie [The other side of health. Starting points of a systematic illness and therapeutic theory]. Heidelberg, Germany: Carl-Auer-Systeme.

Simon, F. B., Clement, U., & Stierlin, H. (1999). Die Sprache der Familientherapie. Ein Vokabular. Kritischer Überblick und Integration systemtherapeutischer Begriffe, Konzepte und Methoden. [The language of family therapy. A vocabulary. Critical summary and integration of system therapeutic terms, conceptions, and methods]. Stuttgart, Germany: Klett-Cotta.

Spencer-Brown, G. (1997). Laws of form. Gesetze der form. Lübeck, Germany: Bohmeier.

Ulfig, A. (1999). Lexikon der philosophischen Begriffe [Dictionary of philosophical terms]. Wiesbaden, Germany: Fourier.

Watzlawick, P. (1969). Menschliche Kommunikatione. Formen, Störungen, Paradoxien [Human communication. Patterns, pathologies, paradoxes]. Bern, Switzerland: Huber.

Welsch, W. (1993). Unsere postmoderne Moderne [Our postmodern modernity]. Berlin: Akademie.

Willke, H. (1993). Systemtheorie. Eine Einführung in die Grundprobleme der Theorie sozialer Systeme [Systems theory. An introduction in basic problems of the theory of social systems]. Stuttgart, Germany: Fischer/UTB.

Woltmann, B. (1991). Planen, Autopoiese und Sozialpädagogik—Ausführungen zu einer Epistemologie didaktischer Wirklichkeitskonstruktionen [Planning, autopoeisis and social pedagogy—Explanations on an epistemology of didactic construction]. In T. M. Bardmann, et al. (Eds.), *Irritation als Plan. Konstruktivistische Einredungen* (pp. 64–107). Aachen, Germany: Kersting.

CHAPTER 9

Existentialism and Phenomenology in Nursing Theories

Hesook Suzie Kim

Existentialism and phenomenology have been providing important influences on the development of nursing knowledge, especially since the early 1980s. However, Paterson and Zderad (1976) were the pioneers in nursing who adopted the philosophies of existentialism and phenomenology in their proposal for humanistic nursing and "nursology." Their work, premised on the rejection of determinism, positivism, and reductionism was ahead of its time, because nursing in the 1970s was very much preoccupied with the idea of legitimatizing the discipline as a science in the traditional positivistic mode. The republication of *Humanistic Nursing*, by the National League for Nursing in 1988, indicates a change in the mood in which the theoretical and empirical sectors of nursing have become stirred for a reexamination of nursing's subject matter and its methodology during the last two decades.

Nursing literature of the last two decades is full of philosophical expositions, theoretical proposals, and research that are based on existentialism, phenomenology or both (see, for example, in more recent works, Benner, 1994; Bishop & Scudder, 2003; Caelli, 2000; Crotty, 1996; Jones, 2001; Lopez & Willis, 2004; Omery, 1995; Paley, 1997; Sadala & Adorno, 2002; Todres & Wheeler, 2001). However, philosophical orientations and methodological adoptions in nursing studies are as diverse and disparate as the diversity that exists within both existentialism and phenomenology as general philosophies. Hence, we find in the nursing literature the works identifying Husserl, Heidegger, Merleau-Ponty, and Schutz (1966) as providing phenomenological foundation, and those citing the existential philosophy of Kierkegaard, Jaspers, Marcel, Nietzsche, and Sartre. The term *existential phenomenology,* however, was introduced in a nursing theory by Parse in 1981. Besides Parse and her colleagues whose works are based on Parse's theory, we are beginning to see specific references to existential phenomenology in nursing literature. For example, Häggman-Laitila (1997) examined health as an individual way of existence from an existential phenomenological perspective, and Jones (1998) examined the application of an existential-phenomenological method of clinical supervision in palliative-care nursing. Among the nursing theorists, Margaret Newman (1990, 1994) has been revising the assumptions undergirding her theory of "health as expanding consciousness" to align with existential phenomenology in her recent writings.

Existential phenomenology as an ontological focus in itself is claimed by various scholars to be based on different philosophical sources. It can be traced to Husserl, Heidegger, Merleau-Ponty, Sartre, Jaspers, and Binswanger. The versions of existential phenomenology coming from these philosophers interweave the tenets of existentialism and phenomenology selectively and in various ways. Hence, it is necessary to examine the ontological features of both existentialism and phenomenology before extricating the major themes in existential phenomenology.

PHENOMENOLOGY AND EXISTENTIALISM

As philosophies, phenomenology and existentialism are modern European developments, in response to the philosophical traditions of the time that are entrenched in and threaded with the philosophies of Descartes, Kant, and Hegel. These were inwardly directed turns that address ontological questions regarding human consciousness and human existence. These developments took place mostly in Germany and France until the middle of the twentieth century, contrasted with the developments of analytic philosophy, positivism and neo-positivism, and pragmatism in England and America.

Phenomenology and existentialism, as developed through the nineteenth and twentieth centuries, are not single, unified philosophies. Leading phenomenologists (such as Husserl, Heidegger, and Merleau-Ponty) and existentialists (Kierkegaard, Nietzsche, Jaspers, Marcel, and Sartre) offer somewhat diverse views regarding human experiences, consciousness, existence, and human lot. The relationship between phenomenology and existentialism is elusive, and paradoxical as well. Both philosophies are concerned with the existential content of life; address the role of consciousness as central to the questions of experience, perception, and existence; and are against quantitative methods and causality explanations. However, in focusing specifically on human existence some existentialists reject the appropriateness of applying phenomenological analysis to the study of human existence, which is thought not to be objectifiable, whereas phenomenology is concerned not only with human existence but with all phenomena that are consciously constituted. It means that they focus on the ontological questions of existence from different angles: phenomenology is concerned with modes of phenomenal existence, while existentialism focuses on the meaning of human existence. Furthermore, the paradoxical relationship between the two is rooted in the apparent opening offered by Husserl for the germination of existentialism, the identity of Heidegger and Merleau-Ponty as both phenomenologists and existentialists, and Sartre's commitment to phenomenology (Barrett, 1962).

Turning to phenomenology, it is necessary to begin the exposition with the phenomenology of Husserl, and then provide some insights regarding the alternative views advanced by two other leading phenomenologists, Heidegger and Merleau-Ponty. This is important because the phenomenological movement originated with Husserl, who remained committed to both Decartes and Kant, although moving beyond their doctrines regarding *mathesis universalis* and transcendental philosophy (Natanson, 1966).

The major tenets of phenomenology are founded upon Husserl's expression, *"Zu den Sachen selbst:* "To the things themselves." This notion is tied to the concept of "things," or phenomena as acts of consciousness, that is, constituted in consciousness. Hence, Husserlian phenomenology encompasses three major ideas: the theory of intentionality, essences *(eidos)* or the essential structures of things, and phenomenological method as reduction, all of which are interrelated. Husserl's theory of intentionality is concerned with how things are constituted in the life-world *(lebenswelt)*, the ordinary world as shaped within the immediate experiences of each person and constituted through human subjectivity and consciousness. Because it is through consciousness that things come to have meanings or exist as such, human acts are also constituted through consciousness and are experiences of meaning. Thus, for Husserl, "intentionality is seen phenomenologically as foundationally given; it is neither deduced from other elements of consciousness or experience nor postulated from observed elements. Consciousness *is* intentionality" (Natanson, 1966, p. 15). This means that experiences are intentional, and that they are constituted to have meanings as essences or essential structures. The essences *(eidos),* or essential structures of things, acts, and experiences, are invariant features constituted through consciousness to them. As Moran (2000) states, phenomenology is concerned with what is given in intuition, which is self-validating, and counts as a valid source of knowledge "only what is given in experiences and all of what is given in experience" (p. 127).

The phenomenological method developed by Husserl for phenomenological investigation integrates these two ideas, the theory of intentionality and the concept of essences. Phenomenological method is the mode of investigation for phenomena that exist as consciously constituted affairs. It involves both description and analysis. Spiegelberg (1982) identifies seven features of phenomenological method, only three of which are thought by him to be accepted widely by phenomenological proponents:

1. investigating particular phenomena
2. investigating general essences
3. apprehending essential relationships among essences
4. watching modes of appearing
5. watching the constitution of phenomena in consciousness
6. suspending belief in the existence of the phenomena
7. interpreting the meaning of phenomena

This statement suggests that phenomenological method, as it is being understood and developed within the school of phenomenologists, is united by certain basic procedures and premises, but is also differentiated in important ways. What is important here is that phenomenology cannot be considered without referring to phenomenological method because it is both philosophy and science, and is rooted in Husserl's epistemological focus.

The key features of phenomenological method as advanced by Husserl are (a) phenomenological reduction, (b) eidetic reduction, and (c) *epoché*. The main idea of phenomenological method is *reduction*. Reduction to Husserl means "a radical shift in attention from factuality and particularity to essential and universal qualities" (Natanson, 1973, p. 65). The phenomenological reduction focuses on consciousness as the essential feature of constituting the world. The aim of the phenomenological reduction is to understand the world as the intentional correlate of transcendental subjectivity, by changing the world into a phenomenon that is known in and by consciousness. In order to do this, it is necessary to "bracket" and suspend all things, as Husserl (1931) put it:

> . . . we set all these theses "out of action", as take no part in them; we direct the glance of apprehension and theoretical inquiry to *pure consciousness in its own absolute Being*. It is this which remains over as the "phenomenological residuum" we were in quest of: remains over, we say, although we have "Suspended" the whole world with all things, living creatures, men, ourselves included. We have literally lost nothing, but have won the whole of Absolute Being, which, properly understood, conceals in itself all transcendences, "constituting" them within itself. (pp. 154–155)

The eidetic reduction, on the other hand, focuses on "essences." In the eidetic reduction, the investigator must grasp the essences of phenomena—the universal and invariant structures—by peeling away the factual and incidental features that are inherent in variations and attending to essences by means of intuition *(Wesensschau)*. To Husserl, phenomenology is "to be a science of pure essences" extracting from "the merely contingent, factual features of our experience in order to isolate what is essential to all experiences of that kind" (Moran, 2000, p. 132). This is accomplished through the eidetic reduction.

Underwriting these two forms of reduction and the phenomenological method itself is the concept of *epoché*, meaning "suspension of judgment." It is the means by which phenomenological description aims to achieve descriptive neutrality and the phenomenological attitude of investigation is attained. Husserl (1931) specifies the role of phenomenological *epoché* as follows:

> *We put out of action the general thesis which belongs to the essence of the natural standpoint,* we place in brackets whatever it includes respecting the nature of Being: *this entire natural world therefore which is continually "there for us," "present to our hand,"* and will ever remain there, is a "fact-world" of which we continue to be conscious, even though it pleases us to put it in brackets. If I do this, as I am fully free to do, I do *not* then *deny* this "world," as though I were a sophist,

> I *do not doubt that* it is there as though I were a skeptic; but I use the
> "phenomenological" *epoché,* which *completely bars* me *from using
> any judgment that concerns spatio-temporal existence.* (p. 107)

Phenomenology as developed by Husserl (the Husserlian version
often termed as transcendental phenomenology in a narrow sense)
has culminated in a philosophical tradition with many variants of significance, among which are Heideggerian hermeneutic phenomenology and Merleau-Ponty's phenomenology of perception as notable
influences in nursing.

Martin Heidegger moved away from the Husserlian tenets of phenomenology by focusing on the meaning of 'Being'. In his *Sein und
Zeit (Being and Time,)* published in 1927, Heidegger offers the concept
of *Dasein* (being there), or being-in-the-world, as the pivotal point for
analyzing the meaning of 'Being'. Heidegger rejects Husserl's ideas of
transcendental consciousness and his phenomenological reduction as
the descriptive and analytic methods for understanding phenomena.
Instead, Heidegger turns to interpretation as a way to understand the
meaning of 'Being'. Hence, Heidegger's main concern was not the
meaning of experiences per se, but the meaning of existence. Heidegger (1962) conceives *Dasein* (being there, or being-in-the-world) for
each human existence in two possible modes: authentic existence
(eigentliche) or inauthentic existence *(uneigentliche),* in which authen-
ticity is taking up of one's existence through one's own choices,
whereas inauthenticity is submitting one's choices to others. In addition, Heidegger (1962) discloses that the basic structures of *Dasein* are
primordial moodness *(Befindlichkeit),* understanding *(Verstehen),* and
language or discourse *(Rede);* and that temporality, encompassing past,
present, and future, grounds the 'being' of human being. To Heidegger, being-in-the world means being in relation with things: (a) with
mood as a way of being tuned to the world, (b) with preunderstanding
of things, which comes both from the things themselves in our experiences of them and through our understanding of ourselves, and (c)
through discourse (or expression) that is interpreting and interpreted.

Hence, Heidegger reformulated phenomenology as a study of ontology in terms of what exists as it appears, transcending the objec-
tive-subjective and real-ideal distinctions. To Heidegger, then, things
are experienced by the self through *Dasein's* concernful engagement
with things in the environment. All experiences are relationships between *Dasein* and other things, which are seen as certain things projecting certain sets of expectations. Hence, our relation with things
"is primarily interpretive, or *hermeneutical*" (Moran, 2000, p. 234).

Maurice Merleau-Ponty, a contemporary of Sartre and Simone de Beauvoir and an existentialist, was also the most eminent French phenomenologist. Although greatly influenced by Husserl, Merleau-Ponty rejected Husserl's idea of human consciousness and transcendental ego as the foundation of human experiences. Instead, he proposed that perception is the source of knowledge, and that human beings are subjects with bodies that are experienced and experience the phenomenal world through perceptions (Merleau-Ponty, 1962). Hence, human existence in the world is through the lived body's involvement with the world through perception. Unlike Heidegger, Merleau-Ponty affirmed the phenomenological method that focuses on "lived experiences," or *Lebenswelt* (life-world), as the sources of knowledge, but doubted the possibility of bracketing as a means to gain complete insight into meanings. In both Heidegger and Merleau-Ponty, phenomenology is turned toward existentialism, moving away from transcendental ego as the source of all meanings and experiences.

Although it is a twentieth century philosophy, existentialism is deeply rooted in two nineteenth-century philosophers, Friedrich Nietzsche and Sören Kierkegaard. Existentialism, as a philosophic movement addressing the question of 'being', is traced by Barrett (1962) as the central and common thread in recasting the individual's relation to the meaning of religion and religious question, and elevating the centrality of human choice in the question of existence. Barrett (1962) identifies the following leading existentialists: Jean-Paul Sartre, Simone de Beauvoir, Albert Camus, and Gabriel Marcel among the French; the Germans Karl Jaspers, Martin Heidegger, and Martin Buber; Vladmir Solovev, Leon Shestov, and Nikolai Berdyaev from Russia; the Spaniards Miguel de Unamuno and José Ortega y Gasset; and the pragmatist William James of the United States. These names, of course, reveal the variant nature of existential thinking, especially in terms of human beings' relationships to religion and God. In existentialism, the human person is the one being in the world that as a free agent exists in the present but also is open to a future that is determined by one's own choices and actions. Human beings become themselves through their choices, choices of ways of life (Kierkegaard, 1959), or choices of actions. Human existence through choices is the reality in which the self is embroiled in the choices and the life is projected.

To existentialists, human choices are not framed in any sort of rational grounds but are determined by human freedom, so that choices are the responsibility of the self. Hence, humans are open to right or wrong ways of choosing: For Kierkegaard the choice is among the three levels of existence—the aesthetic, ethical, and religious; for Heidegger, it is the choice between the authentic or inauthentic existence; and for Sartre, the choice leads to an action that is performed either with sincerity or with bad faith.

Human existence, thus, is not only living with one' choices but also living with choices that are projected into a future, thus requiring humans to commit themselves to the choices that are made freely with accompanying self-responsibility. Because human existence is viewed as being situated for each individual and in a concrete, temporally situated context, existentialism opposes objectivism, positivism, and idealism. Thus, existentialism is found to be closely related to phenomenology on two accounts: humans' existential reality is grounded in situation, and human beings themselves determine their own existence.

EXISTENTIAL PHENOMENOLOGY

It is difficult to identify clearly the exact nature of existential phenomenology, because this label is attributed to various existentialists and phenomenologists in a rather casual manner in the literature. Sattler (1966) suggests that existential phenomenology as a philosophical orientation for psychology has begun to penetrate the American psychological scene by the 1960s. Sattler (1966) identifies existential phenomenology as an approach that is based on the existential notions about human existence, combined with the phenomenological idea of temporality. He states that the basic thesis of existential phenomenology is "man is in his inherent nature continually in the process of becoming. In becoming, man also transcends his physical limitations and is not simply a spatiotemporally defined entity. Temporality implies that knowledge of the future is incorporated into man's present action" (pp. 291–292).

More specifically, three versions of existential phenomenology may be identified in association with the philosophical orientations of Sartre, Heidegger, and Merleau-Ponty. Existential phenomenology with a strong identification to Sartre, as seen in Gordon's work (1995), is characterized by its commitment to the study of human existence in which human freedom and consciousness projects the self with choices.

The existential phenomenology of Heidegger is based on his notion of *Dasein* as a fundamental ontology by which humans are "already" involved in an ongoing world. For Heidegger, phenomenology is an exact study of 'being', the method of ontology. Moran (2000, p. 239) claims that existentialists, especially Sartre, accepted Heidegger's notion that "humans can make themselves who they are by seizing their possibilities," that are embedded in their understanding of themselves. On the other hand, Merleau-Ponty's existential phenomenology is grounded in his phenomenology of perception and his rejection of transcendental ego.

It is clear from these identifications that existential phenomenology in general is grounded in the ontology of existentialism and the method of phenomenology. However, the phenomenological method adopted by existential phenomenology is not that of Husserl, because existentialists reject the key tenets of Husserl's phenomenology, such as *eidos,* transcendental ego, bracketing, meaning constituted by consciousness, and phenomenological reduction.

PARSE'S THE HUMAN BECOMING THEORY

Parse first proposed the Human Becoming theory in 1981 as the Man-Living-Health theory, changing its name in 1992 to the current version. Parse claims that her theory is a human science theory, with the principal orientation to the concept of "human becoming" as "a unitary construct referring to the human being's living health" (Parse, 1997, p. 32). She particularly specifies that the assumptions of the theory have been constructed by synthesizing ideas from Rogers' science of unitary human beings and existential phenomenology (Parse, 1981, 1992, 1997). Existential phenomenological thoughts are drawn primarily from Heidegger, Sartre, and Merleau-Ponty (Parse, 1997). She also cites Kierkegaard as providing the concept of human subject (Parse, 1981).

Parse provides nine philosophical assumptions for the theory, which resulted from the synthesis of selected ideas from Rogers' science of unitary human beings and existential phenomenology. These are as follows:

1. The human is coexisting while coconstituting rhythmical patterns with the universe.
2. The human is open, freely choosing meaning in situation, bearing responsibility for decisions.

3. The human is unitary, continuously coconstituting patterns of relating.
4. The human is transcending multidimensionally with the possibles.
5. Becoming is unitary human living health.
6. Becoming is a rhythmically coconstituting human-universe process.
7. Becoming is the human's patterns of relating value priorities.
8. Becoming is an intersubjective process of transcending with the possibles.
9. Becoming is unitary human evolving. (Parse, 1997, p. 32)

Undergirding these philosophical assumptions are two tenets of existential phenomenology, intentionality and human subjectivity; and three principles (resonancy, helicy, and integrality) of Rogers' science. These provide concepts that are directly or indirectly inferred from the philosophical assumptions. The concepts are coconstitution, coexistence, and situated freedom from existential phenomenology; and energy field, openness, pattern and organization, and multidimensionality from Rogers. In addition, from these philosophical assumptions Parse draws out three major themes of her theory: *meaning, rhythmicity,* and *cotranscendence,* which lead to three principles of the theory as follows (Parse, 1981):

1. Structuring, meaning multidimensionally, is cocreating reality through the languaging of valuing and imaging.
2. Cocreating rhythmical patterns of relating is living the paradoxical unity of revealing-concealing, enabling-limiting while connecting-separating.
3. Cotranscending with the possibles is powering unique ways of originating in the process of transforming. (p. 69)

According to Parse, the concepts drawn from existential phenomenology and Rogers are embedded in all nine philosophical assumptions. This means that each of the assumptions has ideas from both sources integrated into a unified set. Hence, fundamentally, two distinct but interrelated questions are raised in viewing Parse's theory within the ontological orientation of existential phenomenology: (a) Are the assumptions advanced for the theory coherently and heuristically in alignment with the major tenets of existential phenomenology? (b) Can the ideas drawn from existential phenomenology be articulated with the ideas of Rogers' science of unitary human beings to form the foundation for the Human Becoming theory?

Parse's articulation of the two tenets of existential phenomenology (*intentionality* and *human subjectivity*) comes mostly from Heidegger. She then concludes that these two tenets lead to the assumptions about humans that "man coconstitutes situations with the world, man experience existence as coexistence, and man has freedom in situation" (Parse, 1981, p. 20). How would existentialists (especially those cited by Parse, such as Heidegger, Merleau-Ponty, and Sartre) interpret the *co-* in coexistence and coconstitution? From Heidegger at least, *Dasein* is structured existentially by moods *(Befindlichkeit)*, understanding *(Verstehen)*, and logos *(Rede)*, maintaining the self and the world both in diametrical connections and in embeddedness. It appears then that the terms starting with *co-*, when used in reference to humans and the universe, also must mean existential structuring of the universe in and with the humans in a side-by-side fashion. This does not seem to align with the ontology of existentialism, because existentialism is a philosophy of human existence, not of universal existence. Hence, in order for Parse to create the concepts of coexistence and coconstitution as foundational for her theory, it is necessary for her to develop an ontology that will encompass the *co-* notion of existence.

The second question concerns the appropriateness of articulating the philosophy of existentialism with Rogers' science. The principles and concepts from Rogers' science that are articulated and retained in the assumptions are openness, human-universe mutual process, rhythmicity, patterning, and multidimensionality. Rogers' concept of openness refers to the openness of humans and environments in relation to each other, and is closely related to the concept of human-universe mutual process. These two concepts in Rogers' science of unitary human beings provide the principles by which human beings and their environments are interpenetrating and moving along together, which are counter to existential phenomenology. This is because the focal point of 'being' in existential phenomenology is the humans who have the subjectivity, are making choices, and are the ones structuring their existence in the world, although not apart and away from the world but not in a mutual sense except with other humans. The concepts of rhythmicity and patterning, although drawn originally from Rogers, have been revised and defined uniquely in Parse's theory. Although these concepts definitionally do not violate the major tenets of existential phenomenology, it is important that the theory does not presuppose the existence of "essential" types or forms of rhythm and pattern. In addition, the concept of multidimensionality is brought in from Rogers' science and indicates an existential realm that goes beyond the spatiotemporal boundary. It is in line with the thought in existentialism that considers human existence not just as a spatiotemporal one.

This exposition suggests that the articulation of existential phenomenology in Parse's theory of Human Becoming is both illuminating and force fitting, mainly because she tried to reconcile this philosophical foundation with the Rogers' science of unitary human beings. Coming from the background of holism, Rogers' theory of unitary human beings assumes mutuality of humans and their universe. This foundation puts humans not at the core but on the same plane with the environment (or the universe) in examining human matters. Quite different from existential phenomenology's centering of humans and human existence, this seems to be the irreconcilable, fundamental contradiction between the two foundations that are said to be the major sources of philosophical assumptions of Parse's theory.

PHENOMENOLOGY IN NURSING RESEARCH

Knowledge development in nursing from the phenomenological tradition has been very active during the past two decades, as shown by numerous research articles and books published under this heading. It is possible to categorize the publications in nursing related to phenomenology mainly into four groups: (a) research regarding human experiences examined from the Husserlian phenomenological perspective, including works with the Merleau-Pontyian orientation, applying various phenomenological methods; (b) work with the interpretive phenomenological orientation of Heidegger; (c) work related to the existential phenomenological orientation of Parse and others; and (d) debates on phenomenology as a philosophy and phenomenological methods.

Nursing studies from the phenomenological perspective most often have applied the phenomenological methods developed within the psychological tradition specified by Giorgi, Collazzi, and van Manen, usually identified as descriptive phenomenology. Examples of recent works include studies on women's experiences related to pregnancy and delivery, as in Cote-Arsenault and Morrison-Beedy (2001) on perinatal loss, Lawler and Sinclair (2003) on postnatal depression, and Beck (2004a, 2004b) on posttraumatic stress disorder due to childbirth; and descriptions of illness-related experiences as in Beitz (1999) on having an ileoanal reservoir, Adams (2003) on being a diabetic, Johnson (2004) for critical care experiences, and Appelin and Bertero (2004) on experiences of palliative care. The issue is how such studies may culminate in middle-range descriptive theories of various human experiences, a question rarely raised by the researchers in phenomenological studies.

The work in interpretive phenomenology in the tradition of Heidegger in nursing took off with Benner's early work (1984). Though the majority of work from this perspective focuses on nurses' practice (for example, Darbyshire, 2004), it has also dealt with ordinary life experiences and practices as suggested by Benner (1994b) and Johnson (2000). Although there have been pointed critiques about the appropriateness and interpretive correctness regarding Heideggerian phenomenology in nursing (see Crotty, 1996, 1997; Holmes, 1996; Paley, 1998), the problem lies in differing notions regarding the nature of knowledge obtained from this perspective. Context and history are viewed in hermeneutic phenomenology as the frames within which knowledge of people's everyday practices and experiences is gained through interpretations, thus making the knowledge tentative and oriented to understanding. The literature is rather confusing in many of the researchers' framing of context and history.

Most worrisome in phenomenological research is the imprecise use of language both in expression and interpretation, especially in using terms such as *meaning, life-world, experience, lived,* and *themes.* Furthermore, epistemological differences that are fundamentally grounded in the two traditions of phenomenology have not been well-addressed in nursing studies. Researchers continue to use the same terms to describe their findings, possibly with different meanings and perspective. Theory development from the phenomenological perspective in precise terms requires a definition of descriptive theory that is appropriate in the tradition, and an identification of methodologies specifically suited for theory development as the primary step.

CONCLUSIONS

The foregoing exposition provides the background for considering existentialism and phenomenology as possible ontological focus for nursing theories. In order to take existentialism, phenomenology, or both as an ontological focus for a nursing theory, it is necessary to pose the following questions:

- What is the meaning of human health within the tenets of existentialism and phenomenology?
- How is the experience of human health and health care interpreted in terms of human subjectivity, freedom of choice, existential meaning, temporality, situatedness, and historicity?
- What is the meaning of human health existentially and phenomenologically?
- What does it mean to be in human practice existentially and phenomenologically?
- How is the role of researcher (investigator) articulated for existential and phenomenological knowledge of human health, suffering, and practice?
- How is it possible to distinguish existential or phenomenological researcher from existential or phenomenological practitioner?

Theories emerging from such foundations must assume a different format from those based on other ontological foci, which permit explanation or prediction or both. Basically, theories with the ontological focus of existentialism or phenomenology will need to be oriented either to the specification of methodology or the descriptive features regarding the realm of human life, such as human health.

REFERENCES

Adams, C. R. (2003). Lessons learned from urban Latinas with type 2 diabetes mellitus. *Journal of Transcultural Nursing, 14,* 255–265.

Appelin, G., & Bertero, C. (2004). Patients' experiences of palliative care in the home: A phenomenological study of a Swedish sample. *Cancer Nursing, 27,* 65–70.

Barrett, W. (1962). *Irrational man: A study in existential philosophy.* Garden City, NY: Doubleday Anchor Books.

Beck, C. T. (2004a). Birth trauma: In the eye of the beholder. *Nursing Research, 53,* 28–35.

Beck, C. T. (2004b). Post-traumatic stress disorder due to childbirth: The aftermath. *Nursing Research, 53,* 216–224.

Beitz, J. M. (1999). The lived experience of having an ileoanal reservoir: A phenomenologic study. *Journal of WOCN, 26,* 185–200.

Benner, P. (1984). *From novice to expert: Excellence and power in clinical nursing practice.* Reading, MA: Addison-Wesley.

Benner, P. (Ed.). (1994a). *Interpretive phenomenology: Embodiment, caring, and ethics in health and illness.* Thousand Oaks, CA: Sage.

Benner, P. (1994b). The tradition and skill of interpretive phenomenology in studying health, illness, and caring practices. In P. Benner (Ed.), *Interpretive phenomenology: Embodiment, caring, and ethics in health and illness* (pp. 99–127). Thousand Oaks, CA: Sage.

Bishop, A. H., & Scudder, J. R., Jr. (2003). Gadow's contribution to our philosophical interpretation of nursing. *Nursing Philosophy, 4,* 104–110.

Caelli, K. (2000). The changing face of phenomenological research: Traditional and American phenomenology in nursing. *Qualitative Health Research, 10,* 366–377.

Cote-Arsenault, D., & Morrison-Beedy, D. (2001). Women's voices reflecting changed expectations for pregnancy after perinatal loss. *Journal of Nursing Scholarship, 33,* 239–244.

Crotty, M. (1996). *Phenomenology and nursing research.* Melbourne, Australia: Churchill Livingstone.

Crotty, M. (1997). Tradition and culture in Heidegger's being and time. *Nursing Inquiry, 4,* 88–98.

Darbyshire, P. (2004). 'Rage against the machine?': Nurses' and midwives' experiences of using Computerized Patient Information systems for clinical information. *Journal of Clinical Nursing, 13,* 17–25.

Gordon, L. (1995). *Bad faith and antiblack racism.* Atlantic Highlands, NJ: Humanities Press.

Häggman-Laitila, A. (1997). Health as an individual's way of existence. *Journal of Advanced Nursing, 25,* 45–53.

Heidegger, M. (1962). *Being and time* (J. Macquarrie & F. Robinson, Trans.). New York: Harper & Row. (Original work published in 1927)

Holmes, C. (1996). The politics of phenomenological concepts in nursing. *Journal of Advanced Nursing, 24,* 579–587.

Husserl, E. (1931). *Ideas: General introduction to pure phenomenology* (W. R. B. Gibson, Trans.). New York: Macmillan. (Original work published in 1913)

Johnson, M. E. (2000). Heidegger and meaning: Implications for phenomenological research. *Nursing Philosophy, 1,* 134–146.

Johnson, P. (2004). Reclaiming the everyday world: How long-term ventilated patients in critical care seek to gain aspects of power and control over their environment. *Intensive and Critical Care Nursing, 20,* 190–199.

Jones, A. (1998). 'Out of the sighs'—An existential-phenomenological method of clinical supervision: The contribution to palliative care. *Journal of Advanced Nursing, 27,* 905–913.

Jones, A. (2001). Absurdity and being-in-itself. The third phase of phenomenology: Jean-Paul Sartre and existential psychoanalysis. *Journal of Psychiatric and Mental Health Nursing, 8,* 367–372.

Kierkegaard, S. (1959). *Either/or* (Vol. I–II). (D. F. Swenson & L. M. Swenson, Trans.). Princeton, NJ: Princeton University Press.

Lawler, D., & Sinclair, M. (2003). Grieving for my former self: A phenomenological hermeneutical study of women's lived experience of postnatal depression. *Evidence Based Midwifery, 1,* 36–41.

Lopez, K. A., & Willis, D. G. (2004). Descriptive versus interpretive phenomenology: Their contributions to nursing knowledge. *Qualitative Health Research, 14,* 726–735.

Merleau-Ponty, M. (1962). *Phenomenology of perception* (C. Smith, Trans.). London: Routledge and Kegan Paul. (Original work published in 1945)

Moran, D. (2000). *Introduction to phenomenology.* London: Routledge.

Natanson, M. (1966). Introduction. In M. Natanson (Ed.), *Essays in phenomenology* (pp. 1–22). The Hague, The Netherlands: Martinus Nijhoff.

Natanson, M. (1973). *Edmund Husserl: Philosopher of infinite tasks.* Evanston, IL: Northwestern University Press.

Newman, M. A. (1990). Newman's theory of health as praxis. *Nursing Science Quarterly, 3,* 37–41.

Newman, M. A. (1994). *Health as expanding consciousness* (2nd ed.). New York: National League for Nursing.

Omery, A., & Mack, C. (1995). Phenomenology and science. In A. Omery, C. E. Kasper, & G. G. Page (Eds.), *In search of nursing science* (pp. 139–158). Newbury Park, CA: Sage.

Paley, J. (1997). Husserl, phenomenology and nursing. *Journal of Advanced Nursing, 26,* 187–193.

Paley, J. (1998). Misinterpretive phenomenology: Heidegger, ontology and nursing research. *Journal of Advanced Nursing, 27,* 817–824.

Parse, R. R. (1981). *Man-living-health: A theory of nursing.* New York: Wiley.

Parse, R. R. (1992). Human becoming: Parse's theory of nursing. *Nursing Science Quarterly, 5,* 35-42.

Parse, R. R. (1997). The human becoming theory: The was, is, and will be. *Nursing Science Quarterly, 10,* 32–38.

Patterson, J. G., & Zderad, L. T. (1976). *Humanistic nursing.* New York: Wiley.

Patterson, J. G., & Zderad, L. T. (1988). *Humanistic nursing* (2nd ed.). New York: National League for Nursing.

Sadala, M. L. A., & Adorno, R. D. C. (2002). Phenomenology as a method to investigate the experience lived: A perspective from Husserl and Merleau Ponty's thought. *Journal of Advanced Nursing, 37,* 282–293.

Sartre, J. (1956). *Being and nothingness* (Special abridged ed.). (H. E. Barnes, Trans.). Secaucus, NJ: Citadel Press.

Sattler, J. M. (1966). The existential-phenomenological movement and its impact on contemporary American psychology. *Journal of Existentialism, 6,* 289–294.

Schutz, A. (1966). Some leading concepts in phenomenology. In M. Natanson (Ed.), *Essays in phenomenology* (pp. 23–39). The Hague, The Netherlands: Martinus Nijhoff.

Spiegelberg, H. (1982). *The phenomenological movement: A historical introduction* (3rd ed.). The Hague, The Netherlands: Martinus Nijhoff.

CHAPTER 10

Humanism in Nursing Theory: A Focus on Caring

May Solveig Fagermoen

The philosophies of humanism and caring have been foundational to nursing throughout its history, shaping the basic character of nursing, namely, that nursing inherently is a moral practice. Viewed as a service to humankind, nursing always has been guided by a moral motivation to act in the best interest of those in need of nursing care.

In modern nursing, Florence Nightingale, a true humanist, stands out as a warrior in her fight for patients' dignity and decent care, first during the Crimean War and later when she worked to improve nursing care and the conditions within hospitals. In her view, caring for patients implied providing the best possible environment to promote reparative processes in patients and to help them meet their physical needs in an individualized manner. Both action orientations were to be based in astute observations and knowledge. From this perspective, several theorists have expanded on her ideas of what nursing is all about, what constitutes good nursing care, and how to think and act to provide the best possible care within a humanistic tradition. For example, Abdellah, Henderson, and Orem explicated further our understanding of nursing as complementary assistance toward fulfilling patients' basic needs when they are lacking the knowledge, strength, or will to carry out the necessary activities themselves and in a manner that upholds and restores their independence and self-care. Other theorists, such as Peplau, Travelbee, and Watson, have all developed the ideas about individualized care, specifically in relation to the interpersonal domain of nursing, while Leininger's concept of transcultural care has extended our vision of what nursing care is all about.

To understand their theoretical perspective in advancing nursing, it is useful to examine their foundational ideas. A basic building block in these and other nurse-theorists' work is the idea of humanism. Therefore, in this chapter humanism will be traced from a historical perspective, how it is developed within other disciplines, how it has influenced nursing's disciplinary culture, and finally, Watson's theory of human care will be viewed within this general frame. The chapter will conclude with what humanism and caring means for nursing practice and the advancement of nursing knowledge.

HUMANISM—TRACING THE DEVELOPMENT

Today, the word *humanism* has many connotations. Generally, humanism is understood as the tendency to emphasize humans and their status, importance, powers, achievements, or authority. Humanism is also referred to as a school of thought, as a philosophical movement, and as a worldview, which assign human beings a special position in the world at large. In the literature we find that different strands of humanism are distinguished by descriptive adjectives such as religious humanism, secular humanism, Renaissance humanism, Enlightenment humanism, and so forth. This reflects that humanism as we understand it today has been a movement over time, molded by a theological or atheistic worldview and variously constructed in different historical contexts. The common ontological characteristics across different denominations are the centrality of humans, their powers and potentialities. The presentation of humanism is not aimed at covering every aspect of humanism in philosophic writings, but to select and include those ideas that to my knowledge have had the greatest impact on the development of nursing science.

Although the word humanism came into usage at a later time, the movement or philosophical idea of humanism was rediscovered in Italy in the second half of the fourteenth century at the advent of the Renaissance era. Thinkers in this period sought to reintegrate humans into the world of nature and history and to interpret them in this perspective. This movement was the renaissance of antiquity, "the preservation and cultivation of the ideals and culture in the classical world" (Luik, 1991a, p. 17). Through the study of the classical literature and art, the "rebirth" of a spirit that humans had possessed in that age and had lost in the Middle Ages could be realized. It denoted a move away from God to humans as the center of interest, which allowed for "a spirit of freedom that provided justification for man's claim of rational autonomy, allowing him to see himself involved in nature and history and capable of making them his realm" (Abbagnano, 1972, p. 70).

The central theme of humanism was the potentialities of humans, their creative powers. These powers, including the power to mold oneself, were latent, to be brought out, and the means to that end was education. The humanists saw education as the process by which humans were lifted out of their natural condition to discover their *humanitas* (humanness). At the end of the fifteenth century, *humanista* (humanist) was used to describe the teacher of the classical languages and literatures, in contrast to *legista,* the teacher of law (Kolenda, 1995). The Renaissance term for what they studied was *Studia humanitatis,* which represented grammar, rhetoric, poetry, history, languages, politics, and moral philosophy. Here we find the root of the fields of study that today are known as the humanities.

The privilege accorded to the humanities was founded on the conviction that these disciplines alone could educate humans and put them in the position to exercise their freedom effectively. Andic (1991) summarizes the mood of the Renaissance era:

> [W]e need to understand and realize ourselves in our humanity and to cultivate those humane virtues that makes us fully human beings—then where better place to begin this self-study than with the . . . [writings] from outstanding men and women drawn from the treasury of Latin and Greek history and literature, in order to learn by imitating their deeds and avoiding their failures to become such as they are? (p. 90)

God remained the creator and supreme authority, but His activities were seen as less immediate, more a general control than a day-to-day interference. This change in belief, combined with an emphasis on humans' power of reason, encouraged their ability to find out about the universe through their own efforts, and more and more to control it. Hence, this worldview enabled a scientific outlook to arise that saw the universe as governed by general laws, albeit laws laid down by God.

> When the fourteenth and fifteenth century humanists and philoso-
> phers said that man is placed in the center of the world and can be-
> come what he himself chooses, they did not mean that everything is
> permitted to him; they said that he is the middle, not as the *measure*
> of all things but as the *mediator* of the divine vision and love. . . . They
> thought that God is fully divine only in man. (Andic, 1991, pp. 92–93)

The breach between art and science had not yet taken place. Humans, seen as natural beings whose interest is to make nature their domain, were given tools, that is, their senses, through which they could
question and understand nature. Humanity with all its facets and
distinct capabilities, problems, and possibilities was examined in
paintings and poetry. The great artists of the time, Michelangelo and
Leonardo da Vinci, who both also studied anatomy and physiology,
rediscovered the human body through drawings and paintings. Bullock (1985) made this comment: "The combination of the observation, description and representation of nature has been claimed as one
of the indispensable prerequisites for the burst of scientific innovation
which begins with the humanist-scientist Galileo" (p. 39). Hence,
Renaissance humanism is generally considered to be one of the conditions that contributed to the birth of modern science.

In Renaissance humanism, the insistence on the value and centrality of human experience was reflected in the core idea of "*dignitas*—
the proper relationship between God and nature" (Madigan, 1991,
p. 327). This Renaissance concept—the dignity of "man"—reflects a
confidence in the value of humans and their work and is grounded in
the latent power women and men possess. The ability to create and
communicate in language, the arts, and institutions, and also to observe themselves, to speculate, imagine, and reason "enable men and
women to exercise a degree of freedom of choice and will, to change
course, to innovate and thus to open the possibility . . . of improving
themselves and the human lot" (Bullock, 1985, p. 156). The concept
of human dignity was recovered and restated later, as in the Enlightenment, when human dignity no longer was seen as being linked to
humans' divine origin, but to their rational possibilities in this world.
The concept of human dignity and what it implies is the foundation
for human rights as we know them today.

Humanism in the Enlightenment is linked to the eighteenth-century
thinkers "who believed that the central concern of human existence
was not the discovery of God's will, but the shaping of human life and
society according to a set of universally acknowledged rational principles" (Luik, 1991b, p.118). The Enlightenment humanists' enormous

confidence in, and commitment to, human reason was reflected in their belief in the centrality of science and the scientific method. One of the great philosophers at that time, Immanuel Kant (1724–1804), claimed that "Enlightenment is man's emergence from his self-concurred immaturity," with the "motto of enlightenment therefore: *Sapere aude!* Have the courage to use your *own* understanding!" (cited in Luik, 1991b, p. 119).

Reason was not only the discovery of facts, but also a base from which one, in part, could create moral principles, that is, give a grounding for morality. Two foundational principles in Kant's ethics are still recognized today: (a) persons as ends in themselves, that is, all rational beings exists as an end in themselves and not merely as means to be used arbitrarily by this or that will; and (b) the centrality of freedom, that is, only human persons can freely set and achieve ends, and the unique value of human persons is to be found in their self-determining ends. Enlightenment humanism may be defined by the confidence in human autonomy, "an autonomy secured through the creative and ordering power of reason" (Luik 1991b, p. 118). Among others, David Hume (1711–1776) was a strong opponent of Kant's in regard to the grounding of morality in reason. He did not reject that reasoning is important in morality, but rather disputed its primacy. According to Baier (1987), Hume held that "morality rests ultimately on sentiment, on a special motivating feeling . . . our capacity for sympathy with other's feelings" (p. 41). The interdependence between persons requires collaboration and accordingly, for Hume, morality depends on "a *reflective* sentiment, and on self-corrected self-interest and corrected sympathy" (Baier, 1987, p. 47). Hume's thoughts on morality are relevant today in view of the increased emphasis on relational ethics and the ethics of caring.

As in the Renaissance era, individual freedom was a central value, in addition to equality and tolerance, which were emphasized and reflected in the Enlightenment humanists' beliefs in the moral sense of responsibility and the possibility of progress. Although they believed in the primacy of reason, it was to be used in the service of social and political reform. These characteristics were later revived in pragmatism, which was the most influential philosophy in America in the first quarter of the twentieth century. (Humanism in pragmatism will be addressed later in the chapter.)

The belief in the centrality of science—its method and orderly explanations formulated in propositions and laws—proliferated in the next centuries and expanded into all aspects of human life. Darwinism was a major force that stimulated the extension of scientific explanations beyond the natural sciences to social sciences. It is also with Darwinism that humanism first acquired its modern association with atheism and agnosticism. Wilhelm Dilthey (1833–1911), a German philosopher, was one of the first to criticize this single-science conception and opposed the strategy of applying the scientific method on human phenomena other than the natural ones because it was inappropriate: such phenomena required different methods. Hence, humans' unique position in the world of nature was reemphasized.

Dilthey did not believe that human life could be understood by using the explanatory model that classifies events according to the laws of nature (Nerheim, 1995). Human life is lived in a cultural world created by human beings. This, a shared world of ideas, values, beliefs, languages, symbols, and institutions, can be grasped accordingly and understood from the inside, that is, as humans we can enter into them. This conception of the common ground is basic to the introduction of hermeneutics in the social sciences. Dilthey argued that the methods needed to uncover these phenomena that constitute an inner world of purpose and meaning have to be of an interpretative nature and cannot be revealed by the methods of natural sciences (Skirbrekk & Gilje, 1987).

Purpose and meaning cannot be explained, only understood, and understanding *(Verstehen)* requires a common ground, that is, human beings can understand what human beings have created. Understanding in this context is conceived as a mental act—it is an activity, not merely an experience. Hence, Dilthey insisted on a difference between *explanation* and *understanding;* the first can be sought by the scientific methods, the latter by the hermeneutic method. This general method of comprehension of meaning is central to the *Geisteswissenschaften* (translated as *human sciences* in America; see Polkinghorne, [1983, pp. 283–289] for a clarification on the choice of English words). However, Dilthey did not see the hermeneutic method as the only and exclusive method in the human sciences. Humans are not pure *Geist* (spirit) only, and therefore other methods may be needed: It is the topic at hand that decides the choice of method (Skirbrekk & Gilje, 1987). Thus, the human sciences must conceive of humans as both subject and object. As subject, humans must be understood as creators of their own world and as beings controlling their actions, because humans are creative, strive for meaning, and act intentionally. To understand humans as object, their actions can be conceived in causal terms; however, there are limits to causal explanations because humans are creative beings and can change. Thus, Dilthey underscored the relativistic nature of humans and human life; everything is dependent on time and place.

In contrast to Dilthey's exposition of hermeneutics as a method central to the *Geisteswissenschaften,* Heidegger (1889–1976) considered hermeneutics primarily as a process fundamental to human life, that is, his position is ontological. Heidegger argued that *understanding (Verstehen)* is a basic form of human existence: It is not the way we know the world; it is the way we are. To be human is to be interpretative; humans are hermeneutic beings whose whole lives are forever interpretation. Hence, Heidegger saw hermeneutics as the basic pattern of human understanding: We vacillate between the known and the unknown, between the parts and the whole, continuously seeing new sides, gaining new insights, possibly seeing better and more clearly, but always as imperfect humans in our search (Skirbrekk & Gilje, 1987). Hence, the act of interpretation is linked with being, for "interpretation is the activity that enables us to experience the world. . . . everything that exists in the world exists for people through the act of interpretation and understanding" (Thompson, 1990, p. 237). This distinction between hermeneutics based in ontology and hermeneutics discussed from an epistemological position (as Dilthey espoused) is important, yet not always recognized. Thompson (1990) called these two of the "three conversations in hermeneutics," the third one being the methodological discussion that voices questions about the proper methods for data collection and analysis in an interpretative study.

In his philosophical analyses, Heidegger sought answers to the overriding question of the meaning of 'being' (Nicolaisen, 1997). In his major work, *Being and Time,* Heidegger argued that the answer to what makes reality meaningful must be sought from the perspective of what is particular to the being of 'man', his being in the world. One result of this analysis—human living as a continuous interpretative process—was discussed above. Foundational to this answer is Heidegger's position that meaning is not something created by ideas, but is evolving as we involve ourselves in the world. Humans are relational beings, from the moment of birth; thrown into the world, humans are in relation to other beings and other things. Humans are not conceivable without relationships. The concept of *Sorge* (translated to *care* or *caring* in English), is used by Heidegger to characterize the basic principle of humans' 'being'. This being is constituted as a *being-in-the-world* and as a *being-together-with-others* (Nerheim, 1995).

Hence, our being presupposes the being of others. Our existence is communion: Our foundational characteristic is that we are living because of and for others for our own sake. Consideration and care for others in *their* interest are in our own interest. "Our task in this world is one: we are and have to be" (Nicolaisen, 1997, p. 529). This is human freedom, to choose who to be. Furthermore, the human interpretative nature is a premise for the comprehension of (a) what is in the other's interest and (b) what is seen from the other's perspective. However, the presence of an attitude *(Befindlichkeit)* in which one acknowledges the other's personhood is required in order for care to be authentic. The concept of *Sorge* emphasizes that authentic self-understanding can only be found by relating to the world through "practical" work and at the end, the answer to who you are has reference to the world in which you live and act, the human life-world (Nerheim, 1995, p. 291).

Heidegger was a critic of the humanisms of the past, which he saw as resting on the notion that the dignity of humans was tied to the assumption that humans are the rational animals (Goicoechea, Luik, & Madigan, 1991). He posited that for humans to live in their highest dignity it is not enough to think of themselves as rational animals, and argued for a return to "original humanism which [he] refers to as 'mediating and caring, that man be human and not inhuman, that is, outside his essence'" (cited in Goicoechea et al., 1991, p. 21). In this, we see traces of Hume's standpoint in regard to the foundation of morality.

In North America, humanism is clearly reflected and developed further in the philosophical movement of pragmatism, which emerged toward the end of the nineteenth century. This movement. which is linked foremost to the ideas of Charles S. Pierce (1839–1914), William James (1842–1910), and John Dewey (1859–1952), "is best understood as in part, a critical rejection of much traditional academic philosophy and, in part, a concern to establish certain positive aims" (Thayer, 1996, p. 430). Pragmatism sought to reconcile incompatibilities between philosophical idealism and realism, that is, it was struggling with the following question: Does reality exist only in human experience and in the form of perceptions and ideas, or does reality exist in the form of essences or absolutes that are independent of human experience? (Maines, 1992). According to Francis (1991), the basic pragmatist thought is as follows:

> There exist no permanent essences of any kind, including none of humankind. Everything is in a constant reorganization by interacting and transacting with something. . . . Basically all that exists is change,

and the interactions and complexity or diversity of change. . . . human existence, life, and all experience, including the intellectual, are contingent, tentative, developing aspects of change. (pp. 238–239)

Hence, such dualisms as matter and mind, object and subject, and reality and thought collapse (Diggins, 1994).

Strongly influenced by the evolutionary theory of Darwin, pragmatists focused on human beings' struggle for existence in an ever-changing world in which they themselves are changing, individually and socially. *Experience* is a fundamental term in pragmatism, conceived as "an active, interacting, undergoing, undertaking, and reconstructing of life's events" (Francis, 1991, p. 236). Hence, humans' capacity for problem solving is central to the pragmatic school of thought. Rather than being passive responders to stimuli, humans are active, creative organisms, empowered with agency. Human 'being' is embedded in an ongoing complex nature and is engaged continuously in learning-by-doing, to make sense of things, and to solve problems. Hence, human life "is [seen] as a dialectical process of continuity and discontinuity and therefore [as] inherently emergent" (Maines, 1992, p. 1532). In an interactive relationship, humans and society are constantly shaping and reshaping themselves, sustained by symbolic communication and language. In the pragmatic school of thought, this interdependence between the individual and the society included also the individual's responsibility for social reform and moral conduct for the public good. The pragmatic method, synonymous with the method of science, was hailed as supreme in solving problems of both social and moral character, as expressed by Dewey (1976/1916).

Social questions are capable of being intelligently coped with only to the degree in which we employ the method of collected data, forming hypotheses, and testing them in action which is characteristic of natural science, and in the degree in which we utilize in the behalf of the promotion of social welfare the technical knowledge ascertained by physics and chemistry (p. 343). . . . The social interest, identical in its deepest meaning with a moral interest, is necessarily supreme with man. (p. 345)

Pragmatism also represented a critique of society, and both Dewey and Mead, together with other pragmatists, engaged in programs for social change in Chicago.

The basic principle of pragmatism, whose Greek root *pragma* means action, is that "ideas must be related to practical consequences and must be responsive to the broader problems of civilization"

(Kurtz, 1972, p. 88). Education was seen as synonymous with democracy, providing liberation from oppressive authorities. In education and social life generally, the pragmatic principle was the ideal, that is, all ideas should be submitted to a threefold procedure: cooperative inquiry, experimental testing, and judgment arrived at through public consensus. Mead (1964a) outlined the procedure of a discourse ethics based on the same principle.

Hence, pragmatist thoughts can be seen as roots of diverse movement of today, such as problem-based learning, Habermas's critical theory, and the corresponding action research. The philosophical movement of pragmatism has been influential in many fields, especially in education, psychology, and sociology. Many of the theories adapted into nursing can be traced to pragmatism, such as Mead's thoughts reflected in symbolic interactionism and Glaser and Strauss' grounded theory, Dewey's educational theory, and humanistic psychology.

HUMANISM REFLECTED IN PSYCHOLOGY AND SOCIOLOGY

As outlined earlier, a basic humanistic thought in pragmatism is the linkage between humans' self-generating powers and social reorganization. Although both concepts were developed further within American sociology and social psychology, the founders of humanistic psychology adopted primarily the former concept, in their shared view that a person is a "being-in-the process-of-becoming." DeCarvalho (1991) summarized their views in this manner:

> Each human being . . . is a unique organism with the ability to direct and change the guiding motives or "project" of life's course. In the process of becoming, one must assume the ultimate responsibility for the individualization and actualization of one's existence. To reach the highest levels through the process of becoming, a person must be fully functioning (Rogers) or functionally autonomous (Allport); the self must be spontaneously integrated and actualizing (Maslow); there must be a sense of self awareness, centeredness (May), and authenticity of being (Bugental). (pp. 83–84)

The view of the person as being in a process of becoming was an attack by these psychologists on, and their answer to, the dominant psychology at that time, namely, behaviorism. Thus, the reflection is evident of the pragmatists' emphasis on humans as active and creative, shaping their world and not being passive and mere responders to stimuli. These psychologists also introduced phenomenology and existentialism into a traditional positivist milieu. In this, one can see the influence of the pragmatist philosopher William James, who according to Diggins (1994) "gave philosophical legitimacy to all kinds of experience, personal and spiritual as well as physical and factual. . . . making room for the subjective as well as the objective, [he] paved the way for making American philosophy receptive . . . to existentialism and phenomenology" (p. 126). An American psychologist often referred to in nursing, Amadeo Giorgi (1970), is also based in phenomenology and existentialism. He was the first to argue that psychology ought to be understood as a "human science" considering its subject matter: the person-in-becoming. His position also was taken as a reaction against behaviorism and its ideal of natural science as the proper and only method of psychological research (Polkinghorne, 1983). Giorgi has developed his own method for phenomenological study, which is frequently used and referred to by nurse researchers.

As seen, in psychology the tension between experimental and experiential paradigms of understanding human nature was introduced just after World War II. These paradigms, as discussed by Dilthey 100 years earlier, refer to the contrast between explanation and understanding as the goal of scientific work. This has been an issue of discussion in the social sciences also (Fay & Moon, 1994) and in medicine (Schwartz & Wiggins, 1985). The former argued the benefit of and need for both in furthering knowledge development in their fields, while the latter called for a humanistic approach in medicine, "Without humanism of medicine we remain blind to the complexities and details of the human evidence. . . . Only this enlarged understanding of the humanness and individuality of patients can provide the evidential context for a medical science of health and illness" (p. 359). Humanism has a long tradition in nursing; however, only since the late 1970s has there been growing evidence for its impact on methodology in nursing research.

Two of the early theorists in pragmatism, Charles Cooley (1864–1929) and George Herbert Mead (1863–1931) explicated further the ideas of humans' self-generative powers and social reorganization. Both rejected the dualism between mind and society and developed theories about the interdependence between the two. Their theories have had profound influence in social psychology and sociology in regard to the understanding and studies of roles, social groups, conflicts, negotiations, organizations, for example, as reflected in the work of Erving Goffman, Anselm Strauss, and Herbert Blumer. Concepts such as the *looking-glass self* (Cooley), and *I* and *Me* and *role-taking* (Mead), are foundational to other theories in sociology, especially within interactionism. The looking-glass self refers to Cooley's theory on the development of self-concepts, that these are behaviorally derived through reflected appraisals of the actions of others in which the primary groups are especially important as they link the person to society. Society, on the other hand, "is an interweaving and interworking of mental selves" (Maines, 1992, p. 1533).

Mead held that mind and selves developed in the social act as humans, by imaginatively placing themselves in the position of others, taking the role of the other, and learning the symbolic meanings embedded in society. This involves "a conflation of subjective and objective processes through which persons adjustively contend with the facts of their environments and simultaneously create new situations" (Maines, 1992, p. 1533). Hence Mead, in his analysis of role-taking, or the construction of shared meanings, was concerned with "intersubjectivity," a core concept within phenomenology that was later discussed and developed further by the sociologist Alfred Schutz (Turner, 1986). Mead explored the concepts of subjectivity and objectivity, represented in the terms *I* and *Me,* also in regard to the methods of science (Mead, 1964b). Thus, Mead laid the basis for the development of a research method in which both subjectivity and objectivity are combined rather than competing, namely, that of grounded theory (Glaser & Strauss, 1967).

When reviewing the names of theorists in psychology and sociology whose thoughts are rooted in pragmatism and humanism, most can be recognized as central to the development of nursing as a discipline, especially in North America. The founders of humanistic psychology have had great impact on all writings on the interpersonal relationship between nurses and patients, such as those of Travelbee, Peplau, Orlando, Zderad and Paterson, and Watson, who also refers to Giorgi, the phenomenological psychologist. Giorgi is frequently mentioned when research methods within the qualitative paradigm are discussed or outlined in the nursing literature. Interactionism in sociology has had an impact on nursing through its theories of socialization, role development, organizational issues, and also through the grounded theory approach in research. One may conclude that humanism and pragmatism are at the center of modern nursing.

HUMANISM OF TODAY

A critical remark was made in a recent publication that explored traces of humanism in the ideas of philosophers from antiquity to the present time: To consider everyone a humanist "who are interested in the best life of human beings" is not a useful definition of humanism (Goicoechea et al., 1992, p. 36). What, then, can be said of humanism of today?

In general, humanism is not considered one philosophical system but rather a continuing debate in which the central issues are the many different views on humans' place in the order of things and humans' being in the world. Several sources reviewed for this chapter argue that a central tenet of humanism is "to acknowledge the humanity in everyone, the capacity of every person to think and act of himself" (Andic, 1991, p. 86). Furthermore, humanism is most often contrasted with other competing positions, such as the supernatural transcendent position, which considers humanity to be radically dependent on divine order, and the scientific position, which treats humanity scientifically as part of the natural order, on a par with other living organisms. In this cleavage, humanism is placed in a middle position as it discerns in human beings unique capabilities and abilities to be cultivated and celebrated for their own sake. Humanism focuses on humans and the human experience.

> That does not rule out either religious belief in a divine order or the scientific investigation of man as part of the natural order but it makes the point that, like every other belief—including the values we live by, and indeed all our knowledge—they are derived by human minds from human experience. (Bullock, 1985, p. 155)

Accordingly, humanism accepts that there is more than one way to the truth.

Another characteristic of humanism of today are the contrasts between theological and secular underpinnings of the basic values expressed in humanism. One overriding value in humanism is that of *human dignity*, which from the theological position is founded on the belief that humans are created by God and in God's image, while from a secular position this value is held high because of humans' unique capabilities, particularly their ability to reason, as expressed by Protagoras: "Man is the measure of all things." Similarly, the value of individual *freedom* is from a secular position arising from humans' reasoning power, in contrast to the theological belief that freedom is based in free will, given by God. Equality and tolerance are two other esteemed values in humanism, which may be seen as values derived from human dignity. Hence, these values are given different grounding from these two types of humanism. Both values underscore the interdependence between human beings. This is the foundation for a moral sense of responsibility, and is an impetus for social and political engagement to better the world of humans. Social reconstruction is a central concept in humanism, as well as self-realization. Central to these concepts is education, which is seen as a cornerstone for social change. Education is aimed at awakening the possibilities, drawing out the humanness and the all-around development of the personality and the full range of individual talents.

CARING AS THE PHILOSOPHICAL FOCUS

Caring as a phenomenon is as old as humankind. There has always been someone within the family or close social network who was given the responsibility to take care of those not able to do so themselves. To take care of one's own was a duty, and others were left to caring for themselves. When presenting caring as a philosophical focus, it seems reasonable to start with the advent of Christianity. In his own acts and in his teachings, Christ emphasized the need for and importance of caring for those who were sick, weak, or fallen or who were outcasts, regardless of family or social ties. A great contrast to the common practice in the community, Christ's primary commandment to "love Thy neighbor as Thyself" was a provocation as was his story of the good Samaritan. However, these became the ideals of his followers, upon which they developed a system of service for those in need, later established as cloisters. Until the Renaissance, nursing as a social service was closely associated with these institutions and carried out by nuns.

In reintroducing humanism with its emphasis on the unique powers of humans, the Renaissance was the period that also introduced the weakening of the Catholic Church and its power over minds and people. Some of the consequences were that in many places Church hospitals were closed, the sick and helpless were left to their own care, and the ideal of the individual's responsibility for the weak, the sick, and so forth was generally weakened. Institutional care became low-grade work for uneducated women and the quality of care was minimal. Generally, this was the situation when modern nursing saw the light with the founding of a nursing school at Kaiserswerth in Germany in 1836, and later through Florence Nightingale's work in the Crimean War and the establishment of her nursing school at St. Thomas Hospital in London.

The caring philosophy of Florence Nightingale evolved from her Christian beliefs and materialized in hands-on care, first for the soldiers in the war and later for those most unfortunate of London. Hers was a war on behalf of the sick to better their conditions. Nightingale's theory on nursing, published in *Notes on Nursing* (1859/1992), reflects a caring philosophy in which caring for the patient implies attending to basic needs individually through careful and considerate nursing "to put the patient in the best condition for nature to act upon him" (Nightingale, p. 75). She saw the patients' experience of discomfort and suffering as related to inadequacies in the environment, be they physical (stale air, dirty linen, etc.) or the nurse herself (noisy shoes, loud talk, etc.). Nightingale's focus of care was essentially actional not interactional and the action orientation was toward the environment: to provide the proper use of warmth, light, air, cleanliness, quiet, and a sufficient and useful diet, with the least expenditure of energy for the patient. Thus, to Nightingale caring implied a moral imperative in nursing, realized in actions that assisted the reparative processes in patients and decreased suffering.

Care has been at the core of service since the emergence of modern nursing. The centrality of the concepts of care and caring is evident in the vast amount of literature on these subjects. The elaboration on these concepts in the nursing literature, however, is diversified and lacks conceptual clarity. For example, caring is discussed as a generic value; as a trait or an attitude of the nurse; as a characteristic of the nurse-patient relationship; as an intervention; and as philosophy or an ethic of nursing (Morse, Bottorff, Neander, & Solberg, 1991; Morse, Solberg, Neander, Bottorff, & Johnson, 1990).

Earlier in this chapter, several sources have been referred to who see care as fundamental to human life and as such they have addressed the philosophy of caring. To Heidegger, his concept of *Sorge* (care or caring) characterizes the basic principle of humans' 'being', that is, care or caring are foundational to human life; being-in-the-world and being-together-with-others constitute humans' 'being'. Such interdependence requires that each and every one care, in order to maintain and enhance life and society at large. This illustrates one of the major contradictions in human life, namely, that a life characterized by self-rule is also a life lived in interdependent relationships with others. This was a theme also discussed by Mead. "We are what we are through our relationship to others" (1934, p. 379). Hence, consideration of others' interests and well-being is in one's own interest. Along the same line, Hume, in his dispute with Kant's ethics based in rationality, argued that morality rests on the ability to "*reflective* sentiment", and on a balance between sympathy for the other and self-interest.

Similarly, the basic premise for the ethics of care developed by Noddings (1984) is that every human being is "existentially" dependent on others; one is both free and bound. Noddings traced the value of caring to our earliest memories of both caring and being cared for. These memories, the "longing for goodness" (p. 2); "our longing for caring—to be in that special relation . . . provides the motivation for us to be moral" (p. 5). It constitutes the ethical ideal by which to live. Thus, caring is seen as a relation that according to Noddings is characterized by receptivity and reciprocity. The notion of receptivity is linked to the *one-caring*, "I see and feel with the other" (p. 30) which motivates a person to be "at the service of the other" (p. 33). Reciprocity is linked to the *one-cared-for:* "being himself, this willing and unselfconscious revealing of self, is his major contribution to the relation" (p. 73). Thus, the reciprocal "gift" from the one-cared-for can be seen as the trust he or she bestows on the one-caring. In Nodding's explication of an ethic of caring, caring appears as a relational value, "as a mark of a valuable kind of relation . . . [and] a characteristic way of being in the world" (Noddings, 1990, p. 28).

The concept of *transpersonal caring* developed by Watson (1988a) appears to be closely related to Noddings' concept of caring as a foundational and relational value. Watson also argues that caring is a moral ideal of nursing "whereby the end is protection, enhancement, and preservation of human dignity" (p. 29); however, she also discusses caring as a characteristic of the nurse, as an approach, and as a personal response, that is, as nurses' acts or behavior on behalf of the patient.

WATSON'S THEORY OF HUMAN CARING

Jean Watson, with her book *Nursing: The Philosophy and Science of Caring* (1979), was one of the first nurse theorists to address the concept of caring as the focus of a nursing theory. In a recent article, Watson (1997) described this work as emerging from a "quest to bring new meaning and dignity to the world of nursing and patient care" (p. 49). The influence of biomedical sciences and the medical paradigm, she argued, limited the scope of care and also was in dissonance with "nursing's paradigm . . . of caring-healing and health" (p. 49). The *ten carative factors* provided the organizing framework of this first book and are developed further in her later work (Watson, 1988a, 1988b). The carative factors are seen as a combination of interventions and include the following:

1. The formation of a humanistic-altruistic system of values
2. The instillation of faith-hope
3. The cultivation of sensitivity to one's self and to others
4. The development of a helping-trust relationship
5. The promotion and acceptance of the expression of positive and negative feelings
6. The systematic use of the scientific problem-solving method for decision-making
7. The promotion of interpersonal teaching-learning
8. The provision for a supportive, protective, and (or) corrective mental, physical, sociocultural, and spiritual environment
9. Assistance with gratification of human needs
10. The allowance for existential-phenomenological forces. (1979, pp. 9–10)

According to Watson, these carative factors make up the *core of nursing*, which "refers to those aspects of nursing that are intrinsic to the actual nurse-patient/client process that produce therapeutic results in the person being served" (Watson, 1979, p. xv). Considering nursing as a therapeutic interpersonal process, as both scientific and artistic, Watson in her theory sought "to combine science with humanism" (p. xvii). The theoretical perspectives brought to the formulation and her explication of the carative factors were humanistic psychology, phenomenological philosophy, and existentialism (Watson, 1979, 1997). Furthermore, the value system on which these factors rest "was humanitarian, aesthetic, and spiritual" (Watson, 1997, p. 50). She argues that the carative factors provide "a structure and order for nursing phenomena" (p. 50), implying that these are to be viewed as a nursing theory. Her concern is the human dimensions of nursing care, thus emphasizing the human-to-human relationship, characterized as a caring and healing relationship.

In *Nursing: Human Science and Human Care* (1988a), Watson posited her theory as reflecting an alternative worldview of nursing that "will place nursing within a metaphysical context and establish nursing as a human-to-human care process with spiritual dimensions" (p. 37), which is aimed at helping "persons gain higher degree of harmony within the mind, body, and soul [i.e., health]" (p. 49). Accordingly, in this book, more emphasis is put on the moral, spiritual, and metaphysical dimensions of caring, for both patients and nurses. The caring relationship is seen as one that affects both the cared-for and the one caring, as "in the caring transaction both are in a process of being and becoming" (p. 58), and "the nurse can enter into the experience of another person, and another can enter into the nurse's experience" (p. 60). In a recent publication, Watson (1997) comments on the development of this concept of *transpersonal caring:*

> [It] ultimately evokes and invites ontological development, a transformation of self . . . an integration of mind, body, and spirit . . . which is connected with all, elicits the spiritual and expanded views on what it means to be human: embodied spirit, both immanent and transcendent. (p. 51)

It is clear that human beings, whether patients or nurses, now are viewed from a spiritual and metaphysical perspective. In accordance with this Watson comments that her work "can be read as philosophy, ethic, or even paradigm or worldview" (p. 50). Thus, her carative factors, rather than providing a structure for nursing phenomena, as in 1979, are developed into a philosophical foundation from which nurses (and others) can develop a caring-healing relationship. However, because Watson only attributes these carative factors as the essential characteristics to be held and processed by the nurse in this so-called transpersonal caring, her position has not moved away from the notion of caring in nursing as a one-sided, normative approach. This position can be viewed as humanitarian, but is not in full agreement with the major tenets of the generic notions of humanism. However, Watson (2003, 2004) has revised her model of caring science of self and community, bringing the model in line with the ethical philosophies of Levinas and Løgstrup, in which caring is seen more as relational. She specifies its foundations in terms of moral and philosophical commitments to existential humanity, "Caritas/Love" and "Communitas/Connectedness" as relational processes of caring, and interpenetration of selves, others, and environments in caring. In this newer model, Watson has infused both the principle of interrelatedness of human existence and the ethical imperative of caring as the basis of relationship and being human.

Watson's theory is eclectic, that is, she has pulled ideas from several sources in building her theoretical expositions. In addition to those already mentioned, major thoughts from pragmatism are evident, such as seeing humans as experiencing subjects (subjective dimension) in ongoing change (interactive dimension), and the interconnectedness between humans and the world (interdependence dimension). Also, the influence of European philosophers, for example, Heidegger and Merleau-Ponty, is reflected in the use of concepts such as *being-in-the world* and *the embodied spirit.* Thus, many of her position statements reflect thoughts from pragmatism and humanism generally; however, her theory departs from mainstream humanism in the sense that major ideas from this philosophy are not reflected. The way this theory now is developed, it might be better named an ontology of spirituality or spiritualism argued as a foundation for nursing practice, rather than being seen as a humanistic nursing theory. Since the Enlightenment era, humanism has opposed metaphysics and major strands of humanism are secular in their character. In humanism, rationality is seen as the definite characteristic of human beings, as a unique ability that furthers free will, decision making, and self-determination. The aspects of nursing care that deals with how to preserve and facilitate patients' autonomy in decisions about their care are not reflected in the theory as it is now presented. Thus, the core value within humanism is now overshadowed by spiritualism in Watson's theory. However, Watson's newer model infuses ethical and moral perspectives from Levinas (1985, 1998) and Løgstrup (1997), bringing in ideas from existential, phenomenological ethics that focus on the ethics of belonging and becoming, but remaining metaphysically oriented.

HUMANISM AND CARING IN NURSING— AN EXPOSITION

The philosophies of humanism and caring have been foundational to nursing throughout its history, shaping the basic character of nursing, namely, that nursing inherently is a moral practice. This practice is carried out in relation to persons in vulnerable and often dependent positions vis-á-vis the nurse. Thus, the nurse, being responsible for the patient's well-being while in the nurse's care, is implicitly a moral agent and nursing practice is grounded in moral values. In this perspective, three core values in humanism—human dignity, equality, and freedom/autonomy—will be discussed as to their conceptualization in nursing, as well as the concept of care. It will be argued that in nursing, care must be seen as a moral motivation to act, with human dignity as a core value from which the values of autonomy and equality are derived.

The humanistic belief of the inherent worth of each person, his or her uniqueness, is a value held in high regard in nursing as reflected in the first injunction in the American Nursing Association's *Code for Nurses* (2001), which states that the nurse unrestrictedly "provides services with respect for human dignity and the uniqueness of the client." Within humanism the fundamental status of persons, human dignity, is associated with the value of autonomy. This position within humanism can be traced to Kant, who argued that "respect for autonomy flows from the recognition that all persons have unconditional worth, each having the capacity to determine his or her own destiny" (Beauchamp & Childress, 1989, p. 71). Autonomy is considered one of the most central values of a free society and is defined as "the condition of living according to laws one gives oneself, or negatively, not being under the control of another" (Haworth, 1986, p. 11). Kupfer (1990) argued that autonomy, conceived as a natural trait of human beings, as embodied in people, demands that every person be respected. This is an unearned respect, in contrast to the respect bestowed when one has done something extraordinarily well or beneficial to others. Respecting a person implies considering that person to have the same rights, privileges, or status as oneself. Hence, the value of equality is closely related to the value of autonomy. Furthermore, respecting a person requires that one help the person to secure what is needed to realize these values in this person's life situation. Also, "respect implies a realistic regard for the individual" (Kupfer, 1990, p. 51) that encompasses acceptance of and a willingness to take the other's point of view with regard to the individual's own interests, values, and purposes.

In humanism generally, it is held that competence and rationality, the capacity for reasoning, is necessary in order to be considered a person, that is, having unique individual value (human dignity). Furthermore, that rationality is a prerequisite for a person to be considered autonomous (Beauchamp & Childress, 1989). In the nursing context, the position that respect for persons is linked only to their rational capacity is highly problematic. Often patients in nurses' care are in situations where their competence and reasoning capacity are limited either temporarily (unconscious patients) or permanently (patients with senile dementia).

Therefore, the position taken here is that in nursing, respect must be, or rather is, grounded in the inherent worth of individuals as human beings regardless of their capacities and characteristics (a nonsecular position). As stated by Kupfer (1990), a person is respected not "*because* of his individuality, we do respect him *in* his individuality. We take his interests, purposes, and degree of autonomy itself into account in the particular way we treat him" (p. 48). Because nurses respect the inherent worth of each patient, they uphold the value of equality by acting and interacting in regard to the degree of autonomy that is present. Looking at nursing practice, one finds that nurses speak a normal language with patients who are demented; allow patients to decide issues within their capacity; interact with and give nursing care to unconscious patient in the way they themselves would want to be treated in a similar situation. As seen in nursing practice, the value of the inherent worth of persons (human dignity) is not founded solely on the capacity to reason. Furthermore, as the examples illustrate, in nursing, autonomy and equality must be seen as rights that are derived from human dignity, rather than be regarded as foundational to human dignity, as within humanism.

The value of equality has two dimensions in nursing, one associated with the relation between nurse and patient. Basic to nurses' acts and interactions with patients is the belief that patients and nurses have equal value as human beings; they are fellow human beings. In this the value of equality is an absolute right to be actualized in the nurse-patient relationship. The other dimension has to do with the relation between patients in regard to their rights to an equal share of privileges. The question of priorities has always been a part of nursing practice; however, because of cuts in economic resources to health care, ethical dilemmas related to actualizing the value of equality are more pressing than ever. Equality cannot be seen as an absolute right in this regard, for it is not possible to realize in the nursing service of today. The value of autonomy also has two dimensions in nursing. One is associated with the nurses' own autonomy to exercise the right to decide issues of patients' care that are in the nurses' domain and to be heard as a competent partner in decisions that are common ground for doctors and nurses. This is a right that needs to be negotiated in a health care system in which physicians still dominate the power of decision making. The other dimension is the actualization of the patients' right to autonomy through collaboration and patients' active participation in decisions that concern them. In nursing, however, autonomy cannot be seen as an absolute right of patients. In the interest of some patients' own good, the nurse may have to execute some form of paternalism, for example, forced suctioning of suicidal patients, overriding a patient's decision when it is harmful, and gentle prodding to change patients' minds when it is in their best interest.

This issue brings in the value of altruism, which has been at the core of nursing throughout its history and lately has reemerged as the value of care. Care is a relatively new concept within contemporary moral philosophy and ethics (Blum, 1992). The reintroduction of care as a moral value came with Gilligan's (1982) research on women's reasoning and solutions to moral dilemmas, which identified a "moral voice" different from that of justice—the "voice of care." Historically, care was not used as a concept, nor seen as a value as such, but as a moral orientation, or rather as the foundation of morality, that which motivates one to act morally. Among some philosophers, such as Schopenhauer, Hume, and Kierkegaard, altruism/compassion is regarded at the "cornerstone of ethics" (Blum, 1992). Although compassion is considered a sentiment underlying morality, altruism is generally defined as the regard for the well-being of others. A pertinent and significant question, then, is, How does one know what is good for the other?

In the nursing context, in which the good sought is the patient's health, well-being or peaceful death, the nurse's professional knowledge and experience provide the basis from which to judge what is good for the actual patient. This is not sufficient, however. In nursing an understanding of what is good for the other from the patient's perspective is also needed, either directly from the patient, the patient's relatives, or through reflective imagination, because without this understanding the desire for the patient's good may not be served. Hence, in nursing the moral foundation of altruism "activates" the realization of the values of equality and autonomy.

In the philosophy of caring explicated by Noddings, a reciprocal relationship between trust and caring is seen as foundational to human life. That is, the interdependence among individuals requires that everyone both care and trust to maintain and enhance life and society at large. One question surfaces however: Are these explications of caring and trust in general human relationships a sufficient moral basis for nursing? One will argue that they are not. In contrast to caring and trust as ideals for conduct between people in general, in nursing these values have to be upheld and actualized by the nurse independent of patients' participation and contribution to the relationship. Nurses are also responsible for nursing care to patients who lack the ability or sufficient capacity to be actively involved in the relationship, for example, patients on ventilators or unconscious or dying patients. That is, the conditional interdependence so basic to these values in general human relationships cannot always be upheld in the nursing context.

In conclusion, the philosophies of humanism and caring provide a foundation for nursing as a moral practice. However, the basic values of these philosophies have to be reconceptualized to reflect and meet the realities of nursing practice as discussed above. Hence, care is best seen as a moral motivation to act in regard to the patients' well-being rather than as a relational value, that is, altruism is reintroduced in nursing. In nursing, respect for the patient as a person also must be founded in the inherent worth of the individual regardless of capacity and competence, rather than in the notion of the rational autonomous individual. Furthermore, this value of human dignity is considered the core value in nursing (Fagermoen, 1995, 1997). Hence, in nursing the values of equality and autonomy flow from the value of human dignity. Several studies of nurses have reported that nurses focus and purposely act through nursing care to preserve patients' dignity when it is in jeopardy and to restore it when diminished. The value of human dignity in nursing, then, can be considered as more than holding an attitude of respecting the individual's worth, but as a value actualized in concrete acts to restore and maintain the health and well-being of patients. Accordingly, the required physical care will in certain situations be primary to the relationship as such, and in emergency situations, for example, actions required to restore health and preserve dignity may conflict with other values, such as autonomy and reciprocal trust. Thus, in nursing these values are subsumed under the value of human dignity.

Finally, one moral imperative in humanism—to strive to understand the perspective of the other—is emphasized in professional nursing. To fulfill the aim of delivering care that is in the best interest of patients, professional nurses use a diverse base of knowledge. Taken together, professional knowledge, an understanding of what is good for the patient from the patient's perspective, previous experiences with other patients, intuition, and reflection on the specific patient's situation provide a basis for a general understanding of "what it is like" for patients. These sources of knowledge are constructing the foundation on which decisions will be made in the patients' best interest, with the core value, human dignity, giving direction to how the values of autonomy and equality are to be actualized in nursing care guided by an altruistic motivation.

So far, the ontology embedded in the philosophy of humanism and its consequences for nursing practice have been addressed. Epistemological issues also have to be outlined in relation to the advancement of nursing knowledge. Accepting that humans are experiential, self-determining, and interpretative beings whose understanding of themselves, of others, and of situations is ongoing in interaction with the social and cultural context, has definite implications in regard to how to investigate the human realm.

From the perspective of humanism, it is not possible or desirable to obtain objective knowledge untangled by personal bias and personal perspective, that is, the knowledge to be uncovered is relativistic in nature and the knowledge described is considered approximations of truth. This position rests on two epistemological positions of pragmatism and hermeneutics. First, knowledge of a person's lived life is embedded in meanings that are individually constructed, that is, this knowledge is subjective and situated. Second, knowledge is also embedded in social and cultural values, artifacts, and practices; such knowledge is constructed as intersubjective meanings. Third, these views on human understanding and meanings of course also apply to the investigator and not only to the person being investigated. Research in the human realm, then, requires a high degree of self-reflection by the investigator both in preparing and conducting a study, to be attentive to foreknowledge, values, and attitudes that may color perceptions and interpretations. Further, multiple forms of inquiry are needed to uncover such knowledge whether it is the patients' or nurses' experiences and meanings or nursing practice as such. Phenomenological, ethnographic, grounded theory and critical theory approaches employ methods of data collection, analysis, and interpretation that are in line with foundational ideas in humanism, each however with different emphasis on which dimensions of understanding and meanings are focused.

Humanism in the new century has to embrace not only the idea that humans must be allowed to exercise the power of self-determination but also at the same time realize that in doing so there is a great danger of alienating ourselves from the basic values of humanity. Thus, knowledge development in general, and more specifically in human practice disciplines such as nursing, must be oriented to value identification and value determination as well as understanding and explanation. Nursing theories within the perspective of humanism should begin with this paradoxical struggle in human nature.

REFERENCES

Abbagnano, N. (1972). Humanism. In J. Edwards (Ed.), *The encyclopedia of philosophy* (Vol. 4, pp. 69–72). New York: Macmillan.

American Nurses Association. (2001). *Code of ethics for nurses with interpretive statements.* Silver Spring, MD: American Nurses Association.

Andic, M. (1991). What is Renaissance humanism? In D. Goicoechea, J. Luik, & T. Madigan (Eds.), *The question of humanism. Challenges and possibilities* (pp. 83–98). Buffalo, NY: Prometheus Books.

Baier, A. (1987). Hume, the women's moral theorist? In. E. F. Kittay & D. T. Meyers (Eds.), *Women and moral theory* (pp. 37–55). Totowa, NJ: Rowman & Littlefield.

Blum, L. (1992). Altruism. In L. G. Becker & C. B. Becker (Eds.), *Encyclopedia of ethics* (Vol. 1, pp. 35–39). New York: Garland.

Bullock, A. (1985). *The humanist tradition in the west.* New York: Norton.

Beauchamp, T., & Childress, J. (1989). *Principles of biomedical ethics* (3rd ed.). New York: Oxford University Press.

DeCarvalho, R. J. (1991). *The founders of humanistic psychology.* New York: Praeger.

Dewey, J. (1976/1916). Physical and social studies: Naturalism and humanism. In C. D. Sclosser (Ed.), *The person in education: A humanistic approach* (pp. 336–347). New York: Macmillan.

Diggins, J. P. (1994). *The promise of pragmatism: Modernism and the crisis of knowledge and authority.* Chicago: University of Chicago Press.

Fagermoen, M. S. (1995). The meaning of nurses' work: A descriptive study of values fundamental to professional identity in nursing. *Dissertation Abstracts International,* 56/09 B, 4814.

Fagermoen, M. S. (1997). Professional identity: Values embedded in meaningful nursing practice. *Journal of Advanced Nursing, 25,* 434–441.

Fay, B., & Moon, J. D. (1994). What would an adequate philosophy of science look like. In M. Martin & L. C. McIntyre (Eds.), *Readings in the philosophy of social science* (pp. 21–35). Cambridge, MA: MIT Press.

Francis, R. P. (1991). The human person in American pragmatism. In D. Goicoechea, J. Luik, & T. Madigan (Eds.), *The question of humanism. Challenges and possibilities* (pp. 234–243). Buffalo, NY: Prometheus Books.

Gilligan, C. (1982). *In a different voice. Psychological theory and women's development.* Cambridge, MA: Harvard University Press.

Giorgi, A. (1970). *Psychology as a human science.* New York: Harper & Row.

Glaser, B., & Strauss, A. (1967). *The discovery of grounded theory.* Chicago: Aldine.

Goicoechea, D., Luik, J., & Madigan, T. (Eds.). (1991). *The question of humanism.* Buffalo, NY: Prometheus Books.

Haworth, L. (1986). *Autonomy: An essay in philosophical psychology and ethics.* New Haven, CT: Yale University Press.

Kolenda, K. (1995). Humanism. In R. Audi (Ed.), *The Cambridge dictionary of philosophy* (pp. 340–341). Cambridge, UK: Cambridge University Press.

Kupfer, J. H. (1990). *Autonomy and social interaction.* Albany: State University of New York Press.

Kurtz, P. (1972). American philosophy. In J. Edwards (Ed.), *The encyclopedia of philosophy* (Vol. 1, pp. 83–93). New York: Macmillan.

Levinas, E. (1985). *Ethics and infinity* (R. Cohen, Trans.). Pittsburgh, PA: Dusuqesne Univerity Press.

Levinas, E. (1998). *Entre nous: Thinking-of-the-other.* (M. B. Smith & B. Harshav, Trans.). New York: Columbia University Press.

Løgstrup, K. (1997). *The ethical demand.* Notre Dame, IN: University of Notre Dame Press.

Luik, J. (1991a). The question of humanism and the career of humanism. In D. Goicoechea, J. Luik, & T. Madigan (Eds.), *The question of humanism. Challenges and possibilities* (pp. 15–25). Buffalo, NY: Prometheus Books.

Luik, J. (1991b). An old question raised again: Is Kant an Enlightenment humanist? In D. Goicoechea, J. Luik, & T. Madigan (Eds.), *The question of humanism. Challenges and possibilities* (pp. 117–137). Buffalo, NY: Prometheus Books.

Madigan, T. (1991). Afterword: The answer to humanism. In D. Goicoechea, J. Luik, & T. Madigan (Eds.), *The question of humanism. Challenges and possibilities* (pp. 326–334). Buffalo, NY: Prometheus Books.

Maines, D. R. (1992). Pragmatism. In E. F. Borgatta & M. L.Borgatta (Eds.), *Encyclopedia of sociology* (pp. 1531–1536). New York: Macmillan.

Mead, G. H. (1934). *Mind, self, and society.* Chicago: University of Chicago Press.

Mead, G. H. (1964a). Philanthropy from the point of view of ethics. In A. J. Reck (Ed.), *Selected writings: George Herbert Mead* (pp. 392–407). Chicago: University of Chicago Press.

Mead, G. H. (1964b). The definition of the physical. In A. J. Reck (Ed.), *Selected writings: George Herbert Mead* (pp. 25–59). Chicago: University of Chicago Press.

Morse, J. M., Solberg, S. M., Neander, W. L., Bottorff, J. L., & Johnson, J. L. (1990). Concepts of caring and caring as a concept. *Advances in Nursing Science, 13*(1), 1–14.

Morse, J. M., Bottorff, J. L., Neander, W. L., & Solberg, S. M. (1991). Comparative analysis of conceptualizations and theories of caring. *Image: Journal of Nursing Scholarship, 23*(2), 119–126.

Nerheim, H. (1995). *Vitenskap og kommunikasjon* [Science and communication]. Oslo, Norway: Universitetsforlaget.

Nicolaisen, R. F. (1997). Eksistensialismen [Existentialism]. In I. T. Tollef-sen, H. Syse, & R. F. Nicolaisen (Eds.), *Tenkere og ideer* (pp. 524–537). Oslo, Norway: Ad Notam/Gyldendal.

Nightingale, F. N. (1992). *Notes on nursing: What it is and what it is not.* Philadelphia: J. B. Lippincott. (Originally published in 1859)

Noddings, N. (1984). *Caring. A feminine approach to ethics and moral education.* Berkeley: University of California Press.

Noddings, N. (1990). Private caring and public care-giving: A proposal for synthesis. *Nytt om kvinneforskning, 2,* 25–34.

Polkinghorne, D. (1983). *Methodology for the human sciences.* Albany: State University of New York Press.

Schwartz, M. A., & Wiggins, O. (1985). Science, humanism, and the nature of medical practice: A phenomenological view. *Perspectives in Biology and Medicine, 28*(3), 331–361.

Skirbrekk, G., & Gilje, N. (1987). *Filosofi historie.* Bind 2 [History of philosophy. Vol. 2]. Oslo, Norway: Universitetsforlaget.

Thayer, H. S. (1996). Pragmatism. In P. Edwards (Ed.), *The encyclopedia of philosophy* (Vol. 6, pp. 430–436). New York: Macmillan.

Thompson, J. L. (1990). Hermeneutic inquiry. In L. Moody (Ed.), *Advancing nursing science through research* (Vol. 2, pp. 223–280). Newbury Park, CA: Sage.

Turner, J. H. (1986). *The structure of sociological theory* (4th ed.). Belmont, CA: Wadsworth.

Watson, J. (1979). *Nursing: The philosophy and science of caring.* Boston: Little, Brown.

Watson, J. (1988a). *Nursing: Human science and human care.* New York: National League for Nursing.

Watson, J. (1988b). New dimensions of human caring theory. *Nursing Science Quarterly, 1,* 175–181.

Watson, J. (1997). The theory of human caring: Retrospective and prospective. *Nursing Science Quarterly, 10*(1), 49–52.

Watson, J. (2003). Love and caring: Ethics of face and hand—An invitation to return to the heart and soul of nursing and our deep humanity. *Nursing Administration Quarterly, 27,* 197–202.

Watson, J. (2004). Caritas and communitas: A caring science ethical view of self and community. *Journal of Japan Academy of Nursing Science, 24,* 66–71.

CHAPTER 11

Pragmatism, Nursing, and Nursing Knowledge Development

Hesook Suzie Kim and Björn Sjöström

Pragmatism as a philosophy is known to have its roots in America. It is viewed by most to be influenced first and foremost by the works of Charles Sanders Peirce of the late nineteenth century, with its label and perspective proclaimed by William James in his lectures and writings at the turn of the century, and reinforced and reiterated by John Dewey during the early years of the twentieth century. Pragmatism as a movement is often thought to have its origins in the discussions and interactions that went on at the Metaphysical Club at Harvard University, which included members such as Charles Sanders Peirce, Oliver Wendell Holmes, Jr., John Fiske, James Chauncey Wrights, and William James. However, the pragmatism that exists currently as a philosophy bears a variety of positions regarding truth, knowledge, science, and practical life. Pragmatism is not a unified philosophy, but its adherents do share a common understanding and belief that the focus of human effort is to make the human lot as good as possible by creating advantages, and taking advantage of, emerging possibilities and opportunities in human potential. Although pragmatism is often identified with utilitarianism and instrumentalism, pragmatism has a broader philosophical base and meaning than those two positions. Hence, in this chapter we take up pragmatism as the focus.

During the past two to three decades, pragmatism has infiltrated every sector of contemporary life, not only in the United States but also in Europe and the rest of the world, as a philosophy and vision. The naïve and populist form of pragmatism especially has been hailed as the cornerstone for technological advances and political success, and many persons hold it as a "motivating force" for modern advances and achievements. On the other hand, there are also many critiques, especially within the philosophical and scientific circles, that depict pragmatism as lacking philosophical rigor in projecting its positions and suggest that it has neither helped to systematize knowledge development nor form a unified worldview to tackle serious problems of this new century.

Pragmatism as a philosophy went through a rather tortuous route in its development into the present forms as Dickstein (1998b) describes in the Introduction to *The Revival of Pragmatism*. To begin with, after William James in 1898 asserted pragmatism in his lectures as a philosophic movement and a method, citing much of Peirce's work, Peirce (1904/1997), in protest of popularization and misuse of the label in the literature, proclaimed "pragmaticism" to express his version. Dickstein (1998b) illustrates several different currents of the twentieth century as either promoting (e.g., evolutionary naturalism and social Darwinism, liberalism, humanism, and pluralism) or deterring (e.g., conservatism's revival during and after World Wars I and II, logical positivism, analytic philosophy, and popularization of existentialism) the development of pragmatism. The demise of pragmatism during the middle decades of the twentieth century was followed by its revival and reconfiguration during the last two decades in the United States, especially in the form of neopragmatism and by its transplantation into the European cultural scene. Dickstein writes that "pragmatism has come to be seen as an American alternative, an escape from the abstraction of theory and the abyss of nihilism" that resulted from "the mixture of European theories from Marxism to poststructuralism," and considers pragmatism "a constructive skepticism" (1998b, p. 16) oriented to searching for methods that would make it possible to find answers among the rubble of the crumbled foundations that are based on rationalism, idealism, and absolutism.

Currently pragmatism is the foundation for specific perspectives within different disciplines such as law, literature, history, politics, ethics, education, and sciences. Philosophers, scientists, and professional practitioners advocate pragmatism as representing their views on truth, knowledge, scientific methods, human conduct, and communal life. The debates and discussions regarding pragmatism in nursing also take several different directions, arising from those concerned with the questions within the philosophy of science perspective to those specifically oriented to the nature of nursing practice. In this chapter, our exposition will address three areas viewed by the philosophic lens of pragmatism: (a) the questions of truth and reality; (b) the issues in epistemology and the philosophy of science such as aims of knowledge and science, scientific methods, and scientific theories; and (c) the conceptions of human conduct and everyday practice, especially pertaining to the concept of nursing practice. The discussions on these three topics will be presented following a brief description of the philosophy.

MAJOR TENETS OF PRAGMATISM

It is not easy to provide in one sweep what the major tenets of pragmatism are, as there are different depictions of it not only by the early pragmatists such as Peirce, James, and Dewey but also by more current scholars such as Bernstein, Putnam, and Rorty. In addition, pragmatism can be discussed from different orientations such as historical, ethical, legal, scientific, or literary perspectives. The birth of the term *neopragmatism* also points to the emergence of different orientations this philosophy has been identified with by various proponents.

Kloppenberg, a historian, points out the differences between the early pragmatists and the contemporary pragmatists as follows: (a) "the early pragmatists emphasized 'experience,' whereas some contemporary philosophers and critics who have taken a 'linguistic turn' are uneasy with that concept"; and (b) "the early pragmatists believed their philosophical ideas had particular ethical and political consequences, whereas some contemporary thinkers who call themselves pragmatists consider it merely a method of analysis" (1998, p. 84). As Kloppenberg (1998) and others describe, the lineage of pragmatism can be traced to the original pragmatism by Peirce, James, and Dewey who together and separately opposed the idea of absolutes and foundationalism, and insisted on emphasizing human experience as the bedrock for knowledge and human understanding. Their philosophy was an attack against positivism, absolute objectivism, and foundationalism, and was attacked by those in the camps of logical positivism (Carnap) and analytic philosophy (Russell). The revival of pragmatism was occasioned by the rise of postmodernism in the latter half of the twentieth century by diverse camps such as the hermeneutic human science movement led by Gadamer, Ricoeur, Taylor, Winch, Geertz, and Giddens; the critical philosophy of Habermas; and poststructuralism by Foucault, Derrida, and Lyotard. Pragmatism in the 1980s and 1990s found its voice in such scholars as Richard Bernstein, Hilary Putnam, and Richard Rorty. Because pragmatism has come to be identified with scholars holding various philosophic positions such as relativism, antirealism and realism, critical philosophy, and hermeneutics, there is a great deal of confusion regarding exactly what its major philosophical tenets are. This diversity among the adherents exists, Morgenbesser (1998) argues, because pragmatic theories of inquiry, truth, scientific theories, and nature are independent of each other.

It is therefore necessary to clarify the major tenets of pragmatism that are fundamental to this philosophic movement at a bare-bones level by taking up the ideas from the initial proponents of pragmatism. The seeds of pragmatism are found in Peirce's work (1878/1997) as expressed in such statements as the following:

- The essence of belief is the establishment of a habit; and different beliefs are distinguished by the different modes of action to which they give rise (p. 33)
- [E]very purpose of action is to produce some sensible results (p. 35)
- [W]e come down to what is tangible and conceivably practical, as the root of every real distinction of thought, no matter how subtle it may be; and there is no distinction of meaning so fine as to consist in anything but a possible difference in practice (p. 35)
- Consider what effects, that might conceivably have practical bearings, we conceive the object of our conception to have. Then, our conception of these effects is the whole of our conception of the object (p. 36).

These ideas turn the focus to human thoughts as what they do rather than what they are, thus shifting the philosophy's attention to what humans did with thinking and thoughts. James (1907/1981) summarizes this idea of Peirce by stating that "our beliefs are really rules for action, said that, to develop a thought's meaning, we need only determine what conduct it is fitted to produce: that conduct is for us its sole significance" (p. 26).

Peirce's ideas were taken up further by James (1907/1981) who made pragmatism a philosophic movement by proposing a theory of truth that is grounded in "practicality." James's pragmatism comes from his statements that

> what difference would it practically make to any one if this notion rather than that notion were true? If no practical difference whatever can be traced, then the alternatives mean practically the same thing, and all dispute is idle. Whenever a dispute is serious, we ought to be able to show some practical difference that must follow from one side or the other's being right. (1907/1981, p. 26)

James further states that "the whole function of philosophy ought to be to find out what definite difference it will make to you and me, at definite instants of our life, if this world-formula or that world-formula be the true one" (1907/1981, p. 27). From this, James offers a theory of truth in which truth is viewed to be a "leading" that is worthwhile or an idea that must have a practical value derived from the practical importance of its object to people.

Pragmatism focuses on consequences, "last things" as James termed them, and on ideas that are translated into actions. By focusing on consequences, human "workings," including thinking, conceptualizing, and doings, are only significant to the extent of what they produce and what differences they make to our lives. Diggins affirms this by a statement that "pragmatism purports to reconcile theory and practice by making the latter the test of genuine ideas" (Diggins, 1994, p. 161). All other conceptions of pragmatism stem from this fundamental orientation.

Bernstein (1988/1997) most succinctly characterizes the "pragmatic *ethos*" in the following five themes in his examination of historical as well as current philosophical traditions for their impacts on the development of pragmatism:

1. Anti-foundationalism that opposes the notion of fixed foundations as both the goal and content of knowledge, for which Peirce provided the initial arguments as a pragmatist and which has been refined and redefined by Quine and Sellas;
2. Fallibilism, which grounds pragmatism's orientation to the openness in inquiry and tentative nature of knowledge;
3. The need for a critical community of inquirers to act as disciplined arbiters and regulators for inquiries and knowledge-claims;

4. Contingency and chance as the "pervasive features of the universe" and the need for humans to be ready and capable in responding to them;
5. Plurality of "traditions, perspectives, philosophic orientations" (1997, pp. 385–389).

PRAGMATIST'S LENS FOR TRUTH AND REALITY

The concept of truth has been a central issue in various philosophical schools, and has eluded not only philosophers but also lay persons in their efforts to find answers to the meanings of life, the workings of what we encounter, and the nature of human ideas. The question "What is truth?" entails the statement that there is truth and falsity and that there must be a way to judge the difference of one (truth) from the other (falsity). Along with this statement, then, there is the question regarding whether or not truth refers to a condition of absolutes and permanency as opposed to transient and changeable ones. This is the question taken up by pragmatists, especially William James, as central to pragmatism.

Countering the notion of absolute and fundamental truth embedded in the nature of things, pragmatism views truth as transient, provisional, and evolutionary. Furthermore, it views that attempting to seek absolute and fundamental truth, even if it were viewed to exist as such, is a futile exercise that would bring us to a confusing maze from which it is impossible to escape. To pragmatists, truth is a passage or a process through which we are able to gain an ever-better understanding of our lives and put forward outputs in response to our purposes.

James (1907/1981) uses the instrumental view of truth, citing Ferdinand C. S. Schiller and John Dewey to project his theory of truth. To him, "the true is the name of whatever proves itself to be good in the way of belief, and good, too, for definite, assignable reasons" (James, 1907/1981, p. 37). He emphasizes the plasticity of truth by stating that individuals' beliefs or scientific theories are revised in order to fit into novel facts and also to bring about greater success in solving problems. The growth of truths not only involves adding new truths and revising old ones, but also the "rearrangement" of stock beliefs. Hence, he holds that because truth is the character of an idea that evolves into it through facts, our efforts must be to seek truth through experiences (James, 1907/1981). Although there are different views regarding the ultimate existence of absolutes and fundamental truths among pragmatists, this provisionary idea of truth has become a somewhat unified theory of truth within various schools of pragmatism. For example, Peirce (1905, p. 416) believes that the notion of truth can only be taken to have a meaning in terms of "doubt" and "belief" and in the course of experience, not in the sense of absolute fixity. To Peirce, truth is a state attained "of belief unassailable by doubt" (1905, p. 416). James presents a similar position by statements that "'the true'... is only the expedient in the way of our thinking, just as 'the right' is only the expedient in the way of our behaving" and "experience ... has ways of boiling over, and making us correct our present formulas" (1907/1981, p. 100). Truth in pragmatism is sought through "a deliberative, social process aimed at identifying what works in a given situation" (Brendel, 2003, p. 571). Dewey goes even further by stating that "truth, in final analysis, is the statement of things 'as they are,' not as they are in the inane and desolate void of isolation from human concern, but as they are in a shared and progressive experience. ... Truth is having things in common" (1911/1978, p. 67). These ideas are summarized well by Diggins (1994) as follows:

> A pragmatist need not make his ideas copy reality or cohere with a larger structure of thought. For truth is not a possession in the form of an abstract mental idea. Instead it is the outcome of an action that is meant to confirm or disconfirm a proposition. ... In a world that is forever changing truth itself becomes the result of change, a consequence of experience and a product of human action. ... To the extent that true ideas enable us to adapt to situations, and to the extent that they result in greater fulfillment and "satisfaction," the pragmatist regards the true not only as the useful but also as the good. (p. 133)

Rorty on the other hand goes further in asserting a linguistic turn for pragmatism and insists that it is neither necessary nor possible to distinguish the notions of "truth-by-correspondence-to-reality" and "truth-as-what-it-is-good-to-believe" (1982, p. xxxvii), and abandons the notion of discovering the truth. He states that "it is the vocabulary of practice rather than of theory, of action rather than contemplation, in which one can say something useful about truth" (Rorty, 1982, p. 162). Thus the question of truth is put squarely and more centrally on "doing" rather than on content.

Although the concept of truth is intrinsically connected to the ideas regarding reality, the concept of reality has been controversial among pragmatists from its beginning. Currently there are pragmatists who espouse realism, antirealism, relativism, and constructivism, pointing out various ways of viewing and conceptualizing what exists in reality and how facts are viewed to have certain meanings.

Peirce connects the conceptions of truth and reality as "the opinion which is fated to be ultimately agreed to by all who investigate, is what we mean by the truth, and the object represented in this opinion is the real" (1878/1997, p. 45). He further notes that although "the characters of the real depend on what is ultimately thought about them" (1878/1997, p. 45), it is independent of specific individuals' thoughts. In stating "the reality of that which is real does depend on the real fact that investigation is destined to lead, at last, if continued long enough, to a belief in it," Pierce (1878/1997, p. 46) expresses his idea of reality as partially known and knowable, and provisional. To Peirce, the reality can be progressively better known and increasingly approximated through various modes of investigations involving logic and science. He is thus thought of as a realist rather than a constructivist in this respect.

James emphasizes another point by stating,

> Realities mean, then, either concrete facts, or abstract kinds of thing and relations perceived intuitively between them. They furthermore and thirdly mean, as things that new ideas of ours must no less take account of, the whole body of other truths already in our possession. (1907/1981, p. 96)

Hence, to James a reality is guided by human ideas so that it can be dealt with in order to fit into our lives, but at the same time is experienced or experienceable. James proposes a radical empiricism in which the reality is solely viewed to exist in experiences, and both materialism and idealism are rejected as dualisms having only one-dimensional views on reality. However, he was called a nominalist by Peirce, who noted his position on reality in relation to individual consciousness and experience, while Putnam claims that James was "the first philosopher to present a well worked out version of direct realism" (Putnam, 1998, p. 37).

These two variations on the concept of reality diverge further among the more recent pragmatists, ranging from realism to antirealism, constructivism to relativism, depending on their commitments in specific theories of truth. The most vocal of the positions on this is from Putnam who is committed to what he calls "internal realism" that views reality represented by the interface of our minds and the external world, which is expressed in this statement: "The mind and the world jointly make up the mind and the world" (Putnam, 1981, p. xi). This multiplicity of positions regarding reality in pragmatism has created confusion and may be understandable only by accepting the argument that philosophical positions regarding truth, reality, science, and values are independent of each other in pragmatism (Morgenbesser, 1998). It thus is tenable to assume realism (a variety of it), antirealism, relativism, and constructivism within the broader philosophy of pragmatism.

PRAGMATISTS' LENS FOR EPISTEMOLOGY AND PHILOSOPHY OF SCIENCE

Pragmatism's orientation in epistemology has always been more on the process, that is, method, than on substance. Peirce first proposes pragmatism as a method by identifying the procedures for the analysis of concepts (or ideas), and includes in it a maxim of logic that is prescribed for a precise and full definition of concepts by tracing out "in the imagination the conceivable practical consequences—that is, the consequences for deliberate, self-controlled conduct—of the affirmation or denial of the concept" (Peirce, 1904/1997, p. 56). This sets out for James and Dewey to extend and elaborate on the pragmatic method. To James, the pragmatic method is a method to interpret different ideas and notions by tracing their practical consequences in order to judge the notions' being right, and by turning "towards concreteness and adequacy, towards facts, towards action and towards power" (James, 1907/1981, p. 28). By this he claims that science and metaphysics work together hand in hand. On the other hand, Dewey, in embracing the instrumentalism, proposes the experimental method "as a systematized means of making knowledge," which involves an examination of the power of tentatively entertained hypotheses, theories, and ideas in producing changes in things through our activity, and which permits the anticipation and predictability of future consequences based on present observations (Dewey, 1916/1997, pp. 210–213). Haack (1996a) extends this by emphasizing (a) empirical justification that depends on individuals' experiences supported by specific evidence, and (b) engagements of many persons in cooperative and competitive contributions as the hallmarks of inquiry in pragmatism.

Knowledge is sought not to settle an argument or to "possess the universe itself," but "to set it to work within the stream of your

experience" (James, 1907/1981, p. 28). James called theories "instruments" to be put to work and to correct or change the nature or the reality. This is extended by later pragmatists such as Laudan who states that "the aim of science is to solve problems, and if two rival theories solve different problems, then it is a subjective matter to decide which theory is best, depending on our preferences as to which problems are more important to solve" (Laudan, 1990, p. 27). Hence, in pragmatism, scientific theories are not absolutes but are tools to get at the business of human life as satisfactorily as possible.

The neopragmatism of Rorty, however, takes pragmatism's epistemology to a different direction, first by rejecting epistemology. This is basically grounded in his characterization of pragmatism in terms of (a) "anti-essentialism applied to notions like 'truth,' 'knowledge,' 'language,' morality,' and similar objects of philosophical theorizing"; (b) the rejection of "any epistemological difference between normative truth and existential truth, any metaphysical difference between facts and values, or any methodological difference between morality and science"; and (c) the acceptance of inquiry not constrained by the nature of the objects, of the human mind, or of language, but only by the responses from other inquirers (Rorty, 1982, pp. 162–165). Rorty (1982) specifically states that

> Pragmatism . . . does not erect Science as an idol to fill the place once held by God. It views science as one genre of literature—or, put the other way around, literature and the arts as inquiries, on the same footing as scientific inquiries. Thus it sees ethics as neither more "relative" or "subjective" than scientific theory, nor as needing to be made "scientific." Physics is a way of trying to cope with various bits of the universe; ethics is a matter of trying to cope with other bits. Mathematics helps physics do its job; literature and the arts help ethics do its. Some of these inquiries come up with propositions, some with narratives, some with paintings. The question of what propositions to assert, which pictures to look at, what narratives to listen to and comment on and retell, are all questions about what will help us get what we want (or about what we should want). (1982, p. xviii)

This conversationalist version of knowledge rejects the privileged position of the so-called scientific knowledge in relation to other sorts of knowledge. This position holds that inquiries provide the epistemic privilege regarding the nature of the world and human activities only through consensus among the community of language users. Rorty holds that human solidarity is the hallmark of science, and that objects of inquiry (scientific or otherwise) is not their nature but what

they do since "all objects are always already contextualized" (1991, p. 97). This has created a great deal of controversy in the revival of pragmatism in the recent two decades (See, for example, Haack, 1996b; Ramberg, 2002; Rockwell, 2003, among others).

PRAGMATISM AND EVERYDAY LIFE:
CONCEPTIONS OF HUMAN CONDUCT
AND EVERYDAY PRACTICE

Pragmatism's orientation in human experience as both the basis of truth and the goal makes it imperative to consider the notion of everyday life central to this philosophy. Furthermore, linguistically the terms *practical* and *pragmatic* express the groundedness of human experience and activity in specific situations and for specific needs or goals. Everyday life and human activities in specific *situ* are the central concerns of pragmatism, because the focus of attention in this philosophy are how things are accomplished and how our engagement in life ends up in certain consequences. To pragmatists, "what one does" is the key concern from both the individual and the collective (community) perspectives. Because individuals' lives are viewed as entrenched in societies, human activity cannot be viewed simply in the subjectivist's, existentialist's, or phenomenologist's orientations, but is considered in the context of society that provides "a cohesive basis of identity, meaning, and value" (Diggins, 1994, p. 360). The central place of society and communality within pragmatism, especially in understanding (or explaining) human activities, has placed in the camp of pragmatism the symbolic interactionism of Charles Horton Cooley and George Herbert Mead, the critical philosophy of Habermas, and Bourdieu's work. Although the notion of society and its interpenetration into individuals' actions are viewed differently by these philosophers, the paradox and fear apparent in the loss of selfhood in human life from this connection is troublesome to all of them and has been the major point of deliberations. A more conservative view regarding the connection between individual and society is found in early Dewey (1930), who supported the dependency of an individual's experience on the nature of social life, from which he later shifts his emphasis on individuality and individual determinism by stating that "individuals are the finally decisive factors of the nature and movement of associated life" (Dewey, 1939, p. 347), and "it

attaches fundamental importance to the activities of individuals in determining the social conditions under which they live" (1939, p. 348). This interconnectedness between individuality and society is taken up by symbolic interactionism, especially by Cooley (1909/1962) and Mead (1934), by emphasizing mutual perspective-taking in interactions as the central process of individual-society interpenetration; by Habermas (1971; see also, Aboulafia, Bookman, & Kemp, 2002), who focuses on communicative action as the basis for communality with an emphasis on mutuality; and by Bourdieu (1977), who has proposed mediation and evolutionary reciprocity between individual's actions and social conditions. Individual experience and actions in the context of society connect them not only to political life but also to the concerns related to ethics, values, and morality.

In his book *Human Nature and Conduct,* Dewey (1922/1957) sets out human actions in terms of habit and deliberation and in relation to morality and sociality. To Dewey, human conduct is oriented to harmonizing and resolving conflicts that exist within multitudes of habits, impulses, and preferences; is social based on the belief that "man is a being who responds in action to the stimuli of the environment" (1922/1957, p. 187); and involves morals because human conduct emerges from possible alternatives that entails deliberation regarding reflective choices. Morals, to Dewey, are not absolutes but are revisional and growing resulting from experiences, that is, growing "out of specific empirical facts" (1922/1957, p. 271), and from coordinated engagements of individuals in social life. Dewey (1922/1957) states that

- all moral judgment is experimental and subject to revision by its issue (p. 258);
- morality is a continuing process not a fixed achievement. Morals means growth of conduct in meaning; at least it means that kind of expansion in meaning which is consequent upon observations of the conditions and outcome of conduct . . . morals is education. It is learning the meaning of what we are about and employing that meaning in action (p. 259); and
- [m]orality depends upon events, not upon command and ideals alien to nature. (p. 286)

In this sense, the appropriate method for addressing the problems of human conduct, including moral problems, is an empirical method involving intelligence that "treats events as moving, as fraught with possibilities not as ended, final," in which the present is not used "to control the future," but instead "the foresight of the future is used to refine and expand present activity," and through which freedom is actualized "in the use of desire, deliberation and choice" (Dewey, 1922/1957, p. 286). The concept of intelligence for Dewey is not the same as the intellectual capacity that is thought of as inert to individuals, but is bound up "with community life of which we are a part" (1922/1957, p. 287), making it social through and through. From this, Dewey proposes the concept of democracy as a way of life not only from the political orientation but, more important, from the orientation of shared life in an ordinary, everyday sense. Democracy involves an approach of cooperation in testing hypotheses and working out solutions to problems of experience. Diggins (1994), however, is disturbed by Dewey's elevation of intelligence "to the status of an absolute or 'key value,' an entity that not only functioned to bring about good but is good in and of itself" and considers the endowment of intelligence with the status of authority for "the power of self-legitimation" to be circular (p. 247).

From the perspective of pragmatism then, humans are in full control of and responsible for their conduct through the use of their intelligence that is embedded in social life, because humans are thought to be involved in events that are not fixed but contextually determined, different, and changing. General rules of behavior or universal standards of conduct are thought to stifle and inhibit the intelligent adaptation of human conduct to such changing environmental conditions. This position taken by Dewey and other pragmatists regarding values, morals, and ethics has led the insurgence of "pragmatic bioethicists," who have adopted the importance of consensus and experience and the denial of authoritative norms or foundational principles as the basis for moral decision making. More specifically, "clinical pragmatism" has been advanced as a new method of moral problem solving in clinical practice by applying the Deweyan experimental method (Jansen, 1998). Furthermore, Rorty's neopragmatism has been hailed by many pragmatic bioethicists as providing the grounds for new approaches that focus on redescription and recontextualization for bioethics. For Rorty, liberalism is the ethnocentric base from which liberty and individual self-expression are encouraged and coercion, cruelty, humiliation, and forced redescription are proscribed in bioethics (Arras, 2003).

In facing various critics against pragmatic bioethics who cite the untenability of "criterionless choice" in moral decisions (MacIntyre, 1966), arbitrariness of consensual agreements (Tollefsen & Cherry,

2003), and nonrational means of persuasion based solely on language and vocabularies (Arras, 2003), many have turned to Habermas's "discourse ethics" as a way to redress the questions of ethical norms and objectivity, and to deal with consensus in communicative openness and respect (Cooke, 2003).

PRAGMATISM IN THE NURSING CONTEXT

Pragmatism has been discussed in nursing from three aspects: (a) pragmatism in its advocacy for pluralism as it is related to nursing knowledge development, (b) pragmatism in relation to methodology, and (c) pragmatism in relation to practice. Discussions of pragmatism in relation to nursing epistemology center around the need to place nursing knowledge development within a coherent philosophy of science in the postpositivistic awakening that has become apparent in nursing during the past two decades. A pragmatic turn has been suggested by Rodgers (1991) in her advocacy for an evolutionary epistemology, by Kim's (1993) treatment of pluralism in nursing knowledge development, in Fry's (1995) espousal of Laudan's approach of science as problem solving, and in the advocacy of Im and Chee (2003) for fuzzy logic as the basis for theoretical development in nursing. The relevance of pragmatism for nursing knowledge development is stressed by these and other scholars on the grounds that (a) nursing is a practice discipline that is goal- and problem-solving-oriented in specific clinical situations, (b) nursing's subject matter is diverse and experientially grounded, and (c) nursing practice has been stifled by grand theorizing that assumes objectivity in knowledge and essentialism. Warms and Schroeder (1999) especially advocate pragmatism for nursing science from the pluralistic needs of knowledge.

In addition, methodologically, action research has been suggested as a way to address situation-specific, experience-based, and revision-oriented theory development in nursing from the pragmatic orientation (Hope & Waterman, 2003). Sjöström and Dahlgren (2002) on the other hand suggest phenomenography as a methodological approach to study phenomena and conceptualizations embedded in experiences and actual practices. Although Rorty's linguistic approach has not been articulated well in the nursing context, the recent emphasis on narratives as a way of knowing in nursing seems to be close to recontextualization and linguistification, which are critical aspects of neopragmatism.

Pragmatism in a naïve, common-sense form is well articulated in addressing issues of nursing practice, especially in relation to theory application in practice. Donaldson (1995) stresses eclectic uses of theories in clinical practice from a utilitarian orientation. This is in line with Brendel's (2003) suggestion for psychiatric practice for which "a pluralistic set of explanatory tools" become available to practitioners, full participation of the patient in treatment is advocated, and the tentative, revisional nature of knowledge and explanatory models is accepted. Doane (2003) on the other hand suggests that philosophic inquiry be used by practitioners as a way of establishing the situation-specific nature of knowing in experiences. The lure of pragmatism for practice discipline is in its emphasis on consequences and experiences as well as the primarily utilitarian focus on the use of knowledge.

Although the revival of pragmatism and development of neopragmatism have potential to impact greatly on nursing practice and nursing knowledge development, such impact has not been apparent on a full scale. The passion with which pragmatism may infiltrate into examining nursing epistemology and nursing practice may need to be censured in order to guard against the blindness that often accompanies any passion. Thus, it may be important to look at the potentially negative sides of pragmatism. Diggins (1994), posing a detached stance, offers some of the following:

- It does not give us objects of knowledge, since it confines itself to providing ways of knowing.
- It does not give us knowledge of truth, since truth has no antecedent existence but instead comes into being in the process of becoming known—and can in fact be transformed by that process.
- It does not give us accuracy of representation, modes of knowledge capable of grasping an independent reality against which we can check our thought, since knowledge of reality cannot be brought to bear upon the very operation of our own thoughts.
- It does not, even though it may claim to do so, give us a means of recognizing imperative moral obligations, since value judgments are arrived at only after we experience the good.
- It does not give us authoritative principles that can regulate human affairs, since human existence is characterized by the inexorable contingencies of experience.
- It does not give us truths that can compel the mind, since the mind itself is incapable of apprehending truths disclosed to the mind.

- It does not give us the basis of making present decisions, since all verifiable propositions can only refer to the future.
- It does not, in short, give us a criterion of judgment, since there is no authority to render it. (p. 248)

Diggins further notes, by citing Santayana (1956), that pragmatism ultimately offers us

> the benign message that it is better to pursue truth than to possess it, and better to regard as knowledge only those ideas that enable us to change things according to our desires, rather than to regard knowledge as a criterion of judgment that stands over and against our drives and desires. (1994, p. 248).

Is pragmatism sufficient and adequate for nursing knowledge development and legitimating nursing practice if it provides a perspective for inquiry (i.e., method) not for substance; for truth understood to be tentative, temporary, and revisional; and for human action circumscribed not by any fundamental authority or principles but by experience and consensus?

REFERENCES

Aboulafia, M., Bookman, M., & Kemp, C. (Eds.). (2002). *Habermas and pragmatism.* London: Routledge.

Arras, J. D. (2003). Rorty's pragmatism and bioethics. *Journal of Medicine and Philosophy, 28,* 597–613.

Bernstein, R. J. (1988/1997). Pragmatism, pluralism, and the healing of wounds. In L. Menard (Ed.), *Pragmatism: A reader* (pp. 382–401). New York: Vintage Books.

Bernstein, R. J. (1998). Community in the pragmatic tradition. In M. Dickstein (Ed.), *The revival of pragmatism* (pp. 141–156). Durham, NC: Duke University Press.

Bourdieu, P. (1977). *Outline of a theory of practice* (R. Nice, Trans.). Cambridge, MA: Cambridge University Press. (Originally published in 1972)

Brendel, D. H. (2003). Reductionism, eclecticism, and pragmatism in psychiatry: The dialectic of clinical explanation. *Journal of Medicine and Philosophy, 28,* 563–580.

Cooke, E. F. (2003). On the possibility of a pragmatic discourse bioethics: Putnam, Habermas, and the normative logic of bioethical inquiry. *Journal of Medicine and Philosophy, 28,* 635–653.

Cooley, C. H. (1909/1962). *Social organization.* New York: Schocken.

Dewey, J. (1911/1978). The problem of truth. In J. A. Boydston (Ed.), *The middle works of John Dewey* (Vol. 6, p. 67). Carbondale: Southern Illinois University Press.

Dewey, J. (1916/1997). Theories of knowledge. In L. Menard (Ed.), *Pragmatism: A reader* (pp. 205–218). New York: Vintage Books.

Dewey, J. (1922/1957). *Human nature and conduct: An introduction to social psychology.* New York: Modern Library.

Dewey, J. (1930). What I believe. *Forum, 83,* 176–182.

Dewey, J. (1939). I believe. In C. Fadiman (Ed.), *I believe: The personal philosophies of certain eminent men and women of our time* (pp. 347–354). New York: Simon & Schuster.

Dickstein, M. (Ed.). (1998a). *The revival of pragmatism.* Durham, NC: Duke University Press.

Dickstein, M. (1998b). Introduction: Pragmatism then and now. In M. Dickstein (Ed.), *The revival of pragmatism* (pp. 1–18). Durham, NC: Duke University Press.

Diggins, J. P. (1994). *The promise of pragmatism: Modernism and the crisis of knowledge and authority.* Chicago: University of Chicago Press.

Doane, G. H. (2003). Through pragmatic eyes: Philosophy and the re-sourcing of family nursing. *Nursing Philosophy, 4,* 25–32.

Donaldson, S. K. (1995). Introduction: Nursing science for nursing practice. In A. Omery, C. E. Kasper, & G. G. Page (Eds.), *In search of nursing science* (pp. 3–12). Thousand Oaks, CA: Sage.

Fry, S. T. (1995). Science as problem solving. In A. Omery, C. E. Kasper, & G. G. Page (Eds.), *In search of nursing science* (pp. 72–80). Thousand Oaks, CA: Sage.

Haack, S. (1996a). Reflections of a critical common-sensist. *Transactions of the Charles S. Peirce Society, xxxii,* 359–373.

Haack, S. (1996b). Pragmatism. In N. Bunnin & C. P. Tsui-James (Eds.), *Handbook of philosophy* (pp. 643–661). Oxford, UK: Blackwell.

Habermas, J. (1971). *Knowledge and human interests* (J. Shapiro, Trans.). Boston: Beacon Press.

Hope, K. W., & Waterman, H. A. (2003). Praiseworthy pragmatism? Validity and action research. *Journal of Advanced Nursing, 44,* 120–127.

Im, E. O., & Chee, W. (2003). Fuzzy logic and nursing. *Nursing Philosophy, 4,* 53–60.

James, W. (1907/1981). Pragmatism: A new name for some old ways of thinking. In B. Kuklick (Ed.), *Pragmatism* (pp. 3–134). Indianapolis, IN: Hackett.

Jansen, L. A. (1998). Assessing clinical pragmatism. *Kennedy Institute on Ethics Journal, 8,* 23–36.

Kim, H. S. (1993). Identifying alternative linkages among philosophy, theory and method in nursing science. *Journal of Advanced Nursing, 18,* 793–800.

Kloppenberg, J. T. (1998). Pragmatism: An old name for some new ways of thinking? In M. Dickstein (Ed.), *The revival of pragmatism* (pp. 83–127). Durham, NC: Duke University Press.

Laudan, L. (1990). *Science and relativism: Some key controversies in the philosophy of science.* Chicago: University of Chicago Press.

MacIntyre, A. (1966). *A short history of ethics.* New York: Macmillan.
Mead, G. H. (1934). *Mind, self, and society.* Chicago: University of Chicago Press.
Menard, L. (Ed.). (1997). *Pragmatism: A reader.* New York: Vintage Books.
Morgenbesser, S. (1998). Response to Hilary Putnam's "pragmatism and realism." In M. Dickstein (Ed.), *The revival of pragmatism* (pp. 54–61). Durham, NC: Duke University Press.
Peirce, C. S. (1878/1997). How to make our ideas clear. In L. Menard (Ed.), *Pragmatism: A reader* (pp. 26–48). New York: Vintage Books.
Peirce, C. S. (1904/1997). A definition of pragmatism. In L. Menard (Ed.), *Pragmatism: A reader* (pp. 56–58). New York: Vintage Books.
Peirce, C. S. (1905). What pragmatism is. *The Monist, 15,* 161–181.
Putnam, H. (1981). *Reason, truth and history.* Cambridge, MA: Cambridge University Press.
Putnam, H. (1998). Pragmatism and realism. In M. Dickstein (Ed.), *The revival of pragmatism* (pp. 37–53). Durham, NC: Duke University Press.
Ramberg, B. (2002, Summer). Richard Rorty. In E. N. Zalta (Ed.), *The Stanford encyclopedia of philosophy.* Retrieved September 10, 2004, from http://plato.stanford.edu/archives/sum2002/entries/rorty/
Rockwell, T. (2003). Rorty, Putnam, and the pragmatist view of epistemology and metaphysics. (Published in *Education and Culture: The Journal of the John Dewey Society*). Retrieved September 8, 2004, from http//:www.california.com/~mcmf/rorty.html
Rodgers, B. L. (1991). Deconstructing the dogma in nursing knowledge and practice. *Image: Journal of Nursing Scholarship, 23,* 177–181.
Rorty, R. (1982). *Consequences of pragmatism.* Minneapolis: University of Minnesota Press.
Rorty, R. (1991). *Objectivity, relativism, and truth.* Cambridge, MA: Cambridge University Press.
Rorty, R. (1998). Pragmatism as romantic polytheism. In M. Dickstein (Ed.), *The revival of pragmatism* (pp. 21–36). Durham, NC: Duke University Press.
Santayana, G. (1956). The irony of liberalism. *New Republic, 135,* 12–15.
Sjöström, B., & Dahlgren, L. O. (2002). Applying phenomenography in nursing research. *Journal of Advanced Nursing, 40,* 339–345.
Tollefsen, C., & Cherry, M. J. (2003). Pragmatism and bioethics: Diagnosis or cure? *Journal of Medicine and Philosophy, 28,* 533–544.
Warms, C. A., & Schroeder, C. A. (1999). Bridging the gulf between science and action: The "new fuzzies" of neopragmatism. *Advances in Nursing Science, 22,* 1–10.

CHAPTER 12

Biography and Biographical Work: An Approach for Nursing*

Barbara Schulte-Steinicke

The topic of biographical work is by no means new in the field of nursing. For some decades now biographical issues have been reflected in this field. On the one side, there are proposals for curricula that deal entirely with questions and aspects of patients' biographies. The reason for this is that professionals have found it easier to understand patients in their states of sickness or disability by investigating the biographical resources or lack of resources that their patients have to cope with. On the other side, nurses themselves are increasingly reflecting on their own biographical paths in order to better understand the interconnections between their own lives, their work in hospital (or in other fields of care), and their careers (Schulte-Steinicke, 2002). Finally, there is the therapeutic aspect: It is not only important for nursing staff to get to know and reflect on their patients' biographies together with patients but it is also important for the patients themselves, who as a result will be able to better understand their situation, remember or cultivate their resources, and cope more effectively with their disabilities (Koch, 2002). And,

---

*Translated from German by Gerald Nixon.

concerning communication between patients and professionals about the patients' biographies, again it is not only the nursing staff that sometimes tries to reflect on and work with the patient in such a way. In the field of health it is also sometimes the doctor, often the psychotherapist, and perhaps even the physiotherapist, the ergotherapist, or the social worker who may work with patients who are sick or disabled by using means that help to anticipate patients' future biographical aspects.

Thus, biographical work is an important medium in the field of health, and in a way, it is also an important medium in the field of self-healing (Koch, 2002). There are many professionals and experts on the topic of biographical work, and it is surely the patients themselves who are the most authentic, and at the same time the most vulnerable, experts. Accordingly, there are many communication options on the subject of biographical work among professionals as well as between professionals and their patients. There is no way of working seriously in nursing today without using the resources of strategies that make use of biographical issues. Nursing today means "holistic nursing in a bio-psycho-social way" (Roper, Logan, & Tierney, 1990), including taking measures that help patients to find their own way of adapting (Schwartz-Barcott, 1999). "Holistic" nursing and forms of nursing that help patients find suitable ways of adapting not only means taking patients' emotions and thoughts as seriously as their bodies; it also means taking patients' personalities, along with their life courses, as seriously as we ourselves would like to be taken (see, for example, Roper's life-span model in Roper et al., 1990).

First, this chapter will give an overview of the therapeutic effects that biographical work has in the field of health and healing. It will include a short overview of the possibilities of biographical work in nursing.

Second, ways of doing biographical work in nursing will be examined. This also presents a number of examples of how to put biographical work into practice.

BIOGRAPHICAL WORK TODAY— WHY AND FOR WHOM?

The therapeutic effects of biographical work in nursing have been observed and appraised for the last 50 years. This has been done in different ways by different fields of study (Friebe, 2004).

The Social Science Perspective

Here, biography is seen above all as an image of the paths people have taken in their individual and social lives. Consequently, human biographies have long been regarded by the social sciences as being divided into childhood and youth as the time of learning; adult life as the time of working; and the senior stage of life. This stage of life differs from the stage of adult life in that it is usually taken to be a period when a person has stopped being part of the working community of societies (Kohli, 1978). In the past this stage of life has hardly ever been considered an interesting period of life. Kohli has also given an overview of research into this period of life during approximately the last 30 years. Especially within the last 16 years, however, things have changed considerably in social life as well as in the social sciences. For one thing, the new science of gerontology has established itself, for which the senior stage of life is an interesting and important period. For another, many theories have been developed about social and individual experience in this stage of life, for example, the theory of disengagement, which postulates that elderly persons no longer wish to remain engaged in their social contexts, let alone seek new opportunities of engagement, but prefer to disengage and take more time for themselves and for reflecting on their past. Moreover, there is the theory of old age being but a myth (cf. Friedan, 1997): To Betty Friedan, old people are the same people they were before; it is merely the body that has changed, along with society's response to this change. If people stopped reacting in a negative way to aging, the problems that exist would virtually be solved. Naegele (1999) differentiates between four periods of adult life: younger and middle adult life as well as the early and later senior period.

All these theories point to a new way of looking at the senior stage of life as a period that has its own tasks as well as its opportunities. However, it is not only the senior stage of life that has gained a new importance today. All the other stages of life, including youth and even childhood, are confronted with new perspectives, responsibilities, and duties (Elkind, 1991; Friebe, 1999). In a society in which unemployment, mobility, and a kind of partnership and family life that consists of living apart are all normal phenomena, the members of this society are obliged to reinvent their everyday life and its meaning almost daily.

Hence, biographies of today are biographies that, in a certain respect, have to be constructed, experienced, and reflected upon over and over again—perhaps for an entire lifetime. It is, furthermore, the phenomenon of growing longevity that is responsible for another new phenomenon, the increase in chronic diseases. More and more people now have to live with diseases and disabilities that were hardly known in the past. And it is a result of research in so-called poetry therapy that reflection upon biographical issues with regard to people's diseases helps them to cope with their state—above all if the disease is one that has either appeared very suddenly or that in the course of time has become chronic. In poetry therapy, this reflection upon people's biographies takes place through the medium of poetry—patients reflect on their own disabilities by reading or writing poetry—but this is only one of many mediums that may be of help in therapeutic reflection.

The Psychological Perspective

In our look at reflection from a social science perspective, we have already touched upon another field in which the value of biographical work in health care has been discussed for some time now. This is the field of psychology, where, in a certain respect, a development has taken place that is similar to the development we have been looking at in sociology: namely, the realization that the different ways in which people go through the various stages of life have become more complex and thus much harder to understand and cope with. For example, when is it a good time in life for people to have children? When is it a good moment to start a new career if the old one is no longer rewarding? Starting a new job, entering a new marriage, having another child or perhaps a first child—all these decisions seem to be possible for a much longer time in life than it was for our grandparents or even our parents. Even growing old or living with a chronic disease or disability may still mean leading an autonomous life: travelling, meeting friends, living alone or together just as a person wishes, if—and this is again the sociological view within the psychological one—there is sufficient money to do so. There are fewer norms that govern our lives, there is more freedom and tolerance for living them in an individual way, and this is not merely the result of social changes. There are also changes in individual experience and psychic processes of integration. And these changes do not yet have their own rules. From a psychological and a sociological point of view, people have to invent their lives and reflect upon them again and again, for an entire life perhaps, with many models but few clear rules. The German psychosociologist Ulrich Beck (2003) calls the result of this phenomenon "modern patchwork biographies."

Thus, biographical work today is perhaps more important than in the past, even though it has always been a tradition of Occidental civilization to try to understand as well as heal oneself by writing down, and in so doing, endeavor to understand parts of one's biography. Hocke (1991), an expert in diary research, sums this up as follows:

> There were two religious and ethical axioms of Greek antiquity in the time after Homer that have awakened an awareness for (the human) personality, which exists in its own right and is indivisible: these are "Know yourself" and "Be who you are." (p. 37, translated by B. Schulte-Steinicke)

The Nursing Science Perspective

There is, finally, the perspective of nursing science. It is Nancy Roper, above all, who has built up a special theory of biographical paths in people's lives: her life-span model. To Roper, all paths of life depend on at least two variables: first, the activities of daily life; and second, people's capacity for independence versus their need for help due to certain dependencies. These two opposites vary in relation to each other all through one's life. Accordingly, people's biographies are always being reconstructed around their capacity to fulfill the different activities of daily life either in an independent way or with a varying degree of dependence (Roper et al.,1990).

It is altogether possible that at a certain time in life a person is dependent in some activities of daily life and independent in others. And it is quite normal that dependence and independence change during life spans. It is normal that children and those who are elderly are more dependent in certain (or perhaps in all) activities than adults or adolescents. And it is normal, too, that people who are ill or disabled are more dependent than people in good health. Hence, dependence itself is a normal phenomenon of human life; but it is an equally normal phenomenon that people try to gain as much independence as they possibly can.

Finally, in some ways growing older in a modern Western society today means staying younger for a longer time. This means that older people today appear to be younger than they seemed 20 or 30 years ago. Naegele (2000) has shown that at the same time people are growing older on average than in the past and living longer before they fall seriously ill, older people also have more money at their disposal on average than used to be the case. This has given rise to a so-called fourth period of life, a period in which people's lives are free from duties like having to work or care for a family, in which they are still independent (Roper et al., 1990) to some extent, and accordingly in which they still have great capacities and ample resources of time and perhaps money for doing and learning whatever they please. Obviously, this brings with it, for one thing, a high degree of liberty for many older people, and for another, a great need to reflect upon life in this period, especially as there are scarcely any models of how to manage one's life in this period.

Authors like Friedan (1997) have shown that this new kind of reflection will also provide the foundations of living a dignified life in this fourth stage as soon as older people form the majority of the populations of Western countries.

BIOGRAPHICAL WORK IN HUMAN SCIENCE RESEARCH

For many years this kind of work was not the object of professional research. During the last four decades, however, research has been undertaken in this field, first of all in the United States and later in Europe as well. In Europe it was primarily during the 1990s that the topic gained importance. At the University of Münster, in particular, many indications have been found that biographical work, for example, biographical writing, has therapeutic effects just like helping depressed, nervous, or anxious people to relax and to better understand their situation and their options (Koch & Kessler, 2002a, 2002b; see also Schulte-Steinicke, 2000).

In Germany, incidentally, there are many people who have not only told and written down their stories of sickness, aging, losing family members, and other traumatic occurrences in their lives but who have also published their experiences. To cite two well-known examples, Karl-Heinz Pantke (1999), with his partner Christine Kuehne, wrote down the story of his locked-in syndrome, describing his feelings during this crucial stage in his life as well as noting his reflections on the new situation and his coping with this experience. Helmut Clahsen (2003) and his wife, Lilo, gave an introspection of her stroke and the following aphasia. Their life without words and the long inner and outer struggle back to normal life are vividly described and reveal enlightening insights into the sufferings not only through the sickness but also the ignorance of the surroundings.

In the Anglo-American field there have been two main paths of research and therapy based on biographical work: that of poetry therapy, which has already been mentioned above; and that of so-called reminiscence training, which is especially popular in Britain.

Poetry Therapy

Poetry therapy entails therapy by reading and above all by writing about one's personal life. Various schools have been founded that teach professionals in the psychosocial and medical fields how to help their patients write down biographical issues in a therapeutic way.

Among others, the following important effects have been noted. First, writing down one's own biographical experiences and questions can help people, especially older people, to deal with depression as well as with social anxiety. Second, professionals may be better able to understand depressive or anxious patients. And finally, it is possible to stay healthier with regard, for example, to hypertonia and resistance to disease by writing down daily personal reflections, feelings, and reminiscences (Schulte-Steinicke, 2000).

Reminiscence Training

Reminiscence training is quite the opposite of this kind of work: People remember not only by being creative—by writing, for example, or by telling—but also by hearing, seeing, or reading things that are associated with memories, particularly things of former daily life.

This underlies the work of nurses and social workers at the London Health Exchange Centre, who make use of various media in order to help people remember, for example, those who are elderly and those who have dementia. The results: dementia is slowed down in its development and almost all older people come to remember more exactly.

WHY DOES IT WORK?

If we ask why—for example, Why should writing down facts and feelings about one's own biography help the healing process?—we should take notice of what diary therapist Kate Adams has found out about these things. Adams (1996) lists these advantages of writing about one's own life in a diary:

1. *The immediacy and availability* of the diary, that is, the means that help to remember and thus help one to try and understand one's own life.
2. *Catharsis* of old feelings and inner states that are perhaps still hurting a person or perhaps hurt again and again whenever something in daily life acts as a kind of associative trigger, bringing an old trauma back to the surface.
3. *Object constancy,* that is, a topic to write about and a capacity for writing are always available, helping to feel trust in a world that sometimes seems to be chaotic.
4. *Repetition.* Former experiences can be remembered again and again by writing and so can be understood better each time.
5. *Reality check.* Things that a person has not dared to think about for a long time become more "real" by being written down. The acceptance of past events as being real, as "having really happened," is an important means of understanding and coping with traumatic events of life like sickness, disability, death, age, conflicts, and so forth.
6. *Self-pacing* means the capacity for, and routine of, understanding oneself and coping with life. Taking a look into one's own inner world by writing as a way of good inner communication.
7. *Communication* has a lot to do with the preceding point: If people are able to communicate well with themselves, they are better able to communicate authentically with others.
8. *Self-esteem* is gained through a better knowledge about the ups and downs individuals have to deal with during their lives and a better knowledge of the resources they possess.
9. *Increasing clarity.* That is, understanding more and more clearly how one's own past has taken place, how one's own development has proceeded, and what the possibilities are for one's own future.

Witness to Healing

This is another important criterion that shows the importance of the various kinds of media such as diaries or old photographs that can help people to remember. These media are, of course, witnesses of the old days; however, they are also witnesses of the process a person has gone through in order to cope with past painful experiences.

Examples of Biographical Work in Nursing

The special benefits of biographical work in nursing are as follows:

1. It helps people to remember, to understand and thus to cope with experiences of their lives, above all with those that have been hurting and perhaps traumatic.
2. It helps people to develop their capacity for coping with old experiences and with new ones, as well as with tasks that still have to be dealt with; in short, helping people to adapt.
3. It helps people to arrange their current lives in an adaptive way (Schwartz-Barcott, 1999).
4. It helps people to make the change from dependence to as much independence as possible in as many activities of daily life as possible (Roper et al., 1990).

Thus, biographical work is a means of helping patients on their way to self-help and self-reliance and, moreover, to work finally in a way that is suited to new models of nursing.

These special approaches need special methods and means that help people in special situations to do their biographical work, assisted by nurses and other professionals. These means are primarily things that help patients to remember, like painting or writing texts. There are also things that help patients do the biographical work—items (such as photographs) of daily life in the past, as in reminiscence training; and perhaps old songs or poems that a person learned a long time ago.

There are also means that help patients remember things they have learned by remembering, such as texts they have written down, as in poetry therapy; or, for instance, maps of visualization that help them to remember new ideas. These maps of visualization especially help those who are elderly and those who are sick to remember what they thought or said earlier.

Two examples of effective ways of visualizing that the author has already worked with are the life-event scale (Figure 12.1) and the mind map.

Life-Event Scale

Generating a life-event scale (LES) begins with entering the facts on personal education and work life, as in a CV (lower part). In the upper part the personal development related to the CV is made visible. If it is helpful, more and other levels can be reflected, such as ideas,

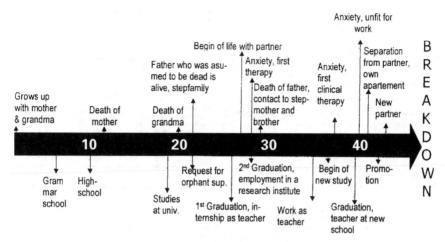

FIGURE 12.1   An example of life event scale of CV (from Kollak, 2004, p. 12).

values, conceptions, or feelings that were important for certain times in life. The LES can be continued over time: personal behaviors, opinions, and emotions become visible as well as relations between events and developments, recurring schemes, and so forth (Kollak, 2004, p. 12).

Mind Map (Schulte-Steinicke)

The mind map is a map of the chapters in the life's novel of a woman named Lucie, 44, who is chronically sick (Figure 12.2). By painting this map, Lucie found some kind of coherence in her life, which had always seemed fragmented to her.

The following is a short poem that Lucie wrote down after painting this map:

Successes and failures
I've always dreamt
Of paradise lost
Even when being sick
Perhaps then more than ever
And the only times
When I seemed to reach it
Was painting
Or holding my baby
For a while.
Then
It seemed to leave
But I still feel it
Somewhere.

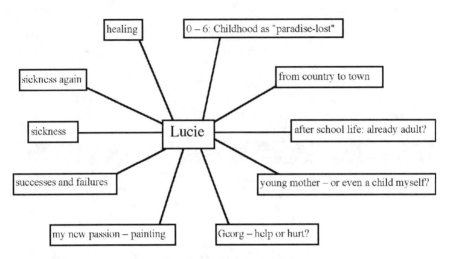

FIGURE 12.2   An example of mindmap of Lucie.

WHERE CAN WE GO?

In the years to come, biographical work will gain increasing importance in the entire field of health care. In this field, nursing science will play a crucial role. It is precisely among the patients and clients of nursing that people are to be found who, more than others, are confronted with (perhaps unexpected) changes in their lives and who experience new ways of coping with their situation: with chronic sickness, with growing old quite differently from other generations, and with many new social situations that there are no well-proven models for handling. Nursing in a biopsychosocial sense means helping patients to discover how to live as independently and self-reliantly as possible at a certain stage of life. At the same time, nursing professionals themselves need help in order to be prepared for this new field of work. At the Alice-Salomon-Fachhochschule in Berlin, a university of applied sciences, we have conceptualized and evaluated a new curriculum of biographical work for people in health care. The modules of the curriculum are as follows:

1. A person's own biography—learning to understand the stages of a person's life: stages of life, remembering, developmental psychology, regarding one's own life as a novel
2. Crises in life and how to understand and handle them by writing as an example of self-coaching

3. People's personal philosophies of life and the self: trying to understand one's own personal philosophy, trying to reflect on and develop it, and trying to understand one's own unconscious hopes about life and death
4. Biographical writing on health and disease, writing healing texts and stories
5 The didactic and pedagogic principles of biographically orientated self-help groups

REFERENCES

Adams, K. (1996). Writing as a powerful adjunct to therapy. *Journal of Poetry, 1,* 31–38.

Beck, U. (2003). *Die Risikogesellschaft—auf dem Weg in eine andere Moderne* [Society of risks—On the way to another modernity]. Frankfurt, Germany: Suhrkamp.

Clahsen, H. (2003). *Mir fehlen die Worte . . . Aphasie nach Schlaganfall—ein Erfahrungsbericht* [I am out of words . . . Aphasia after stroke—A diary]. Frankfurt, Germany: Mabuse.

Elkind, D. (1991). *Das gehetzte Kind* [The pushed child]. Hamburg, Germany: Kernst Kabel.

Friebe, J. (1999). Applying social science concepts to nursing: Systems theory and beyond. In H. S. Kim & I. Kollak (Eds.). *Nursing theories: Conceptual and philosophical foundations* (pp. 105–122). New York: Springer.

Friebe, J. (2004). Der biografische Ansatz in der Pflege [The biographical approach in nursing]. *Pflege und Gesellschaft, 1,* 3–5.

Friedan, B. (1997). *Mythos Alter* [The fountain of age]. Reinbek, Germany: Rowohlt.

Hocke, R. (1991). *Europäische Tagebücher aus vier Jahrhunderten* [European diaries of four centuries]. Frankfurt, Germany: Fischer.

Koch, H., & Kessler, N. (2002a). *Ein Buch muss die Axt sein* [A book must be the axe]. Kiel, Germany: Königsfurt.

Koch, H., & Kessler, N. (2002b). *Lesen und Schreiben in psychischen Krisen* [Readings and writings in psychic crises]. In M. Kohli (Ed.), *Soziologie des Lebenslaufs.* Darmstadt, Germany: Psychiatrie-Verlag.

Kohli, M. (1978). Erartungen an eine Soziologie des Lebenslaufs [Expectations regarding a sociology of biography]. In M. Kohli (Ed.), *Sociology of biography* (p. 12). Darmstadt, Germany: Luchterhand.

Kollak, I. (2004). Lebensläufe sichtbar machen. Biografisches Arbeiten mit Mitteln der optischen Veranschaulichung [Making life-spans visible. Methods of illustrations in biographical work]. *Pflege und Gesellschaft, 1,* 12–14.

Naegele, G. (1999). Vom Dreieck zum Pilz. Der demographische Wandel in Deutschland [From triangle to a mushroom shape. The demographic changes in Germany]. *Senioren als Verbraucher. AgV Forum, 3,* 4–16.

Pantke, K. H. (1999). *Locked-in: Gefangen im eigenen Körper* [Locked-in: Captive in one's own body] (3rd ed.). Frankfurt, Germany: Mabuse.

Roper, N., Logan, W. W., & Tierney, A. J. (1990). *The elements of nursing* (3rd ed.). Edinburgh, UK: Churchill Livingstone.

Schulte-Steinicke, B. (2000). *Bilder werden Worte* [Pictures become words]. Berlin: Schibri.

Schulte-Steinicke, B. (2002). Wissenschaftliche Aufsätze kreativ schreiben [Creative writing for scientific essays]. In K. Reinhard (Ed.), *Das Schreibbuch für Pflegende* (pp. 201–220). Bern, Switzerland: Huber.

Schwartz-Barcott, D. (1999). Adaptation as a basic conceptual focus in nursing theories. In H. S. Kim & I. Kollak (Eds.), *Nursing theories: Conceptual and philosophical foundations* (pp. 9–21). New York: Springer.

CHAPTER 13

Evidence-Based Nursing for Practice and Science*

Martina Hasseler

In health systems all over the world, economic problems are to be observed that are leading to far-reaching changes in the funding, structures, and organizations of these systems. Politicians in charge of health policy are seeking solutions and answers to these problems and, as a rule, the goal they pursue is to achieve a form of health provision that besides being affordable is of high quality and available for all sections of the population. Because of the differences in the systems of health care operating around the world, the solutions to these problems differ to a greater or lesser extent from country to country. In spite of these differences, however, the demand for evidence-based health provision is being asserted almost everywhere. By opting for evidence-based principles and procedures, both health politicians and funding bodies hope to be able not only to remedy errors of provision, whether due to excessive, insufficient, or inappropriate care, but also to increase the quality of provision for care recipients.

Within the health care community the contents of evidence-based provision are discussed predominantly with reference to the medical profession under the heading "evidence-based medicine." Evidence-

---

*Translated from German by Gerald Nixon.

based principles, standards, and procedures with regard to other professions such as nursing play only a minor role, if any. Thus, the concept of evidence-based nursing is rarely to be found outside the profession or beyond the confines of discussions in nursing studies. It is to be assumed that the wider public as well as health system experts either classify evidence-based findings, standards, and procedures in the field of nursing as belonging to that of medicine, or they do not—and take no notice whatsoever of nursing research and studies. Here, one must ask self-critically whether studies in nursing science have been undertaken and published in sufficient numbers to make evidence-based nursing possible.

The necessity in nursing practice, nursing science, and nursing research of debating the concept of "evidence-based health care"—its development, definition and significance as well as its opportunities and limits—derives from the fact that within the health system nursing must become increasingly accountable with regard to the quality, effectiveness, and efficiency of its services and increasingly competitive in its relationships with other professional groups. Although nurses represent the largest group of professionals in most of the world's health systems, it can nevertheless be asserted (as Cochrane put it) that just because one professional group is represented in health provision more frequently than others in terms of numbers, this does not prove in any way that this group makes a difference.[1] The question that can (and must) be answered by evidence-based nursing is whether nursing makes a difference in health provision and the care of patients, and if so, how.

Additional reasons are to be found in the financial constraints and the health policy measures that inform the overall conditions and framework of nursing practice and science. In many health systems, elements of managed care are being introduced that are connected with the development of standardized procedures. Demographic changes and shifts in the spectrum of diseases towards increasing chronic diseases place a wider range of demands on nursing and patient care. The new services being taken over by nursing and care must be judged not only with regard to costs but also with regard to their effects on and benefits to patients. Furthermore, increasing demands are being made for ensuring quality in nursing, that is, the quality of nursing must improve in order to attain better outcomes. It must also be borne in mind that care recipients now have higher expectations of health provision and that health is given an important place in our societies. Future patients will take advantage of the services and facilities of the health system in the expectation that from a qualitative point of view their health will be preserved or their state of health will experience an improvement (Muir Gray, 1997, p. 4ff).

WHAT DOES "EVIDENCE-BASED NURSING" MEAN?

When searching in relevant nursing science databases, what strikes one is that the term *evidence-based nursing* is used in the contexts of both nursing science and nursing practice. According to the literature the question of evidence-based practice is predominantly discussed in terms of financial constraints and change (Muir Gray, 1997, p. 1; White, 1997, p. 175). It is regarded as the new catchword and is a major topic both in journals and at conferences (Dunn, 1998, p. 2; English & Bond, 1998, p. 7).

The word "evidence" does, in fact, have different connotations in different languages. In English usage, it means anything that indicates proof, or "documentation showing the validity of a fact" (Hasseler, 1999, p. 20). The German word *Evidenz,* on the other hand, means the illustration of a fact, clearness, complete certainty, or illuminating information. In contrast to the English sense of the word, this understanding of the term says little about the data on which these facts are based or that these facts have a scientific or rational basis (Hasseler, 1999, p. 20). For an understanding of evidence-based nursing it is the English meaning of "evidence" that must be used, that is, "based on valid facts."

In the English-speaking literature on the subject, the definitions of evidence-based nursing are borrowed to a great extent from those of evidence-based medicine, which is defined by Sackett as "the conscientious, explicit and judicious use of current best external and scientific evidence in making decisions about the medical care of individual patients" (Sackett, 1998, p. 9).

Thus, decisions in medical care are to be made on a rational basis and in accordance with the current state of our knowledge. With reference to nursing, this means that evidence-based nursing is a method of critically selecting and appraising scientific literature and applying the scientific evidence that has been found to a specific nursing situation.

At this point one might ask, How does the individual patient fit into all this? Where is the individual care? For this reason an addition is made to the above definition:

"an approach to decision making in which the clinician uses the best evidence available, in consultation with the patient, to decide upon the option which suits that patient best" (Muir Gray, 1997, p. 9).

The consequence of this is that by using evidence-based procedures, the individual experience of the nurse (clinical expertise) and the preferences of the patient are to be combined with the scientific evidence of clinically-relevant research (Sackett, 1998, p. 9). According to Sackett the individual experience and the expertise of those who are able to apply evidence-based practice are a fundamental and essential requirement for judging whether clinically relevant research should be used in treating a patient (Sackett, 1998, p. 19). Patients' preferences, their social surroundings, and their personal attitudes and outlook should always be taken into consideration. The following conclusions can be drawn from what has been said already:

- Evidence-based nursing is the provision of health care in keeping with the principle that all nursing interventions are based on the best available scientific evidence or data (Shorten & Wallace, 1997, p. 22). It is a form of nursing based on scientific knowledge.
- Evidence-based nursing has nothing to do with what has been called "cookbook" nursing. On the contrary, a scientific basis is sought which is helpful in everyday decision making. External research results must be integrated into the individuals' circumstances, including their preferences and their social environment. Through evidence-based practice, nursing and care become more transparent and patients become involved in the decision-making process. By being informed and enlightened, patients are able to make decisions based on information.
- Evidence-based nursing is not only an instrument for decision-making but also a concept of lifelong learning. Lifelong leaning is reflected in the fact that, by applying evidence-based nursing, nursing procedures are constantly evaluated, working routines reviewed, new treatment plans drawn up and solution options established (Brinker-Meyendriesch, 2003, p. 230).
- The aim is to implement successful and cost-effective nursing and care, to improve the quality of care and to optimize the nursing outcome.
- The consequence of introducing evidence-based nursing is the necessity of a shift of perspective away from a form of nursing and care strongly oriented to the individual towards a form of

nursing and care related to populations (Closs & Cheater, 1999, p. 11). This means that a more epidemiological perspective is necessary since one must proceed from experience of the individual case to systematic studies and vice versa.

Carrying out evidence-based nursing follows a particular pattern (Lühmann, 1998, p. 48; Perleth, 1998, p. 15; Porzsolt & Sigle, 1998, p. 40), as shown in Figure 13.1.

In carrying out the different steps of the evidence-based method, it must be noted that differing degrees of evidence (i.e., a hierarchy of evidence) have to be distinguished. Studies and research must fulfill certain criteria of quality before they can be used as evidence in

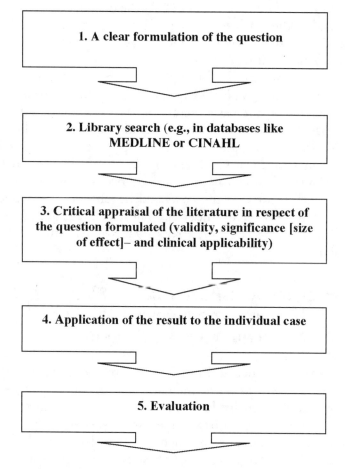

FIGURE 13.1   Steps in the evidence-based practice.

everyday practice. This differentiation of evidence was undertaken by Cochrane as long ago as 1972 (Cochrane, 1972, p. 21ff.), and in the years that followed it was adopted by Sackett and other proponents and advocates of evidence-based medicine (Antes, 1998, p. 21; Sackett, 1998, p. 11).

At the lowest level of the evidence hierarchy are the opinions and convictions of experts, personal experience, and descriptive studies. According to Cochrane evidence at this level is the "simplest and worst" evidence because clinical expertise depends on the experts' ability as well as the depth and breadth of their experience. Furthermore, there are no quantitative measurements or studies to show what would happen to patients if they did not receive the intervention or what further factors might have influenced the effect of a particular intervention (Cochrane, 1972, p. 21). At the next higher level are non-randomized studies such as case control studies or cohort studies. The disadvantage of these kinds of study is generally felt to be their inability to demonstrate the effect of an intervention systematically. Effects and outcomes can be brought about by various factors apart from those studied systematically. The highest level consists of systematic reviews on the basis of randomized studies, or randomized control trials. Cochrane introduced this kind of study as the method of choice when it comes to demonstrating the effectiveness of measures and interventions (Cochrane, 1972, pp. 22–23). In Cochrane's view randomized studies can provide leaders in health systems and institutions with results on the costs and benefits of alternatives to a particular intervention or measure. The advantage of randomized studies is that fewer systematic errors are possible in study design and implementation.

SIGNIFICANCE AND POTENTIAL OF EVIDENCE-BASED NURSING FOR NURSING PRACTICE AND NURSING SCIENCE

Despite nursing science and nursing research, the practice of nursing, that is, the actions performed and the measures taken in nursing, is still dominated by habits and by personal opinions. In the daily decision making in hospitals, most nurses rely on personal experience and information passed on by word of mouth and base their decisions to a large degree on these two sources (Roberts, 1999, p. 3; Thompson, 2003, p. 231). Habits and personal experience, however, are incompatible with evidence-based practice. It is questionable whether habits and personal experience alone guarantee the provision of appropriate and high-quality health care. These are undoubtedly two important factors that are indispensable in daily practical work; nevertheless, studies have indicated that people tend to overestimate their knowledge in respect of its correctness and validity (Thompson, 2003, p. 232). Besides, personal experience alone is insufficient as it is not able to appraise nursing interventions systematically with a view to establishing their benefits, weaknesses, and mistakes (Behrens, 2000, p. 103). One serious problem of personal experience is its particular proneness to ritualizing and habitualizing. Numerous examples from nursing practice can be cited as evidence of this: the old practice of treating decubitus ulcers by cooling with ice and drying with warm air or the still common practice of the 2-hourly change of position and the use of (mostly synthetic) furs in the prevention of decubitus ulcers. These ritualized measures are not only ineffective, inefficient, and unnecessarily costly; for the patients they also involve the likelihood of further inconvenience due to longer periods of nursing or of physical and mental stress.

The potential of evidence-based nursing is to be found in the micro, meso and macro levels of health care. At the micro level, that is to say in the daily routine of nursing and contact with patients, the significance and the potential of evidence-based nursing lie in the fact that nursing decisions and interventions are founded on controlled, empirical experience (Behrens, 2003, p. 107). Self-confidence in performing practical duties can be increased through evidence-based nursing. It can provide the basis for justifying either current practice or necessary modifications (Simpson, 1996, p. 22). The use of verified data enables nursing staff to prevent unnecessary and even potentially detrimental measures. With the help of evidence-based nursing it is possible to select and make use of the most effective measures and interventions. In this way nurses are put in a position to carry out high-quality and cost-effective patient care and to improve the results of their nursing (Simpson, 1996, p. 22). This is pointed out in a study undertaken by Simpson, which reveals that patients who received research-based nursing showed 28% better outcomes than those who received non-research-based nursing and care (Simpson, 1996, p. 22).

Furthermore, evidence-based procedures in nursing provide transparency for patients. It ensures that patients' demands for, and their right to, important information about their treatment are satisfied in order that they are able to make decisions with regard to possible nursing interventions that are based on facts (Berger, 2003, p. 34). Patients can be provided with evidence-based information that outlines the advantages and disadvantages as well as the costs and benefits of possible interventions (Colyer & Kamath, 1999, p. 190). On the basis of such information, guidelines, and standards, they are able to make decisions with regard to the measures recommended and are thus involved to a greater extent in therapy, treatment, nursing, and care (Windeler, 2003, p. 153). Accordingly, the evidence-based approach has the potential for establishing a relationship with patients based on partnership because their preferences and choices are taken into consideration in the care they receive.

At the meso level, important processes take place in which, among other things, interests are negotiated between individual institutions of the health system and funding bodies. Evidence-based procedures, guidelines, and standards can fulfill significant functions at this level. In the future, the implementation of evidence-based procedures will become an important criterion for the financial reimbursement of nursing provision by health-insurance funding schemes.

Besides helping to making sure that money is not being saved in the wrong places and that measures promising success are agreed and funded, evidence-based practice can also contribute towards preventing the introduction of unnecessary innovations despite the lack of evidence (Windeler, 2003, p. 150). By means of evidence-based procedures and standards, decisions can be made by funding bodies that lead to high-quality nursing that is not only effective but also cost-effective.

Evidence-based standards in nursing and care provide transparency for care recipients as well as funding bodies. They can be used in negotiations with funding bodies or in drawing up nursing contracts with patients who require long-term care. They have the potential for ensuring the quality of care and for contributing towards lower costs. For example, prophylactic supplies such as elbow and heel protectors for decubitus ulcers will not have to be procured if studies show that they make no effective contribution in preventing ulcers (Bräutigam, Flemming, Halfens, & Dassen, 2003, p. 75ff).

A further benefit of evidence-based nursing is that it meets the legal obligation of ensuring standards of quality. With the help of evidence-based nursing, guidelines and standards can be formulated that can be implemented in nursing institutions and care services as part of the drive to ensure quality.[2]

Moreover, training courses can be made more effective and more self-active with the help of evidence-based nursing because its origins are founded on the concept of problem-oriented learning (Brinker-Meyendriesch, 2003, p. 23ff). Within the framework of problem-oriented curricula, evidence-based nursing can form the basis of the training strategy. In this way the practical and theoretical experience of participants in training courses can be integrated, resulting in a reconciliation of theory and practice (Brinker-Meyendriesch, 2003, p. 234).

The macro level involves health policy and the decisions and measures taken at the political level. As already mentioned in the beginning of this chapter, there is a growing and louder demand for evidence-based guidelines, standards, and practice on the part of health politicians. The call for a wider application of economic principles in the health system is plainly perceptible in all political manifestos, statements, and measures. There is clear evidence of this in the demand for and introduction of management strategies in health care such as disease management, case management, and clinical pathways, which are all designed to achieve the goal of increased efficiency. It is in this context that the term "evidence-based services" must be seen, which is now appearing in political discussions as if it were already taken for granted. Legislation and measures of health policy require that nurses ensure high standards of quality in patient care and that nursing care is founded on evidence-based practice and information as a guide to decision making. Putting evidence-based nursing into practice in different settings can not only improve nursing practice and make it more transparent but it can also help the largest professional group in health care to take over tasks of responsibility in the new programs, schemes, and models that explicitly require the implementation of evidence-based practice and principles. The important function that nursing performs in the health system can be demonstrated with the help of evidence-based practice, thus generally strengthening the position of nursing within the health system (Dunn, 1998, p. 3).

If the nursing profession fails to become involved in the debate on drawing up and developing evidence-based nursing procedures and standards in the new programs, other professional groups will step in and take over the fields of activity envisaged by these new programs. The result might be that nurses will have to give up even more of their autonomy and their freedom to decide and also some of the more interesting aspects of their work. The underlying hypothesis is that in order not to make itself superfluous in health care, the nursing profession must familiarize itself with the new concepts and models, be ready to adopt them, and lay claim to the fields of activity arising from them. The significance of evidence-based nursing lies in the fact that especially programs like disease management and case management offer interesting fields of work for nursing institutions and facilities, as experience has shown in various countries like the United States, Great Britain, and Australia. The nursing profession should (and must) ask where and how it can cooperate effectively in the new programs with its own evidence-based knowledge and procedures. At the macro level, besides evaluating the potential of new strategies, programs and legal measures and their significance for the nursing profession, the task of nursing management and nursing science must be to develop future options and future visions.

LIMITATIONS AND THE PROBLEMS OF EVIDENCE-BASED NURSING

Evidence-based practice is nevertheless an issue of considerable controversy in nursing literature. One of the main problems discussed is the lack of clinically relevant research and of randomized studies in nursing (English & Bond, 1998, p. 7; Manton, 1998, p. 1). A study undertaken in Great Britain counted 522 randomized controlled trials published in nursing research (Roberts, 1999, p. 17). Considering that nurses represent the largest professional group within the health system, this can be regarded as a relatively small number. It must be assumed, moreover, that no randomized and controlled studies are available in many aspects of nursing (Closs & Cheater, 1999, p. 14).

Many studies carried out in nursing research involve small random samples; as a rule, they are not funded by external sources and are often undertaken in the researcher's spare time (English & Bond, 1998, p. 7). On account of these inadequacies the findings cannot always be generalized (English & Bond, 1998, p. 7). Moreover, although in some areas there is an abundance of research findings, their validity is often very limited with regard to the efficacy of the measures to be taken (English & Bond, 1998, p. 7). Frequently, general recommendations are given on the benefit of nursing interventions but the characteristics as well as the possible effects and side effects of these measures are not taken into consideration (English & Bond, 1998, p. 7). This means that the studies fail to provide any clear criteria for practitioners as to which nursing interventions and measures are appropriate for which groups of patients (English & Bond, 1998, p. 8). Furthermore, many studies in nursing research are carried out on a qualitative basis. Unlike quantitative research, qualitative studies cannot provide any information on cause-and-effect relationships, efficacy, reliability, and so forth, nor can their results be generalized. The advantage of qualitative findings, however, is their greater validity and the fact that they can provide data on processes, meanings, and situations.

Apart from this, however, there is the general lack of research in certain aspects of nursing. In other words, in many areas the efficacy and the benefits of certain nursing interventions and measures have so far not been established, with the result that many questions arising in practical nursing cannot yet be given an evidence-based answer at all (Naish, 1997, p. 65). The lack of research can be partly explained by the fact that nursing still has difficulty in defining itself and its areas of work, so that it is hard to determine nursing measures and nursing outcomes (Naish, 1997, p. 66). In many countries, nurses' tasks and fields of activity have not yet been clearly defined, meaning that the operationalization, definition, and demarcation of nursing interventions and procedures is difficult.

Furthermore, the studies carried out in nursing research vary with regard to fulfilling standards of quality. Not all the studies published have been carried out correctly and with adequate thoroughness (Gerrish & Clayton, 1998, p. 59). Frequently, they display methodological as well as conceptual weaknesses. In many cases their findings are not comparable because of their use of different methods. Especially problematic, according to Panfil and Wurster (2001), are national expert standards, which are to be drawn up at the national level for frequently occurring nursing phenomena and problems, because these are often based on the lowest level of evidence, namely reasoned expert opinions (p. 35).[3]

Yet even if evidence-based information for taking measures of nursing intervention is available to nurses, the regulation of the health system does not enable them to prescribe, let alone carry out, evidence-based interventions on their own. In many health systems, nurses are dependent on doctors' instructions and are not allowed to take appropriate measures independently (Naish, 1997, p. 66). This means that in numerous areas, evidence-based nursing practice is only possible in collaboration with medical staff.

Furthermore, health care provision generally has a multidisciplinary orientation. It may be that evidence exists for a specific medical intervention but there is a lack of evidence generally for the organization of nursing and care, for the effectiveness of nursing and rehabilitation, and for the efficacy and the effects of most routine measures (Roberts, 1999, p. 22). It is these factors that make multidisciplinary, evidence-based health provision and patient care all the more difficult.

A number of obstacles are to be found in nursing practice itself, that is, in the organization and structure of nursing facilities and services. According to an Australian study, one of these problems is that nursing practitioners do not show sufficient willingness to put research findings into practice (Wallace, Shorten, & Russell, 1997, p. 149). The main obstacles named in the literature that prevent the implementation of evidence-based nursing practice are that nurses often lack the time; have difficulty understanding research articles; have a negative attitude towards research; are afraid of staff cuts and only have limited access to databases and journals; and have little experience of library searches and research tools (Nagy, Lumby, McKinley, & Macfarlane, 2001, pp. 319–320; Simpson, 1996, p. 23). The shift away from a nursing practice based on customs and personal experience towards an inquiring and reflective nursing practice is seen as one of the main difficulties in establishing evidence-based nursing (Simpson, 1996, p. 24).

The gap between theory and practice undoubtedly plays a major role in these problems. Carrying out and applying the methods of evidence-based nursing means that greater demands are made of nursing staff. Nurses must possess certain competences in order to be able (a) to formulate the question, (b) to carry out research on the literature in databases, and (c) to undertake an appropriate evaluation of the literature. Besides possessing sufficient knowledge of methods, they must also have the ability to make critical appraisals. They must be able to review the specialist literature with a critical eye as well as to analyze it and make appropriate use of it. A further requirement is that nurses have a certain knowledge of epidemiology, and a third requirement is that they have skills and competences at the personal level: Nurses must be prepared to question their own actions (critical self-evaluation), to change their perspective, and to set priorities. To sum up, this means that nursing staff must be trained in the strategies and procedures of evidence-based nursing practice.

There is evidence indicating that the success of evidence-based nursing and the degree to which it is implemented depends to a considerable extent on how the management of nursing facilities and services encourage and require awareness for, and the use of, research findings in nursing practice (Gerrish & Clayton, 1998, p. 59). An appraisal carried out in Great Britain of the implementation of evidence-based practice has revealed, however, that hospitals and nursing facilities and services often possess neither the time nor the organizational and technical resources—such as information, instruments, books, materials, libraries, and so forth—that are essential for putting evidence-based procedures in place (Gerrish & Clayton, 1998, p. 59).

The demand that clinical decisions be taken according to the hierarchy of the evidence may be a disadvantage. The highest level of the hierarchy is taken up by randomized control trials. The drawback of randomized studies is that only a section of the initially evaluated population is included in the studies. Thus, the evidence is based on a carefully selected population of patients. It may be difficult, therefore, to apply these results to individual patients since comorbidity is not taken into consideration in the studies (Gerrish & Clayton, 1998, p. 59; Hoppe, 2003, p. 822). The focus of clinically relevant studies, moreover, is often very narrow. As a rule, studies of this kind investigate one aspect of an intervention but do not necessarily consider the individual aspects of the patients concerned, which may lessen the efficacy of a measure that is taken (Roberts, 1999, p. 22).

Additionally, putting evidence-based nursing into practice may be made difficult by the patients' lack of compliance. Compliance, that is, following evidence-based recommendations, guidelines, and standards, is based to some extent on patients' personalities. It is quite possible that they alter the measures recommended on their own, whether with regard to the amount, the extent, or even the form of the measure. According to Hoppe it appears particularly difficult to implement evidence-based measures that are related to smoking, eating, and exercising habits (Hoppe, 2003, p. 822).

A large number of tasks and activities in nursing cannot be reduced in every case to evidence-based measures, decisions, and standards. The tasks and activities of nursing are far more complex and are based to a very large degree on interaction, communication, and human care. These are human actions that cannot be measured at all, nor can they be standardized or shown to be effective in any way. This leads to the problem that scientific evidence cannot be gathered for all areas of nursing practice (Roberts, 1999, p. 22). In a number of spheres of health care it is not possible to carry out methodologically well-planned and carefully implemented qualitative and quantitative research. Further, there are certain issues and fields of practical work in which it is not ethically appropriate to undertake studies (Roberts, 1999, p. 22). Nursing has a social duty to perform: It must abide by the principles of caring and of acting humanely according to ethical maxims. Nevertheless, it is possible to examine certain tasks and interventions of nursing practice from the perspective of their effectiveness and their benefits. Acting ethically and appropriately in nursing also means that patients receive the measures and interventions that have proved to be beneficial and effective.

WHAT FORM OF NURSING SCIENCE AND RESEARCH DOES EVIDENCE-BASED NURSING PRACTICE NEED?

It does not suffice to demand merely that evidence-based nursing be put into practice. A major role in implementing evidence-based procedures is played by nursing science and research. In order to implement evidence-based nursing, practitioners need practice-oriented research. Without corresponding research in the specialist fields of nursing, it will not be possible to put evidence-based nursing into practice. This is an overall precondition for the entire field of nursing if this demand is to be met.

In nursing science and research, relevant studies and investigations must be carried out that have to fulfill certain criteria. For this purpose it is essential to develop a culture of research that is concerned with the evaluation, the control, and the efficacy of nursing interventions and measures. Gerrish and Clayton demand that nursing science and research should define its own clear agenda (1998, p. 59). A further task of nursing science consists of thinking over strategies for disseminating the results of this research and how they might find their way into nursing practice. Books and publications are indeed only part of the process of putting theory into practice. It is the task of nursing scientists and researchers not only to make available the knowledge base but also to develop ways and means of transferring this knowledge to nursing practice.

In recent years there has been a general quantitative increase in nursing research in many countries. However, this research has largely been carried out at universities by nursing scientists whose work has been focused on developing nursing as a scientific discipline. In order to be able to carry out evidence-based nursing in practice, though, a much greater extent of clinical research must be undertaken in nursing and care. This means that clinical problems of nursing must be documented, as well as areas of practice in which there is a great need for evidence or in which little or no research at all has been carried out to date (Nagy et al., 2001, p. 319).

Studies are needed that are very carefully planned and carried out and that are closely related to the actual situation of the nursing and care given. They must be reliable and relevant contributions to the concrete shaping of nursing measures and interventions. In their intention, planning, and design they must be capable of having an effect on the provision of nursing and care. From this kind of research, decisions can be taken about the shaping of nursing practice on a well-founded empirical basis (Windeler, 2003, pp. 149–150).

In summary, the following requirements, here briefly stated, must be met by nursing science and research:

1. establishing (also by surveying practitioners) problems relevant to nursing practice and carrying out high-quality studies;
2. investigating the effectiveness and efficiency of interventions (outcomes research);
3. replicating studies to verify results;
4. communicating and cooperating with practitioners;
5. presenting and publishing findings in an understandable form;
6. making research results widely available;
7. publishing consumer-friendly reports on findings with recommendations for practical work (clinical relevance)

POSSIBILITIES OF PUTTING EVIDENCE-BASED NURSING INTO PRACTICE

The question arises, finally, of how evidence-based nursing can be put into practice in facilities and services that provide nursing and care. Using the methods of evidence-based practice, every single nursing practitioner can solve problems on a scientific basis. However, as outlined above, implementation is not always possible since this requires time and human effort as well as technical resources. For this reason, it seems sensible at the level of the institutions themselves to couple questions of implementing evidence-based practice with those of resources. This means that for certain nursing measures, interventions, or problems, a working group could be set up to carry out the steps of implementing evidence-based practice. Such working groups have the additional advantage that there is more likelihood that scientific knowledge will be put into actual daily practice and also more likelihood that the right questions will be asked and answered. In the implementation of evidence-based practice (EBP) in institutions of health care a distinction can be made between **general** and **concrete** options of implementation. Successful implementation, however, presupposes that managers and administrators of institutions of nursing and care pay heed to certain strategies:

1. EBP must become a *corporate goal.*
2. *Supporting a climate for EBP.* Management must promote an awareness for problems among staff. Nurses must be motivated to carry out evidence-based procedures. According to research, an awareness for problems and the use of research findings depend to a large extent on whether, and if so, how institution managers and leaders promote these aspects and also require them from their staff (Funk, Champagne, Tornquist, & Wiese, 1995, p. 44).
3. *Assessing the consequences.* At the planning stage the organizational and financial consequences of an institution's EBP-oriented policy must be considered. Institutions must have answers to the following questions from the very beginning: What are the costs and benefits of EBP for particular problems and for patient care at our institution? What clinical relevance do the problems have? Do they have the potential to help in problem solving and decision making? Has research been carried out on the relevant problems? Do they fit into the setting? Are they reconcilable with the institution's own nursing philosophy? Are there sufficient numbers of patients for these problems?
4. *Creating the technical framework.* Rigorous implementation requires technical resources as a precondition. Accordingly, institutions must be equipped with data-processing facilities so that necessary research can be carried out and so that all members of staff can have access to all information and to evidence-based decisions, standards, and guidelines.
5. *Creating the organizational framework.* The necessary competences of nursing staff mentioned above must be taught, if the need arises, in appropriate courses of in-service training. Institution managements must give staff the time and opportunity to carry out research, analyze the literature, and develop pertinent guidelines.
6. Setting up a *working group* that formulates questions from daily practice and investigates and answers them according to the principles of evidence-based nursing.

As outlined above, the implementation of EBP is carried out according to a certain pattern. In the concrete implementation of EBP the steps might be as follows:

a. A group of nurses with the above-mentioned competencies is formed and formulates questions from daily nursing practice.

b. As a second step, the group searches out and organizes the literature. The search could and should be carried out in peer-reviewed journals such as the *Journal of Advanced Nursing, Nursing Research,* and *Evidence-based Nursing* and in databases like PubMed, Cochrane, CINAHL. First of all, the search is carried out individually and then the findings are compared with each other. The available literature is examined with the help of checklists. As a rule, these checklists are obtainable from associations of evidence-based health care. This means that a critical appraisal is made of articles with regard to validity, reliability, and possible implementation.

c. In a series of group discussions, the practical clinical relevance of the evidence is then talked over and evaluated, and the concrete, practice-related data documented and summarized. Those findings that have proved effective and beneficial are adopted for nursing measures and interventions. The information yielded by the library search can subsequently be incorporated, for example, into written agreements on practice or the institution's guidelines or standards. Using these procedures it is possible to formulate evidence-based guidelines for specific problems of patient care in institutions that provide nursing and care.

d. The institution's nursing staff is informed and, if necessary, the written agreements, measures, standards, or guidelines are discussed with them.

e. When written agreements, guidelines, or standards have been formulated, these will be applied in practice.

f. The efficacy of measures, guidelines, or standards is evaluated (1) for every single patient (case related) and (2) for the whole procedure. The relation to the case can only be checked by the nurse concerned in direct contact with the patient. The parameters that must be taken into consideration here include the following:

1. Do the research findings apply to this particular patient?
2. How great are the benefits and the possible adverse effects for this patient?
3. What are the preferences and the values and beliefs of this patient?
4. How great is the feasibility in this individual case?

The critical appraisal of measures, guidelines, and standards can take the form of patient surveys, for example, or it can be achieved by drawing up outcome parameters. Here, the quality of life, hospital admissions, or complications could be gauged.

The following measures may be formulated as general forms of implementation of EBP in institutions and services:

- Organizing *journal clubs.* At regular intervals, for example, once a month or every 6 months, the latest literature on the specific clinical patterns, nursing interventions, and measures of each institution are analyzed and discussed. Any new findings must be integrated into patient care and, if necessary, into the institution's guidelines and standards. Nursing procedures must be adapted to the latest state of research.
- *Presenting research findings.* By means of in-service training courses and conferences on specialist issues held at the institution or elsewhere, nurses must be familiarized with evidence-based practice along with the latest developments and research findings. It may also be possible to invite researchers to present their own findings on relevant topics. This might help to close the gap between theory and practice, with practitioners supplying researchers with questions from daily practice that require investigation and researchers passing on the results of research to practitioners.
- *Written reports.* In this case the institution's own announcements, directives, books, dissertations, theses, and publications on relevant topics could be made available to all members of staff.
- *Making available relevant journals and materials* so that researchers have easy access to published reports to support their research. Should this option be too expensive because of the high costs involved, cooperation with other institutions in the vicinity, such as hospitals, university libraries, and so forth, might be envisaged in order that journals and specialist publications can be shared.
- *During the development or implementation phase of EBP in nursing institutions* experts could be consulted. They could advise the practitioners, evaluate the process of implementation and provide scientific support.
- *Starting annual reports* on the institution's own progress, on the updating of guidelines, and the appraisal of the innovations in order to ensure transparency and to inform the staff about the success or failure of the measures.

NOTES

1. In his *Effectiveness and Efficiency,* Cochrane wrote, "and the Social Services seem to be evolving in exactly the same unfortunate way as medicine by suggesting that wherever there is a social 'need' a social worker must be appointed whether or not there is any evidence that the social worker can alter the natural history of the social problem" (1972, p. 68).

2. Shorten & Wallace put it this way: According to the law, nurses and carers are obliged to offer patients the choice of whether they wish to be nursed on the basis of precise and relevant information or not (1997, p. 23).

3. For example, guidelines for decubitus ulcer prevention (decubitus standard)

REFERENCES

Antes, G. (1998). EBM praktizieren [Practicing EBM]. In M. Perleth & G. Antes (Eds.), *Evidenz-basierte Medizin. Wissenschaft im Praxisalltag* (pp. 19–26). München, Germany: MMV Medizin.

Behrens, J. (2003). Evidence-based nursing: Pflegerische Entscheidungen in bestverfügbarer Kenntnis ihrer Wirkungen [Evidence-based nursing. Decision making in nursing on a base of available knowledge of health effects]. In M. Landenberger et al. (Eds.), *Pflegepfade in Europa. Neue Forschungsergebnisse und Praxisprojekte aus Pflege, Management und Gesundheitspolitik in Europa* (pp. 92–110). Frankfurt, Germany: Mabuse.

Berger, M. (2003). Am Ende der Aufklärung steht das Goldene Kalb [At the end of enlightenment there is the golden calf]. *GGW, 3*(2), 29–35.

Bräutigam, K., Flemming, A., Halfens, R., & Dassen, T. (2003). Dekubitusprävention: Theorie und Praxis [Pressure ulcer prevention. Theory and practice]. *Pflege, 16,* 75–82.

Brinker-Meyendriesch, E. (2003). Evidenzbasierung: Wissen, Handeln und Lernen in der Pflege [Evidence based: Knowing, acting and learning in nursing]. *Pflege, 16,* 230–235.

Closs, S. J., & Cheater, F. M. (1999). Evidence for nursing practice: A clarification of the issues. *Journal of Advanced Nursing, 30,* 10–17.

Cochrane, A. L. (1972). *Effectiveness and efficiency. Random reflections on health services.* London: Nuffield Provincial Hospitals Trust.

Colyer, H., & Kamath, P. (1999). Evidence-based practice. A philosophical and political analysis: Some matters for consideration by professional practitioners. *Journal of Advanced Nursing, 29,* 188–193.

Dunn, S. (1998). Perspectives on evidence-based practice [Editorial]. *Australian Critical Care, 1,* 2–4.

English, C., & Bond, S. (1998). Evidence-based nursing: Easier said than done. *Pediatric Nursing, 5,* 7–11.

Funk, S. G., Champagne, M. T., Tornquist, E. M., & Wiese, R. A. (1995). Administrators' views on barriers to research utilization. *Applied Nursing Research, 8*, 44–49.

Gerrish, K., & Clayton, J. (1998). Improving clinical effectiveness through an evidence-based approach: Meeting the challenge for nursing in the United Kingdom. *Nursing Administration Quarterly, 22*, 55–65.

Hasseler, M. (1999). Evidenz-basierte Praxis [Evidence-based practice]. *Dr. med. Mabuse, 122*, 20–23.

Hoppe, U. C. (2003). Warum werden Leitlinien nicht befolgt? [Why are guidelines ignored?] *Deutsche Medizinische Wochenschrift, 128*, 820–824.

Lühmann, D. (1998). EBM: Umsetzung von Studienergebnissen in die Praxis [EBM: Realization of research results in practice]. In M. Perleth & G. Antes (Eds.), *Evidenz-basierte Medizin. Wissenschaft im Praxisalltag* (pp. 48–55). München, Germany: MMV Medizin.

Manton, A. (1998). President's message. Validating what we do: A word about evidence-based practice. *Journal of Emergency Nursing, 1*, 1–2.

Muir Gray, J. A. (1997). *Evidence-based health care.* New York: Churchill Livingstone.

Nagy, S., Lumby, J., McKinley, S., & Macfarlane, C. (2001). Nurses' belief about the conditions that hinder or support evidence-based nursing. *International Journal of Nursing Practice, 7*, 314–321.

Naish, J. (1997). So where's the evidence? *Nursing Times, 12*, 64–66.

Panfil, E. M., & Wurster, J. (2001). Professioneller Pflegen geht nicht?! [Professional nursing as good as it gets?!] *Dr. med. Mabuse, 131*, 33–36.

Perleth, M. (1998). Evidenz-basierte Medizin: eine Einführung [Evidence-based medicine: An introduction]. In M. Perleth & G. Antes (Eds.), *Evidenz-basierte Medizin. Wissenschaft im Praxisalltag* (pp. 13–18). München, Germany: MMV Medizin.

Porzsolt, F., & Sigle, F. (1998). EBM: Interpretation von Studienergebnisse zu therapeutischen Verfahren [EBM: Interpretation of research results in therapeutic procedures]. In M. Perleth & G. Antes (Eds.), *Evidenz-basierte Medizin. Wissenschaft im Praxisalltag* (pp. 37–47). München, Germany: MMV Medizin.

Roberts, R. (1999). *Information for evidence-based care.* Abingdon, UK: Radcliff Medical Press.

Sackett, D. L. (1998). Was ist Evidenz-basierte Medizin? [What is evidence-based medicine?] In M. Perleth & G. Antes (Eds.), *Evidenz-basierte Medizin. Wissenschaft im Praxisalltag* (pp. 9–12). München, Germany: MMV Medizin.

Shorten, A., & Wallace, M. (1997). Evidence-based practice. The future is clear. *Australian Nursing Journal, 6*, 22–24.

Simpson, B. (1996). Evidence-based nursing practice: The state of the art. *The Canadian Nurse, 10*, 22–25.

Thompson, C. (2003). Clinical experience as evidence in evidence-based practice. *Journal of Advanced Nursing, 43,* 230–237.

Wallace, M. C., Shorten, A., & Russell, K. G. (1997). Paving the way: Stepping stones to evidence-based nursing. *International Journal of Nursing Practice, 3,* 147-152.

White, S. J. (1998). Evidence-based practice and nursing: The new panacea? *British Journal of Nursing, 3,* 175–178.

Windeler, J. (2003). Medizinische Versorgung gestalten—evidenz-basierte Medizin als Chance [Designing medical services—Evidence-based medicine as a chance]. *Gesundheitswesen, 65,* 149–154.

CHAPTER 14

Transculturality and Nursing[*]

Birgit Rommelspacher

There is a great deal of controversy in the literature regarding the concepts of culture, interculturality, multiculturality, and transculturality. For example, the traditional conception of culture is based on the acceptance of differences and separateness among groups of people, often distinguished by geographic and ancestral belongingness, in terms of organized patterning in the ways of people's lives. This conception emphasizes the uniqueness of people as distinct groups, a setting apart from other groups through "social homogenization, ethnic consolidation, and intercultural delimitation" (Welsch, 1999, p. 194). This notion of culture is currently viewed by many as untenable and inappropriate, because people's affiliations, the forming of life patterns and styles, and acquiring knowledge are influenced greatly by migration, globalization, communication networks, and mobility, which creates and results in a mixing of cultural traditions at all levels of social life. However, the term *culture* is not always used precisely, often referring either to its traditional meaning or to broader, all-encompassing, and common-sense meanings of the word. Uzarewicz (1999) goes further to suggest that "culture is revealed to be a purely notional construct that has no concrete equivalent in empirical reality" (p. 71). Furthermore, the concepts of interculturality,

---

[*]Translated from German by Gerald Nixon.

multiculturality, and transculturality are not used precisely either, sometimes with no differentiation among them and used inter-changeably.

Nonetheless, culture and cultural considerations come to have significance in nursing as nursing is practiced in a rapidly changing cultural scene in which people live, work, and carry on together, though they come from various cultural orientations or backgrounds, from different regional, ethnic, or affiliational origins, and hold commitments to diverse belief systems and customs. What is problematic is that most nursing establishments in Western societies are monocultural and monolingual in orientation in their conceptions and guiding principles, even though many of their staff and their patients come from different cultural backgrounds. In this respect, these nursing establishments mirror society: they provide monocultural answers to a multicultural living environment.

This is seemingly contradicted by quite a number of publications that have taken up the issue of interculturality or transculturality in nursing, for example, *Multikulturelle Pflege [Multicultural Nursing]* (Alban, Leininger, & Reynolds, 2000), in which more than 50 countries from Afghanistan to Vietnam are presented with data on their "geography and demography," their conception of health and illness, as well as the "social" and "physical" elements of life. In the German edition, however, one finds no mention of Germany and its culture. The editors probably assume that the specialist readership the book addresses is of German origin. Thus, from the outset it is not addressed to non-Germans. Yet even if we presume that everyone working in nursing in Germany is familiar with German culture, this experiential knowledge cannot take the place of inward reflection on how, for example, one views oneself in society and how one views "others" and what consequences these views, or the "German" structures in the health service, have on the situation of nursing. That is, the subject of a teaching book on transcultural nursing ought to be the question of how experiential knowledge can be converted into reflexive knowledge. After all, the teaching book referred to above takes it for granted that the acquisition of knowledge about others improves competence in an intercultural nursing environment. Indeed, this too can be called into question.

Accordingly, the purpose of this chapter is to look in more detail at the extent to which such a culture-specific approach is helpful and which new problems might arise from it. I will then examine the question of the advantages and disadvantages that result from this approach as compared to a universalist approach, which highlights similarities and demands the same nursing for everyone, irrespective of origin, appearance, and culture. The basic features of transcultural competence will be developed next along with the conditions required for transcultural change. The final section addresses theoretical ideas regarding transculturality in nursing. I use the German background to illustrate these points of discussion. As in many European societies as well as the United States, Germany has experienced a mixing of many cultures during the past four decades, more actively during the past two. This has raised the questions of culture, interculturality, multiculturality, and transculturality not only at the level of society in general but also within various sectors of social life including health care and nursing.

Culture-Specific Approaches

Culture-specific approaches in nursing are based on a full awareness of heterogeneity and multiculturality in the nursing environment and attempt to respond to this. It is assumed that nursing is a field in which people of different cultures, ethnicities, and nationalities come together and that these differences are accepted and recognized.

However, the question is how these differences are seen, that is, not only which differences are regarded as relevant and how they should be handled but also which differences are not mentioned at all. This means that right from the start it must be clarified whether the differences identified here are in fact the truly decisive ones, namely, whether in certain constellations the different cultures are actually the problem at all. Equally, one might ask whether problems inevitably arise whenever people from different cultural backgrounds interact. Do natural and successful encounters not exist? Or, when there are conflicts, are they really caused by cultural differences?

Culture is the way in which a group of human beings interprets and responds to its physical and social environment and thus the way in which human beings themselves constantly reform and further develop their environment. Culture is therefore a dynamic process and differs from context to context. Culture can be regarded as a set of social practices in which, according to Paul Mecheril (2002), it is not only a matter of implementing norms but also of harnessing resources (p. 22). Consequently, it includes the circumstances in which people live, their way of managing these circumstances, and the resources they have available to do so. In our context, culture means above all how illness and disease are interpreted and which resources we have available—and harness—in order to prevent, alleviate, and cure illness and disease.

However, there always exists a certain relationship between one's own culture and other cultures because cultures only develop in interaction with each other. After millennia of conflict, for instance, collective images form that are imparted to the members of a particular culture by means of legends and stories and through art, literature, and science. That is why there are very different images of the "others" and why, at the same time, these images are clear-cut and unambiguous. In my seminars, for example, when I ask what images my students have of Moslems, Jews, or Roma, they all very quickly agree on what these people look like; at the same time, the images held differ greatly from student to student. Thus, one's own cultural stamp is also revealed in who is perceived to be different and how this otherness is invested with images. (For a more detailed discussion of this, see Rommelspacher, 2002.)

A distinction is also to be made in this connection between the terms *transculturality* and *interculturality*. Although the latter lays greater emphasis on the relationship between two different positions and perspectives, the former focuses on what is similar—and not only the similarities that exist beyond cultural differences but also those that arise as a product of intercultural interaction.

According to the book cited at the beginning of the article, *multicultural nursing* is characterized by the fact that people from one country interact with people from different countries of origin and that the latter are marked by the typical way of life of the particular country from which they come. This has very little to do, however, with the reality of multicultural nursing because most of the people we are talking about have come to the country as immigrants or refugees (or for other reasons, perhaps, such as to marry or study), and in some cases have lived here for generations. Their culture is not identical with what is typical in their country of origin; it is a result of their status as migrants and their own specific migration culture, that is, the process of coming to terms with the circumstances of life they find here. If, however, they are simply identified with the culture or nation of their home country, they are to some extent symbolically forced out of the country to which they have migrated.

Here, finally, a static, self-contained image of culture is built up. Imagine having to describe the attitude of your own country towards health and illness in only a few pages and depicting in short sections the "social and physical elements" of life here. This does not mean that such descriptions cannot also provide useful information and thus sharpen people's awareness that different people have different customs. But this has to be set in relation to the problems that arise from identifying people from different social and cultural backgrounds with the picture that is drawn of them here. Cultures are seen here as systems of meaning that are strictly divided from each other, detached from developments of time and space, and are rigid and homogeneous. And human beings are described as bearing the unique imprint of the culture they belong to. This explains why, for example, Germans or Americans are rightly incensed when they go abroad and are identified as such, with (often negative) clichés. This is felt to be not only incorrect but also highly unfair.

Yet what happens when the "others" do not match the picture one has drawn of them? In a study of bicultural partnerships, Iman Attia (1994) asked German Christian women and men who had Moslem partners how they pictured Moslems. The survey revealed that although they all had a very clear-cut picture of Moslems, their partners—the Moslems they lived with and loved—were quite different from such images. They were not really Moslems, the respondents explained; they had already become "Europeanized." This means that if the people involved do not fit the cliché, they are simply declared exceptions to the rule and turned into non-Moslems. Instead of the cliché's being revised, reality is remolded. The others are then simply not "real" Moslems; it is preferable to deprive them of their identity than to change the cliché. Here, a paradox manifests itself: Through a culturalist prism, the culture of the others is made invisible. For if the others do not come up to one's culturalist expectations, they are, in a sense, expelled from the community. The Turkish woman is not a true Turk any longer because she is emancipated; the Jew is not a real Jew because he is not religious.

Furthermore, it is not to be assumed that clichés that have been stored over the many years of socialization and constantly kept up to date through everyday discussions and media reports can easily be revised by personal encounters, even if these encounters are as intensive as in a partnership. On the contrary, we must assume that everyone encounters the others with certain images in mind. In intercultural situations, therefore, it is not as if totally unprejudiced people from different cultural backgrounds come into contact with each other out of the blue. The opposite is true: They all bring along with them the collective images they have drawn of the others, and these pictures are activated during their encounters. In order to be able to accept others as they see themselves, it is necessary first to take leave of these images. If we really wish to encounter others openly and be curious about them, we must discard certain things we have learned instead of accumulating further images and confirming old prejudices (Castro Varela, 2002).

Frequently, the others have to justify it when they do not match the images we have created. Indeed, not matching can be interpreted as a direct insult by members of the majority group—for haven't they made so much conscious effort to learn something about the culture of the others and haven't they signalled their willingness to attune themselves to the others? If the others ignore this or even feel discriminated against by being identified with a cliché, the members of the majority group are disappointed or infuriated because the others have failed to acknowledge their efforts.

Conversely, the acceptance and recognition of the others means that one sees their perspective and respects their views. This presupposes that one listens to them and that one is also prepared to correct one's own views, thus admitting there are many things one does not know. The others are experts in their own affairs. In this sense Paul Mecheril talks of intercultural competence as being an "interlocking of knowledge and ignorance" (2002, p. 28).

By contrast, *culturalist knowledge*—that is, a knowledge that ascribes a certain, fixed culture to the others—runs the risk of molding them into a "prescribed otherness," which deprives them of their subjectivity and ultimately renders them invisible in their cultural distinctiveness.

Acknowledging the perspective of the others, however, presupposes mutual respect, and this can by no means be taken for granted. As surveys have repeatedly shown, Germans place foreigners, immigrants and asylum-seekers into very different categories. Arabs, Roma, and asylum-seekers from African countries are placed at the bottom end of the scale, while people from western European countries and other highly developed industrial nations are ranked higher. That this categorization is not determined by geographical distance but by economic, political, and cultural prestige can be seen in the fact that eastern Europeans, although they are Germany's neighbors, are ranked much lower than western Europeans or Americans.

This ethnic hierarchy is undeniably present in health care and affects not only individual encounters between nursing staff and patients but also structural measures that an institution implements in the organization of nursing. For why should health care be an exception? Why should other laws apply to nursing than to society as a whole? In virtually all societies, otherness, or foreignness, is always related to social hierarchies. The horizontal (so to speak), neutral plane of difference is linked to the vertical plane of hierarchy. There are scarcely any multiethnic societies in which different groups live with each other side by side in harmony and on equal terms. Hence, as a rule, we must assume that "ethnic strata" exist (Esser, 2000).

In this respect a culturalist perspective, where problems between people from different cultural backgrounds are attributed solely to cultural differences, is inadequate because it fails to take account of this ethnic hierarchy. At the same time, it ignores the fact that we perhaps do not want to know anything about the others because their otherness maintains a distance that helps secure our own status and that gives nourishment to fantasies of superiority.

No doubt there are many people working in health care who sincerely make an effort to treat patients equally and as well as they possibly can, no matter what they look like and what background they come from. However, more than goodwill is necessary in order to counteract the powerful and ubiquitous tendency to form hierarchies. Beyond structural measures, which are examined below, we need reflexive knowledge, that is, knowledge about the motives that underlie our own theory and practice, and knowledge about the consequences this may have for the others. This also includes competence in making analyses in order to recognize more subtle forms of hierarchy building.

In the book on multicultural nursing referred to above, for example, a standard situation is quite naturally assumed to be one in which a German nurse looks after a patient from another country. Apart from the fact, as we have seen, that the majority of cases involve migrants and not foreigners, there is always a clear and unequivocal distribution of roles. The nurse is German and thus belongs to the prevailing, or majority culture while the patient is the foreigner. Yet members of minority cultures are also professionals, that is, agents and subjects. If this had been recognized, the book would also be addressed to them; they ought, for example, to learn something about Germany (or the United States).

It is also possible, however, that members of a minority culture are assumed to possess intercultural competence per se. Even if it can be supposed that in the course of their lives they have had to deal with intercultural situations much more frequently than members of the majority culture, transcultural competence would also be for them a matter of transforming their everyday, experiential knowledge into reflexive knowledge. The "standard situation" in the teaching book also leads implicitly to a reproduction of a power hierarchy in which the needs of the migrants are not satisfied by the nursing staff so that they are also rendered invisible, as it were.

In the following example, too, an ethnic hierarchy within the nursing staff is reproduced. A patient on a ward refused to be looked after by a Black nurse, using a racial slur to let it be known that she would not have a Black person lay hands on her. The nurse in question reported that some of her colleagues were sorry about the incident and several had even rebuked the patient but most of them ignored it. Most of them, however, were also of the opinion that the Black colleague should not take the incident so seriously. The outcome was that a German nurse was assigned to the patient. This seemed to be the most sensible solution for everyone involved—except for the Black nurse herself.

But how would this conflict have been solved if a patient of Turkish origin had refused to be looked after by a German nurse? In all probability such a situation is scarcely imaginable and if it did occur, most people would doubtless advise the patient, without hesitation and in all firmness, to bow to the inevitable—along the lines that "they should be thankful they get such good treatment here."

In both cases the professionals possess a different authority, one taken for granted and unchallengeable, the other questioned and unprotected. Here, it is a question of the distribution of *symbolic power:* the question, namely, of what rank people have in society, who possesses prestige, whose voice is heard, and whose is silenced. Even in the smallest groups, members often have a different standing. One person's word carries more weight than another's. This symbolic power is distributed over many forms of everyday behavior and includes situations in nursing.

In transcultural nursing, therefore, it is not only a matter of cultural differences on the quasi horizontal plane, that is, the diversity resulting from differences in perspectives and habits; it is also always a question of the vertical plane, that is, the differences resulting from the fact that people are classified differently on the scale of social status and have different opportunity of access to social resources. And frequently foreignness is merely used as an excuse in order to justify and to preserve this social hierarchy.

Nevertheless, the culture-specific approach is of great significance for transcultural nursing because it emphasizes that different cultural perspectives exist and that in health care, both institutions and staff have to adapt themselves to this reality. The determining factor, though, is whether respect is expressed for the perspective of the others; or whether, in accordance with a culturalist approach, new certainties are accumulated about the difference of the others, which ultimately eliminates them by assimilating them into one's own conceptions.

Precisely because of the danger of "making differences" as one acknowledges that differences exist, it is important for everyone to treat all people equally.

THE UNIVERSALIST APPROACH

Treating all people equally is a basic concern of human ethics and democratic self-understanding. In order to treat people equally, however, it may indeed be necessary to make differences—that is to say, to treat differently things (or people) that are different. Having the same value is not identical with being of the same kind, hence the distinction between "equality" and "sameness." Thus, the desire to treat all people equally may serve to reinforce differences.

In intercultural encounters, differences always play a role, not only in the perception of the members of the majority culture but also in that of the members of the minority culture. Different associations and emotions are evoked, formed during long years of socialization. These patterns of reaction, furthermore, are not just personal matters or individual false perceptions but are based on cultural stereotypes that in many cases have formed over a period of centuries in a society and are continuously reproduced in current public discourses.

These images, however, also have a function for our own self-image. In my research for a study on anti-Semitism, for example, non-Jewish Germans reported to me that in conversation, the situation changed at once when they learned that the person they were talking to was Jewish. They had the feeling, they said, that suddenly a chasm had formed between them that was almost impossible to bridge (Rommelspacher, 1995). They were no longer neutral and spontaneous, knowing neither how to behave nor what to say or not say.

So-called *interactive tension* arises. From a psychodynamic point of view, this is caused by our preoccupation with warding off prejudices, guilty consciences, and feelings of resentment. The effort needed to repress our own emotions and associations consumes our entire energy. In order to compensate for the ensuing uncertainty, a show is often made of being overly friendly. These are seldom conscious processes. In this respect, the effort made to treat others equally, even when social status factually differs, is often an attempt to protect ourselves from what we do not like to admit about ourselves. Like the young German women who were interviewed, we would not want to belong to a German society of victimizers, preferring—with a neutral, open-minded attitude that embraces all people—to refuse to belong to our own culture. Elaine Pinderhughes (1989) observed a similar phenomenon in encounters between White American nurses and Black patients. Here, too, in their encounters with Blacks, Whites wished to shake off their "whiteness" in favor of a general humanism.

What this implies for counselling situations has been analyzed in detail by the therapist Ursula Wachendorfer (1999, 2000), who takes as her example the relationship between White therapists and Black clients. With the implicit or explicit basic assumption—"I don't make differences; we're all equal"—the therapist signals, on the one hand, a fundamental attitude that is open, humanist, and democratic. This, however, detaches the therapeutic relationship from the prevailing social power structures. Moreover, the White therapist negates the significance of skin color for herself, thus hindering any confrontation with her own ideas about, and feelings towards, Black people, which as a White person she has interiorized in the course of her socialization. In this respect, the postulate of equality or neutrality is to be seen not so much as consideration towards Black clients but rather in its protective function of the White therapist, who tries in this way to fend off her own negative ideas and feelings and protect her "positive self."

In a society that regards itself as democratic, this means that the monocultural perspective is reinterpreted as an egalitarian one. By focusing on what we have in common, the others are assimilated, and if this does not succeed, they are perceived to be obstructions in the nursing routine and considered deficient. The solution then lies in appealing to people's *tolerance*, which endures even the unusual. For the others, however, this tolerance is no guarantee of security but rather puts this security at the mercy of individual and social tolerance levels. When those limits are reached, demands are made that the others adapt and assume their (lower) place in the hierarchy. Thus, on closer scrutiny the perspective that did not seem specifically cultural turns out to be a deculturization of the majority position because it represents the neutral and universally human, the position of tolerance. By contrast, the others become culturalized because if they do not find their place in the system, it must be due to their special cultural affiliation or to their individual inability.

The *practices of monoculturality*, that is, the inability or reluctance to accept different perspectives, are thus reinterpreted and turned into a problem of the others. They are made responsible for the problems because they are "deviant" and it is we who represent the norm. If people from different cultural backgrounds obtain no proper access to nursing facilities and do not claim support in such a way that they also receive it, then it must be their own fault. They cannot make themselves understood, it is then said, or they are simply from a traditional culture that clashes with modern institutions.

This means that in a monocultural outlook, one's own ideas and values are generalized and thus, when applied to the others, naturally gain validity for them, too. An example of this is the individualism underlying Western cultures, which regards individuals as primarily independent of their collective relationships and would like to protect them as such. This is reflected, for instance, in the tendency of nurses to encourage independence among patients or to psychologize illness as personal suffering. And this is also seen, for example, when migrants expect immediate, active, and more symptom-oriented action on the part of nursing staff, which is in contradiction to a problem-oriented and introspective approach. A psychologizing view often fails to take the somatic illness seriously and culminates in the reproach that migrants concentrate on somatic phenomena rather than tackling their psychological problems (Domenig, 2003, p. 89).

Criticism is also raised about the fact that patients are "spoiled" by their families, who try to do everything for them and are continuously there to look after them. The care and attention given to women after childbirth, for example, contradicts the staff's professional aim of enabling patients to regain their personal independence and competences as quickly as possible (Domenig, p. 93). The question that arises here is whether autonomy, in the sense of self-determination, really is the absolute standard by which all other values must be measured; or whether a self-understanding primarily defined through relationships to others is not to be valued equally, provided it does not involve force and pressure. Moreover, the danger of generalizing one's own norms is always present in Western health systems because they are based on the laws of objectivity and empirical demonstrability obtained from the sciences.

Nevertheless, the universalist perspective, which would like to treat all people equally, is of key significance: It stresses that people of different origins also have things in common, for example, with regard to such fundamental existential situations and conditions as pain, disease, and death, as well as their dependence on others and their reliance on help and on human relationships, even if these phenomena may take different forms and be interpreted differently. Furthermore, this perspective expresses the demand that all people have a right to qualified nursing, irrespective of their origin, their appearance, or whether they have entered Germany legally or illegally. As formulated by Domenig, all people have "the right to understand and be understood, the right to inform and be informed, and the right to know the possibilities of treatment and its effects and to have a voice in deciding on the choice of treatment" (Domenig, 2003, p. 88).

The challenge for transcultural nursing lies, therefore, in seeing the similarities without denying the differences—that is to say, in finding the balance between the perception of similarities and the acknowledgement of different experiences and perspectives. This balance requires that the similarities not be so generalized as to fit tidily over the others, nor the differences so narrowly defined that, in a culturalizing view, they render the others invisible in their specific otherness. For this reason one's own perception always needs a corrective in the form of the others, which assumes that the others are recognized as equals and that the power over definitions is shared. In this sense interculturality signifies a constant exchange of perspectives.

PRINCIPLES OF TRANSCULTURAL NURSING

Transcultural competence can be defined, to quote Domenig (2003), as the ability

> to see and understand individual ways of life in special situations and in different contexts and to adapt one's own actions and behaviour accordingly. Transculturally competent professionals reflect on their own way of life and outlook, have the ability to understand and interpret the perspectives of others, avoid the culturalising and stereotyping of certain target groups and have above all a respectful and unprejudiced attitude (or one that reflects on prejudices) towards migrants and other stigmatised target groups. (p. 95)

However—as pointed out by Paul Mecheril (2002)—an intercultural situation does not necessarily require the presence of people of different origins. For instance, it also arises when members of the majority culture talk about people of other cultures and either mutually confirm their images of the others or call the images into question. This means, for example, that when patients of other cultures are discussed at a ward meeting, there is also an intercultural situation because the significance of culture is determined in this context. It also applies to many situations of organizational planning and development at the management level of clinics and funding bodies and in the large nursing federations. As a rule, it is here that the members of the majority culture settle the question (mostly among themselves) of which status the majority and the minority cultures have within the institution. In such situations a certain amount of courage is often necessary to oppose the prevailing consensus. Thus, tension arises not only in direct intercultural contact but also when settling matters in the absence of the others.

Transcultural competence demands, for one thing, *specific knowledge,* namely a knowledge that does not make the others foreign—for example, by transplanting them, symbolically speaking, to their countries of origin—but that sees them in the context in which they are encountered. This necessitates, among other things, knowledge of the living conditions of migrants here in Germany and of how, for example, their morbidity rates and the spectrum of diseases differ from those of the population born and raised in Germany. It is also necessary to know the causes of these differences and how the health risks differ from those of the native population (cf. Borde & Rosendahl, 2003, p. 254).

It is also helpful to know which expectations and which apprehensions can be anticipated on the part of ethnic minorities in their dealings with a "German" institution and to what extent their previous experience of discrimination has led to caution and skepticism. It is also important to discover what knowledge they have of the German health system as individuals, and whether as individuals they have resources and networks they can fall back on, and if so, what these resources and networks are. Finally, it is necessary to know the extent to which their legal status might affect their state of health.

This knowledge is aimed not only at the others and their situation but also at oneself: at the images one has of the others, at the emotional reactions these call forth, and at the implications for one's own position as a member of the majority or of a minority culture. Equally, this means asking oneself what could hinder one from taking leave of stereotypes and clichés. For what is important in connection with this knowledge is less the fact that it is about learning something new and more about discarding what has previously been learned and taken for granted (cf. Castro Varela, 2002).

This presupposes, however, a *specific attitude,* namely openness not only towards the others but also towards oneself. For, as formulated by Paul Mecheril (2002), professional conduct "depends upon being able to enter into a fundamentally reflexive relationship to one's own professional conduct, its conditions and its consequences" (p. 25). One must ask, for example, how one responds, as a member of the majority culture, to being critically appraised by members of a minority culture. In his study on interculturality in counselling and therapy, Charles Ridley (1995) assumes that all Black patients go to therapy sessions with great misgivings at first because they cannot suppose the therapy room is extraterritorial, that is, free of individual or structural racism. Therapists, though, will not normally interpret these misgivings as a useful coping strategy necessary for Black patients' survival that they can make positive use of in the therapeutic process. On the contrary, they will regard it as pathological behavior that must be "therapied," especially when the misgivings are interpreted as questioning the therapists' personal integrity and professional competence.

With regard to one's dealings with the others, the question also arises of whether mutual understanding is at all possible and whether, in spite of the differences, one can empathize with the others to any degree. That is to say, what does the ability to empathize actually mean under conditions of difference and asymmetrical relationships? Empathy is based on the comparison of one's own experienced situations, objectives, and feelings with those of another person. According to Janis Jones (2004) there is always the danger here of assimilation, as she concluded in her analysis of empathy with Black people among White Americans. Jones goes on to propose that this is not entirely due to the fact that White people scarcely ever experience the discrimination to which Black people are constantly exposed but rather that White people by no means desire to experience the Black person's situation. Translated into the standard situation in Germany, this means that German professionals find Turkish patients so hard to understand and so "foreign" because, among other things, they do not wish to conceive of Turkish patients as "native German." They would like to keep their distance, in part not to jeopardize their own exclusive right to the status of "native Germanhood"—that is, the exclusive right to decide which rules prevail in personal dealings—and thus, in part, also to decide who has access to which resources. The precondition of true understanding, however, is the willingness to acknowledge the others as equal and having equal rights, that is, the willingness to *share power*. For whoever decides how a situation is to be interpreted and regulated possesses the power to define as well.

Hence, it is not only a question of cognitive and emotional competences but also of how much interest there is (if any) in training these competences. Thus, the boundaries of the ability to empathize are not solely defined by the limited possibility of comparing life circumstances and situations but also by the interest shown in the others. It must be pointed out, at least, that empathy under conditions of inequality does not have the same meaning as in relationships between equals, in which mutual interest and a genuine exchange of the different perspectives can be assumed.

That a transcultural perspective is closely associated with the sharing of power on the part of the members of the majority culture is also revealed in the fear that one's own social status will be threatened if one supports an intercultural position. Often, one not only upsets the prevailing consensus but one is also concerned with (or about) people who frequently have a lower social status. To a certain extent this reflects back on oneself and reduces one's own standing. In sociology this is called "status diffusion."

Thus, seriously committing oneself to intercultural situations is invariably a risky venture. First, there is the danger of losing one's assuredness about things, namely, that familiar images are questioned and certainties are no longer certain. Then, there is the danger of challenging the community of the like-minded. And finally, there is the risk of endangering one's own status. This must be set in relation to the benefits gained from constantly learning more about oneself and the others, thus developing one's personality in an active process of lively confrontations and acquiring an ever greater confidence as well as a sense of being true to one's own values. There is, of course, sufficient reason not to expose oneself to such dangers, even if one's self-image as a tolerant and open-minded person and one's professional code of ethics demand it. In this respect, particularly on the part of members of the majority culture, a commitment to interculturality remains a precarious undertaking.

For this reason—but also because the efforts of individuals can never counterbalance the weight of an institution—the project of transcultural transformation must direct its energies quite centrally at the structural conditions that leave their stamp on an institution. The demand for a kind of nursing that is culturally aware frequently stands in sharp contrast to a social reality in which there is often no guarantee that people whose mother tongue is not German are even understood. This means that the fundamental requirements of professionally competent work are often lacking, for how can one counsel or provide medical care for a person one does not understand?

The *structural conditions* require, first and foremost, that the institution commit itself to the project of transcultural transformation and that it be anchored in the institution's *mission*. It must make intercultural development a cross-sectional task to ensure in all areas that all clients and patients have equal opportunity of access to the institution's services and resources, irrespective of their country of origin, their appearance, and the culture they belong to.

Such a mission must be fought for, even in the face of a complacent political reality that has thus far failed to recognize the necessity of cultural differentiation. In discussions on German health reform, for example, there is no reference whatsoever to migrants; likewise, the official national and regional health records contain virtually no data on health care among the migrant population (Schultz, 2003). As noted by Basche and Kaouk (2003) among others, the German health system fails to react adequately whenever the norm of the average German patient is deviated from. In this respect the health service, as they express it, is "representative of a society which is only gradually becoming aware of the fact that people of very different cultural types are living in it" (Basche & Kaouk, 2003, p. 203).

The effect of this monocultural orientation is that members of ethnic minorities mostly receive inadequate information about their treatment; they feel that their concerns are not taken seriously; and they repeatedly experience discrimination, prejudice, and racism. "Often the contexts in which they explain their needs do not inspire much confidence in them and they are scarcely able to present their needs and perspectives in such a way that these are heard and understood and given appropriate consideration" (Domenig, 2003, p. 87). This leads to too much, too little, or the wrong kind of care, too much care mainly consisting of the excessive prescription of medicine (Brucks & Wahl, 2003).

In order to enable equal access to all services for everyone, an analysis must first be made of the *barriers* that migrants may face when they come into contact with a "German" institution. With regard to social services, Stephan Gaitanides (2004, p. 6) names the following:

- lack of information about the existence, structure, and usefulness of the services provided
- language difficulties and problems of understanding
- skepticism about the possibilities of intercultural understanding
- anticipation of prejudices against migrants and lack of acceptance
- specialized problem-solving or the referral of part of the problems to other institutions, which is experienced as rejection
- fear of authorities and institutions (including the fear of legal consequences pertaining to immigration laws)
- charges, distance from home, difficulties with applications and appointments, office hours that clash with the daily lives of pressured migrant families
- barriers with regard to institutional "Christian tendencies"

When services are not claimed or have little success, it is always the result of a process of interaction. Here, those who are more powerful—the professionals endowed with institutional instruments of power and superior expert knowledge—bear a special responsibility (Gaitanides, 2004, p. 7). Gaitanides notes that when analyzing the problem of access, one should not focus solely on the users of the institution but should also ask what barriers are put in the way of employing and promoting professionals who belong to ethnic minorities. Above all, this includes the question of the extent to which institutions belonging to the Christian churches—which make up the majority of health facilities in Germany—exclude people of other religions.

The structural conditions thus include the development of user-friendly and effective structures of the services provided, a specific information policy, and special staff recruitment and development. A key feature of a user-friendly structure would be, for example, the availability of an interpreter service. Yet this presupposes structures that enable the staff to make use of these services. If more time is needed, it must be taken into account from the outset. It is interesting to note, for example, that although a central interpreting service is available at the Charité teaching hospital in Berlin, it is scarcely ever made use of. It seems easier to rely on relatives or the cleaning staff in such situations than to put in a request for the service in advance. This may reflect extreme time pressures but it may also be an expression of laziness or even disrespect, signalling that taking special measures for the others (even though warranted) is just not worth the effort.

Transcultural transformation also involves becoming aware of the institutional culture, that is, the atmosphere that an institution radiates and the way it is perceived by the different users. This refers to the present facilities and also to the history of the institution as well as that of the health system generally in Germany, which, as we know, also played a part in creating an inhumane society that marginalized and debased people, and even went as far as to participate actively in their deaths. Looking into how this became possible sharpens our awareness for the extent to which institutions of the health system today play a part in the discrimination of minorities.

Finally, as mentioned above, a conscious policy of employing *professionals from ethnic minorities* is of great importance for structural transformation. There are various reasons for this. First, their transcultural experience is a resource that can be drawn upon, even though it cannot be assumed that this experiential knowledge is converted automatically into intercultural competence, that is, into reflexive knowledge about the significance of ethnicity and culture. Second, these members of staff can facilitate communication with patients who do not speak German and can act as intermediaries between colleagues and patients and between specific ethnic communities. Members of staff with an ethnic minority background often attract patients and clients with a similar background. These patients would be more willing to trust them and would recognize something familiar in the institution, which would make it just a little less alien. It is a fact, at any rate, that when vacancies caused by dismissals are filled with applicants who do not have an ethnic minority background, the proportion of patients and clients with an ethnic minority background usually falls dramatically (Domenig, 2003, p. 100).

However, there is always the danger here of delegating problems of interculturality to the "migration experts," and in doing so, of narrowing their professional competence as well as their professional interests. At the same time, the German majority are more or less relieved of their responsibility of dealing with muticulturality themselves and acquiring more competence in this field.

Hence, the development of intercultural team structures with equal rights must be furthered in order to exploit the synergies produced by the great diversity of the defined problems and the strategies proposed for their solution. At the same time, an ethnic division of labor must be avoided and the acquisition of intercultural competence must be encouraged for all members of staff. Transcultural transformation in institutions is a radical process that must involve all areas and all levels. It means that cultural diversity is acknowledged and that facilities are planned and developed in partnership with all those who will use them.

THEORETICAL IDEAS FOR TRANSCULTURALITY IN NURSING

The foregoing exposition points out potential issues pertaining to nursing practice in relation to culture, ranging from individual to structural ramifications on practice and competence. In this sense, theoretical issues regarding transculturality in nursing are multidimensional and complex. Transculturality is a frame for understanding one's own and others' lives, as well as addressing the similarities and differences all at once in practice, as transculturality encompasses the process with which (a) universalities and particularities and (b) global and local orientations are integrated to form identities and ways of social lives for people. Based on these considerations, it is possible to address transculturality in nursing from at least three theoretical perspectives: (a) the perspective of viewing people's practices having culture-specific and universal bases, (b) the perspective of transculturality as the normative base of human life, and (c) the postmodern perspective of culture in the context of power.

The first perspective is well represented theoretically in nursing by Leininger's theory of culture care diversity and universality (Leininger, 1991; Leininger & McFarland, 2002). Leininger's theory for transcultural nursing emphasizes nursing practice based on the understanding and analysis of culture-specific as well as universal practices of human lives, and articulation of such understanding in designing and providing nursing care to fit an individual's specific life patterns for a culturally congruent care. Leininger's key assumption for this theory is that individuals carry on their lives through "culture care," which refers to multiple aspects of culture that influence and enable people to deal with conditions of their lives including health, illness, and dying (Leininger & McFarland, 2002).

The second theoretical perspective is based on the assumption that transculturality must be accepted as an operative concept of human life, as people's lives are determined by "propagandizing" of specific normative concepts of culture (Welsch, 1999). In this perspective, transculturality posits for an understanding of culture as inclusive and integrated rather than exclusive and separate, and the aim for transculturality is a pragmatic one. Hence, a theory of transculturality from this perspective as a normative theory must specify how people in practice can live harmoniously within transculturality. One approach would be a theory of transcultural interaction as suggested by Welsch (1999). Because nursing is a relational practice, such a theoretical approach may provide a means through which the culturality of both patients and nurses can be acknowledged and shared.

The third perspective of postmodernism on transculturality is applicable in nursing similar to the way feminism as a cultural construct is studied and analyzed from the view point of power and struggle (Harding & Hintikka, 1983). Poststructuralist critiques such as that of Blackford (2003) offer a framework to examine systematic distortions accorded to "otherness" in the cultural context, drawing from the arguments for gender conceptualizations (Fox Keller, 1983, for example). In addition, Habermasian critical philosophy can provide a basis for a formulation of theoretical approach for mutual understanding among people, including between nurses and patients regarding "culture-oriented" practices, as suggested by Holmes and Warelow (1997).

There is a need to move forward to consider transculturality from various theoretical perspectives in order to remedy the limitations offered by the rationalist perspective of transcultural nursing practice as lamented, for example, by Williamson and Harrison (2001).

REFERENCES

Alban, S., Leininger, M. M., & Reynods, C. L. (2000). *Multikulturelle Pflege* [Multicultural nursing]. München, Germany: Urban & Fischer.

Attia, I. (1994). Antiislamischer Rassismus Stereotypen—Erfahrungen—Machtverhältnisse [Anti-islamic racism. Stereotyping—experiences—power structures]. In S. Jäger & N. Räthzel (Eds.), *Rassismusforschung und antirassistische Erziehung*. Duisburg, Germany: Diss.

Basche, J., & Kaouk, M. (2003). Qualitätssicherung durch niedrigschwellige kulturspezifische Hilfen—Möglichkeiten der Mobilisierung informeller Ressourcen am Beispiel der sozialpsychiatrischen Versorgung arabischsprachiger Familien [Quality management through easy-to-access and culturally specific services—Chances of mobilizing internal resources discussed at the example of social-psychological services for Arabic speaking families]. In T. Borde & D. Matthias (Eds.), *Gut versorgt? Migrantinnen und Migranten im Gesundheits- und Sozialwesen* (pp. 203–225). Frankfurt, Germany: Mabuse.

Blackford, J. (2003). Cultural frameworks of nursing practice: Exposing an exclusionary healthcare culture. *Nursing Inquiry, 10,* 236–244.

Borde, T., & Rosendahl, C. (2003). Interkulturelle Kompetenz in Institutionen—eine Fortbildung für interdisziplinäre Arbeitsteams [Intercultural competence in institutions—A manual for interdisciplinary teams]. In T. Borde & D. Matthias (Eds.), *Gut versorgt? Migrantinnen und Migranten im Gesundheits- und Sozialwesen* (pp. 247–264). Frankfurt, Germany: Mabuse.

Brucks, U., & Wahl, W. B. (2003). Über,-Unter-, Fehlversorung? Bedarfslücken und Strukturprobleme in der ambulanten Gesundheitsversorgung für Migrantinnen und Migranten [Over-, under-, and mis-provision. Service deficiency and structural problems in ambulatory services for migrants]. In T. Borde & D. Matthias (Eds.), *Gut versorgt? Migrantinnen und Migranten im Gesundheits- und Sozialwesen* (pp. 15–34). Frankfurt, Germany: Mabuse.

Castro Varela, M. (2002). Interkulturelle Kompetenz—ein Diskurs in der Krise [Intercultural competence and a discourse in crises]. In G. Auernheimer (Ed.), *Interkulturelle Kompetenz und pädagogische Professionalität* (pp. 35–48). Opladen, Germany: Leske & Budrich.

Domenig, D. (2003). Anforderungen an einen transkulturellen Wandel in der stationären Pflege [Requirements regarding on transcultural change in institutional nursing]. In T. Borde & D. Matthias (Eds.), *Gut versorgt? Migrantinnen und Migranten im Gesundheits- und Sozialwesen* (pp. 85–104). Frankfurt, Germany: Mabuse.

Esser, H. (2000). *Soziologie Spezielle Grundlagen Die Konstruktion der Gesellschaft* [Sociology. Special foundations. The construction of society] (2nd ed.). Frankfurt, Germany: Campus.

Featherstone, M., & Lash, S. (Eds.). (1999). *Spaces of culture: City, nation, world.* London: Sage.

Fox Keller, E. (1983). Gender and science. In S. Harding & M. B. Hintikka (Eds.), *Discovering reality: Feminist perspectives on epistemology, metaphysics, methodology, and philosophy of science* (pp. 187–205). Dordrecht, The Netherlands: D. Reidel.

Gaitanides, S. (2004). Interkulturelle Öffnung der sozialen Dienste—Visionen u Stolpersteine [Intercultural accessibility of social service—Visions and pitfalls]. In B. Rommelspacher (Ed.), *Die offenen Stadt—Interkulturalität und Pluralität in Verwaltungen und sozialen Diensten* (pp. 4–18). Berlin: Alice Salomon Hochschule.

Harding, S., & Hintikka, M. B. (Eds.). (1983). *Discovering reality: Feminist perspectives on epistemology, metaphysics, methodology, and philosophy of science.* Dordrecht, The Netherlands: D. Reidel.

Holmes, C. A., & Warelow, P. J. (1997). Culture, needs and nursing: A critical theory approach. *Journal of Advanced Nursing, 25,* 463–470.

Jones, J. (2004). The impairment of empathy in goodwill Whites for African

Americans. In G. Yancy (Ed.), *What White looks like. African-American philosophers on the whiteness question.* New York; London: Routledge.

Kollak, I. (2003). Kultur [Culture]. In *Pschyrembel Woerterbuch Pflege* (pp. 406–408). Berlin: de Gruyter.

Leininger, M. (1991). *Culture care diversity and universality: A theory of nursing.* New York: National League for Nursing Press.

Leininger, M., & McFarland, M. (2002). *Transcultural nursing: Concepts, theories, research and practice* (3rd ed.). New York: McGraw-Hill.

Mecheril, P. (2002). Kompetenzlosigkeitskompetenz. Pädagogisches Handeln unter Einwanderungsbedingungen [Competencelessness. Educational practice under the conditions of migration]. In G. Auernheimer (Ed.), *Interkulturelle Kompetenz und pädagogische Professionalität* (pp. 15–34). Opladen, Germany: Leske & Budrich.

Pinderhughes, E. (1989). *Understanding race, ethnicity and power. The key to efficacy in clinical practice.* New York: Macmillian.

Ridley, C. R. (1995). *Overcoming unintentional racism in counselling and therapy: A practitioner's guide to intentional intervention.* London: Sage.

Rommelspacher, B. (1995). *Schuldlos-Schuldig?* Wie sich junge Frauen mit Antisemitismus auseinandersetzen [Guiltless-guilty? How young women struggle with anti-semitism]. Hamburg, Germany: Konkret Literatur.

Rommelspacher, B. (2002). *Anerkennung und Ausgrenzung. Deutschland als multikulturelle Gesellschaft* [Acceptance and exclusion. Germany as multicultural society]. Frankfurt, Germany; New York: Campus.

Schultz, D. (2003). Kulturelle Kompetenz in der psychosozialen und psychiatrischen Versorgung ethnischer Minderheiten: Das Beispiel San Francisco, Kalifornien [Cultural competence in psycho-social and psychological services for ethnic minorities]. In T. Borde & D. Matthias (Eds.), *Gut versorgt? Migrantinnen und Migranten im Gesundheits- und Sozialwesen* (pp. 167–190). Frankfurt, Germany: Mabuse.

Uzarewicz, C. (1999). The concept of culture and transculturality. In H. S. Kim & I. Kollak (Eds.), *Nursing theories: Conceptual and philosophical foundations* (pp. 71–86). New York: Springer.

Wachendorfer, U. (1999). Inszenierung von Unsichtbarkeit—zur Rolle des Weiss-seins in der Therapie [Staging the invisible—about the role of being White in therapies]. In A. S. Reinhard, C. Hahn, M. Westen, L. Lerch, & R. M. Banda-Stein (Eds.), *Psychosoziale Arbeit im Spannungsfeld unterschiedlicher Kulturen und Lebensformen.* Dokumentation des 22 (pp. 136-148). Berlin: Feministischen Frauentherapiekongresses.

Wachendorfer, U. (2000). WEIß-SEIN—(k)leine Variable in der Therapei. [Being white—small variations in therapies] *Psychologie und Gesellschaftskritik, H1*(93)24, 55–68.

Welsch, W. (1999). Transculturality—The puzzling form of cultures today. In M. Featherstone & S. Lash (Eds.), *Spaces of culture: City, nation, world* (pp. 194–213). London: Sage.

Williamson, M., & Harrison, L. (2001). Dealing with diversity: Incorporating cultural sensitivity into professional midwifery practice. *Australian Journal of Midwifery, 14,* 22–26.

Illness As Risk: On the Genesis and Functioning of Therapeutic Deinstitutionalization[*]

Friedrich Balke

One of the major concerns in nursing science, as a field within the broader domain of health sciences, is conceptualizing health and illness. Conceptualization of health and illness is embedded in the broader context that determines the order of knowledge and the ways power is exercised in a society to deal with the matters of health and illness as social constructions. It is in this perspective that the notions of health, normality, illness, and pathologies as well as how societies develop processes to respond to such notions are examined in this chapter. The focus is in tracing and analyzing the genesis of radically different conceptualizations of health and illness in the modern era with the attendant emergence of power processes that become couched within the health care processes (for example, hospitals) in modern times, and to examine how these are changing in the current scene.

---

*Translated from German by Ellen Klein.

NORMAL AND PATHOLOGICAL:
THE INVENTION OF A NEW OPPOSITION TYPE

Ever since Immanuel Kant, philosophers have liked to pose the question of the condition of possible experience: they retreat, as it were, from what is empirically—that is, concretely—perceived, thought, uttered, and done, and ask what makes it possible for us to perceive, think, utter, or do something in the way we do. This means that there is something present in people's everyday or lifetime actions of which those who carry out the actions are not conscious (just as it is not necessary to know any grammar rules to speak more or less grammatically correctly), but which nevertheless functions in the background and serves as the base that supports a specific practice (practice is to be understood here in the widest sense).

In the following, I shall try, while taking a look at a phenomenon connected with these reflections which I shall call here provisionally "health sciences," to lay bare such a base: a base that begins to take form in the nineteenth century; supplants the classical conception of illness as an "accident," that is, a temporary or lethal defect; and creates a new image of the individual as someone who lives in illness. Illness is always latently present in the individual; even when he is healthy, he is exposed to its *risk* (to the probability of falling ill) and must therefore subject himself to constant and essentially preventive self-observation and self-treatment. What are the changes in the order of knowledge and in the ways of exercising power that are responsible for health gradually ceasing to be the reference point of medicine (insofar as health is defined by the absence of illness and insofar as the body must decide, so to speak, between health and illness, insofar then as there is a real battle being waged between health or "nature" and illness for the body) and normality, or more precisely, the continuity from the normal and the pathological becoming its primary object? Or to put it another way, since we have not stopped distinguishing between healthy and ill: what is meant by this distinction when in the nineteenth century it is given an entirely new content, when it now acquires a sense originating from the horizon of the distinction between normal and pathological, which is of an entirely different nature? In the following, the "conditions for the change or interruption of meaning" will be described, that is, the conditions "under which the meaning fades [in our case: the old meaning of health and illness], thereby allowing something different to appear in its place" (Foucault 1994a, p. 603), namely, the distinction between normal and pathological. In an interview dating from the year 1969, Michel Foucault explains the significance of this distinction for our culture with the following words:

> Every society establishes a series of opposition systems—between good and bad, permitted and forbidden, criminal and noncriminal, etc. All these oppositions, which are constitutive for every society, have been reduced in Europe today to the simple opposition of normal and pathological. This opposition is not only *simpler* than the others are, it also provides the advantage of allowing people to believe that there is a technique with which allows the pathological can be lead back to the normal. (Foucault 1994a, p. 603; italics added for emphasis)

In the following I shall try to answer the question of what makes this new opposition of normal and pathological so attractive, of what lends it its absorbing force. What are the qualities that allow an entire complex of traditional oppositions (good/bad, permitted/forbidden, criminal/noncriminal, etc.) with more or less moral, that is, qualitative, connotations to be translated into merely relative positional values on a graduated scale whose two poles (normality/abnormality) communicate with each other? What is the specific "simplicity" of this opposition in relation to the others spoken of by Foucault? Jürgen Link (1997a), who has presented the first comprehensive study of the archaeology of "normalism," provides the following provisional answer, which will have to be developed further on: The simplicity of this new distinction lies in its *one-dimensionality*. No matter how heterogeneous, discontinuous, or multidimensional a particular range of phenomena is and regardless of its qualitative characteristics, the normalizing strategy consists in ascribing to this multi-fissured territory a parallel level that allows all possible positions, even the most extreme and improbable, to be thought of as homogeneous and continuous. The establishment of such "normal fields" is at the same time the prerequisite for increasing the performance of normalizing interventions, which are to a large extent abstracted from the qualitative peculiarities of their intervention space so as to increase their ability to be technically manipulated.

In a first step the question to be addressed is, What changes in the order of knowledge made this modern normalist perspective possible, which in the nineteenth century began its triumphant advance through the entire realm of human scientific knowledge? Following this epistemological inquiry, which will lead us into the middle of the field of treating and dealing with patients, the way this very new knowledge type interacts with equally new *power processes* will be analyzed. These processes will not only be viewed under the aspect of how normalist knowledge and normalist techniques are applied, but also in particular under the aspect of how such knowledge and techniques are generated, that is, their discursive productivity.

Let us begin with the first question, which requires a brief excursion to the biomedical-knowledge complex that was forming in the nineteenth century. The distinction between normal and pathological conceived in the field of physiopathology undergoes as early as the beginning of the nineteenth century a critical transformation, at the end of which a qualitative difference is replaced by a quantitative difference. Foucault alludes to this process when he emphasizes the "simplicity" of this new opposition, and we shall see that the increasing use of technology involved with it is also connected with this quality. The French science historian George Canguilhem showed in his study *On the Normal and the Pathological,* published originally in 1943, how in medical science of that age classical ontological pathology was replaced by a theory that emphasized the continuity and homogeneity in the sick and healthy states. Although ontological theory envisions "in disease, or better, in the experience of being sick . . . a polemical situation: either a battle between the organism and a foreign substance, or an internal struggle between opposing forces" (Canguilhem, 1978, p. 12), the new conception of illness reduces illness to a mere deviation from health, a measurable change in intensity of the "normal" state. The ill state was conceived by the French doctor Broussais in his treatise *De l'irritation et de la folie,* appearing in 1827 and based on the model of (mental) *irritation,* which according to Broussais is nothing other than "a normal stimulation in an exaggerated form." The phenomena that are the object of pathological examination are not different in nature, but only in degree from those of physiology. This nosology[1] of continuity, developed further with certain modifications and radicalized by Claude Bernard, was taken up by Auguste Comte, the founding father of sociology, who generalized "Broussais's principle" to an axiom also applicable to social processes.

"Our famous fellow citizen, Broussais," should be thanked, said Comte in his fortieth lecture of the 'Cours de Philosophie Positive,' "for his courageously advocated view that the pathological state is not at all radically different from the physiological state, with regard to which—no matter how one looks at it—it can only constitute a simple extension going more or less beyond the higher or lower limits of variation proper to each phenomenon of the normal organism, without ever being able to produce really new phenomena." (Canguilhem 1978, p. 19)

Even philosophers of Nietzsche's caliber were fascinated by the possibilities of knowledge that the qualitative leveling of the former antagonism between health and illness, and the reduction of pathology to the status of a complementary discipline of physiology seemed to afford. Thus we read in an entry from his posthumous works of the 1880s, which is followed by a longer key quotation from Claude Bernard's *Leçon sur la chaleur animale,* translated by Nietzsche: "It is the value of all morbid states that they show us under a magnifying glass certain states that are normal—but not easily visible when normal" (Canguilhem 1978, p. 15). The Bernard quotation translated by Nietzsche reads as follows:

> Health and sickness are not essentially different, as the ancient physicians and some practitioners even today suppose. One must not make of them distinct principles or entities that fight over the living organism and turn it into their arena. That is silly nonsense and chatter that is no good any longer. In fact, there are only differences in degree between these two kinds of existence: the exaggeration, the disproportion, the nonharmony of the normal phenomena constitute the pathological state. (as cited in Nietzsche, 1968, p. 29)

The morbid condition is revealed to modern doctors then as a deviation in a chain of continuity ("differences in degree") from the individual's healthy existence. Modern medicine functions by means of a differential method, a method that differentiates degrees—it is not by chance that "differential diagnosis" has become its most important instrument. The term *normal* is now defined with reference to statistically obtained averages and describes a range of acceptable deviation (obtained by setting limits and tolerance thresholds); *pathological* means in the region on the other side of the normality line, which itself is always dynamic and only temporary, that is, shiftable within a continuum. In any case, no insurmountable wall exists between the two conditions, but only a variable threshold. The process of making a fundamental discontinuity into a continuity consists in constructing a common axis of comparability between two conditions (health and illness) hitherto viewed as qualitatively different. After a period of time in which the field of pathologies had been comprehended with the aid of a taxonomic model that distinguished between perfect realizations of a type and corrupt or "monstrous forms," the doctor's gaze was completely reorganized at the beginning of the nineteenth century:

1. First, it was no longer the gaze of any observer, but that of a doctor supported and justified by an institution, that of a doctor endowed with the power of decision and intervention.
2. The gaze was no longer "bound by the narrow grid of structure (form, arrangement, number, size), but could and should grasp colors, variations, tiny anomalies, always receptive to the deviant" (medicine of deviations instead of medicine of types).
3. It was no longer satisfied with ascertaining what was directly visible or self-evident, but inferred "chances and risks": a calculating, prognosticating gaze. (Foucault 1973, p. 89)

Canguilhem has called attention to the significant etymological circumstance that the term "normal" could be attested as early as 1759, whereas "normalized" was encountered for the first time only in 1834—a time when the debate on the new, positive pathology was at its first peak (Canguilhem 1978, p. 151). We have now reached the point where it becomes clear that there is more to the question with the new distinction of normal/pathological than only acceptance of a changed medical procedure of discovery and treatment. At stake is nothing less than the question of power itself. In order to be able to comprehend our contemporary societies, it is necessary that we divorce ourselves from some of our habits of thought regarding power that we have become accustomed to. Most important is that we abandon the notion of power as something that functions essentially negatively or repressively. According to this conception, the power that is generally localized in the state is essentially concerned with preventing, repressing, skimming off profit, suppressing. It manifests itself in the legal system or in laws whose function consists in formulating prohibitions and threatening sanctions when these rules and regulations are violated. This classic power type, as it was characteristic of the early modern "sovereignty societies," and thus of the founding and establishment phase of the modern territorial states that were equipped with central power, culminates in the right over life and death of its subjects. The symbol of sovereign power is the sword.

However, long before the French Revolution, which swept away the social foundation of absolutistic power, entirely new power mechanisms developed in European societies. Their peculiarity lay in the fact that they were no longer played out at the level of the law—or when this level was entered upon, the way the law functions had been fundamentally changed. We actually live in a society in which the power of the law is not simply diminishing, but the law is being integrated into the mechanism of completely differently functioning power processes: Foucault classifies these new power processes under the heading of *norm* (as opposed to *law*). Symptomatic for this transformation are the difficulties that arise within the heart of justice (criminal justice) itself when the task for which it was created has to be carried out, namely passing judgment, pronouncing a sentence, and determining the punishment for the delinquent. Punishments, of course, continue to be carried out, but in actual practice the function and meaning of punishment have fundamentally changed. This can be recognized by the fact that the status of criminals is being brought closer and closer to that of the ill, or more specifically, to that of the mentally ill, and the sentence for crime is understood as a *therapeutic* prescription.

As the process of arriving at a sentence for crime conforms more and more to medical-psychiatric diagnostics (or these diagnostic procedures attain greater importance in criminal proceedings, noticeably weaken the sharp opposition of guilty/not guilty, and allow all kinds of *reduced* culpability to arise), the ritual of punishing also acquires a new meaning, namely a therapeutic one: "We punish, but this is a way of saying that we wish to obtain a cure. Today, criminal justice functions and justifies itself only by this perpetual reference to something other than itself, by this unceasing reinscription in non-juridical [in fact *normalizing,* F.B.] systems" (Foucault 1979, p. 22). From the moment we begin dealing with a *normalizing society* that interprets the entirety of its moral and legal codes in light of the distinction between normal and pathological, medicine becomes the prime discipline, precisely because it is the science of the normal and the pathological.

As the new power processes become detached from the law, they do not by any means fall back to the level of brute force; to understand them, rather, it is necessary to use language that comprehends them as *forces.* What does it mean then when the central activity of the modern powers is characterized by the term *normalization?* As opposed to normality, which is perceived as a fixed condition that is legally defined and guaranteed by police force, normalization as a category of process accentuates first of all the character of power as a relation between forces: a force does not come into contact with an object or a thing and destroy or change its form, but with another force that it cannot control without making itself dependent on the potency, the inner capacity of that force. Power relinquishes to a certain extent its vertical privilege; it is no longer situated over or in front of its field of activity, but taps into the forces it is trying to command, or more precisely, control. When we say that the new power is a relation between forces, then this simultaneously excludes the notion that it materializes in a sovereign form (for instance, the state). It no longer occurs in the singular (power does not form an opposition to powerlessness), but ceases to be a privilege of the powerful so that the question of who possesses it becomes meaningless. Power is not *possessed,* it is *exercised;* it does not exist in and of itself, it is operative. To stimulate, prompt, produce are the categories of the new power that "has taken possession of the lives of individuals, of individuals as living bodies," and both as individual bodies and as generic bodies. "A power bent on generating forces, making them grow, and ordering them, rather than one dedicated to impeding them, making them submit, or destroying" (Foucault 1981, p. 136). It does this by developing an entire series of *disciplines* for the individual body that serve to "increase its capabilities," "exploit its strengths," and integrate it into effective and economical control systems; furthermore, by subjecting the body of the population to various interventions that are supposed to regulate all aspects of collective life: reproduction, birth and death rates, health standards, life expectancy, migration, settlement, and so on. Nursing would be included within such disciplines.

What Michel Foucault calls the "bio-power" has two sides or two focal points: any *body* and any *population*—the individual physical performance and the collective life processes. A power such as this, which is supposed to guarantee and enhance life

> needs continuous regulatory and corrective mechanisms. It is no longer a matter of bringing death into play in the field of sovereignty, but of distributing the living in the domain of value and utility. Such a power has to qualify, measure, appraise, and hierarchize, rather than display itself in its murderous splendor; it does not have to draw the line that separates the enemies of the sovereign from his obedient subjects; it effects distributions around the norm. (Foucault, 1981, p. 144)

A formulation that makes the norm clearly recognizable as an average value that is derived from a comparative field and statistically obtained.

In his systematic analytics of disciplinary power, that power which selects the individual body as its target, Foucault—following the treatise literature on the subject that he makes use of—now returns to the "repressive" conceptualization of subduing, teaching, training, and so forth. On the other hand it is exactly this disapproval of the "repression hypothesis" that is one of his main concerns. And so he says of "disciplinary power" to which the body is exposed,

It does not link forces together in order to reduce them; it seeks to bind them together in such a way as to multiply and use them. Instead of bending all its subjects into a single uniform mass, it separates, analyses, differentiates, and carries its procedures of decomposition to the point of necessary and sufficient single units. . . . Discipline "makes" *("fabrique")* individuals. (Foucault 1979, p. 170)

The disciplinary power described by Foucault has an *individualizing* effect—and starting with this quality is the best way to approach the concept of normality. For a power can only have an individualizing effect if it assumes a different relationship to deviations from a given norm, if it responds to these deviations not by excluding or perhaps even destroying the deviator, but by employing a complex technique that allows the deviation to be regulated and that possibly even uses it to intensify bodily functions ("immunology") or the function of an institutional connection involving the bodies. To normalize means above all: not to eliminate, but to observe minutely, to differentiate, and to recombine. The new power is attracted to deviations and contributes actively, as shown by the example of the evolution of modern sexuality analyzed by Foucault, to their growth and proliferation. The disciplinary power has an intensifying effect on deviation.

THE BIRTH OF THE HOSPITAL—
FOUCAULTIAN CRITIQUE

Foucault analyzed how discipline functions in a series of typical organizations of modern societies: in addition to the army and factory, also in the school, the prison, psychiatry and the hospital. In the second part of my reflections I would like to take up the particularly interesting case of the hospital and show that the meeting of medicine and hospital, however it is to be judged, is an event whose occurrence is due solely to the new power mechanisms—that a political (and not a medical!) technology forms the basis of what we have known ever since as the hospital. One has the impression nowadays that hospitals are losing their privileged status as a place for treating the ill, a process that, as I expect, many who are involved in patient treatment and care observe with mixed feelings and perhaps even support actively. There is without a doubt a *crisis of the hospital* because there is also a crisis of the other milieus of confinement in whose framework modern power functions. And is not the academic establishment of nursing studies a response to the erosion of the hospital model? Does this not reflect the entire ambivalence of such processes of crisis insofar as some people primarily expect that by turning nursing into a scientific discipline there will be a revitalization of the hospital in the form of economization or increased efficiency (without touching its underlying power type), while others seek to supplement or perhaps even replace it with other forms of patient treatment and care?

A look at the phase of formation of the classic hospital model teaches us that it is not primarily new medical knowledge or knowledge of nursing that will accelerate the transformation of this model, but rather the attempt to use and intensify the crisis of the normalizing power already in process to seek solutions that have neither the character of a big, illusory "revolution" nor that of a reformation in which the goal of stabilizing the old model is pursued by enabling a series of controlled changes (cf. Foucault 1994b, p. 547). The apologists of the status quo have in common with the revolutionary nostalgists that they always make the question of goals the focus of their politics—defining goals is the real strength of the experts of goal reflection, that is, of the intellectuals of the classic type. However, the history of the hospital in particular shows what cannot be made clear enough: No one wanted it, but nevertheless its triumphant progress has been uncheckable. The notion that sociocultural evolution, that is, the emergence and general acceptance of something new in the social world, results from the actions of strongly motivated and unerring individuals has had to be dismissed in the meantime (Luhmann 1997, p. 456). Mutations occur through the exploitation of happy coincidences, and this means they are just as fortuitous as the events by which they are occasioned. Coincidence is not concerned with goals and purposes. The question "What do you really want?" is therefore invariably the question posed by reasonable people, legislators, technocrats, and governments, and addressed to those who want to play a different game (Foucault 1994b, p. 544). History is not an object of the will, but of the coincidence of different factors or forces that none of the participants control. The task of the genealogist, as defined by Nietzsche, is not to go back to the pure origin of things before time, but to their emergence *(Entstehungsherd)*. The beginning is neither true nor good nor beautiful, so it is neither reasonable nor at all simple, but differential, many-faceted, and in a higher sense amoral.

Even those who benefited most from the establishment of the hospital—the doctors—only made it their goal after conditions for making it possible were already given by the coming about of a favorable situation unique in history, a meeting of various "coincidences." In any case, it can be said that the hospital is not an invention of doctors. It can be concluded from this that whatever will come after the hospital or shake the central role this institution plays in the process of medical treatment—and this will not take place without a fundamental change in the established scheme of the division of labor and in the way the participants in the "medical process" (doctors, nursing staff, patients) comprehend their roles—will not be the work of those who have been underprivileged so far in this process. How did the process of the medicalization of the hospital come about? And what developments at the present time justify our suspicion that a loss of the medical privileges claimed by the hospital for itself is not far off? This loss is extremely double-edged in its significance because it can lead to a universalization of the hospital model beyond the walls of the hospital as well as to a turning away from the power mechanisms and their structuring effect on the professions (dominance of medicine over nursing) that made the hospital model possible in the first place.

When I speak of the medicalization of the hospital, then, this means that throughout its history the hospital was not always a place where a specifically medical influence was exerted on the patients. Indeed, until far into the eighteenth century there was in Europe no area of contact between the practice of doctors and the hospital. Around 1760, the idea of using the hospital as an instrument for healing patients came into existence for the first time. In the Middle Ages and in early modern times the hospital did not function as a therapeutic instrument. The hospitals had the function of collecting the sick (and not only the sick) and preventing their coming into contact with their surroundings in order to hinder dangerous processes of infection (of physical as well as of "moral" nature). For the most part, the hospital was even more of a relief institution for the poor than for the sick (and for the sick only insofar as they were poor at the same time). The relief was of both material and spiritual nature. As a rule, it occurred only when a poor person was dying and consisted entirely in providing physical, but above all spiritual relief during the dying process. It was not by chance that the personnel of the hospitals was made up predominantly of members of orders who hoped to promote the salvation of the "patient's" soul as well as that of their own by their activities.

Conversely, at this time medicine is not a hospital medicine and not a hospital profession. The medicine of the Middle Ages takes place outside of the hospitals and is therefore a deeply individualistic practice consisting of three elements: the doctor, the illness, and the "nature." The doctor's intervention in the illness centered around the idea of the *crisis*. The crisis was that moment in which in the sick person's healthy nature and the evil afflicting him stood face to face in battle against each other. In this fight between the (good) nature and the illness, it was the doctor's task to observe the signs, predict the development of the fight, and to do everything within his power to bring about the triumph of health and nature over the illness. Let us recall the words of Claude Bernard translated by Nietzsche precisely regarding that dualistic ontology that makes illness and health into two distinct principles or entities that are involved in an unrelenting struggle, in a real battle from which only one of the two sides can emerge as the victor. "That is nonsense and foolish talk and not good for anything," wrote Bernard without giving an account, however, of the causes leading to the loss of evidence for this polemic schema of medical practice. The treatment, which takes the form of a battle, is invariably reduced to the individual relationship between the doctor and the patient. The idea of making extensive observations in the heart of the hospital to obtain a systematic basis of comparison and thus arrive at a differential ascertainment of the illness was not an element of medical practice for a very long time.

This only changes at the moment as the hospital becomes a political-economic annoyance in the eyes of the representatives of the public order. There is a mixture of all kinds of outcasts collected in it. It is true they are all poor but not all in the same way: beggars, mad people, sick people, prostitutes, and criminals constitute a highly diffuse social ensemble whose control is seen as a growing problem by the political authorities. The first hospital reform, occurring in France in the final years of the seventeenth century, was not of civil but of military hospitals and of hospitals located in the port cities, which above all were places of economic disorder. They were important trading centers for goods smuggled into the country by sailors who feigned illness in order to slip by the customs officials. It was especially the military hospitals, however, that required a new and specifically medical regimen to reduce the high mortality rate of soldiers outside of battle, after the costs for their education and upkeep had become a financial policy issue of the highest order following the introduction of firearms. The reorganization of the military hospitals was not based on a new medical technique, but on a technique that was essentially political, for which Foucault reserved the term *disciplines*. I have already pointed out the essentially productive character of this new power process and its simultaneously differentiating (dissolving impenetrable, complex conglomerates) and homogenizing (creating a new "analytical space") effects, so it only remains for me to specify the most important registers of disciplinary power, while taking into consideration the invention of the hospital as a medical-therapeutic instrument in the following three accounts:

1. Discipline is first of all the art of spatial distribution of individuals: "Each individual has its own place; and each place its individual. Avoid distributions in groups; break up collective dispositions; analyse confused, massive or transient pluralities" (Foucault 1979, p. 143). Medical surveillance of illness and infection goes hand in hand with other controls—first and foremost, the management of things (even before curing patients): registration of medications used, ascertainment of the actual number of patients, regulation of their comings and goings, creation of special categories for certain patients, continuous recording of medical histories, etc. (Foucault 1979, p. 144). In summary: "The first of the great operations of discipline is, therefore, the constitution of *'tableaux vivants'*, which transform the confused, useless or dangerous multitudes into ordered multiplicities. The drawing up of 'tables' was one of the great problems of the scientific, political and economic technology of the eighteenth century" (Foucault 1979, p. 148).

2. Installing discipline requires the establishment of the *coercive gaze:* In the course of the classical period "observatories of human multiplicity" (Foucault 1979, p. 171) come into being. These are realized architecturally so that they enable a vantage point from which one can see without being seen (the ideal of the panoptic view). It is not sufficient merely to observe the patients from time to time, but rather they must be under permanent surveillance because it is only in this way that they can be exposed to knowledge that will change them. The most important instrument of this permanent surveillance of patients therefore becomes the ritual of the visit. Rather than a ritual, it would be more appropriate to speak of an *examination* that establishes over patients a visibility "through which one differentiates them and judges them" (Foucault 1979, p. 184). As Foucault writes,

> [In this] slender technique are to be found a whole domain of knowledge, a whole type of power. The decisive factor for the epistemological 'thaw' of medicine at the end of the eighteenth century was the organization of the hospital as an 'examining' apparatus.[2] The ritual of the visit was its most obvious form. . . . The old form of inspection [which, moreover, was conducted by a physician from outside, who otherwise had no part in the leadership of the hospital, F.B.], irregular

and rapid, was transformed into a regular observation that placed the patient in a situation of almost perpetual examination. This had two consequences: in the internal hierarchy, the physician, hitherto an external element, begins to gain over the religious staff and to relegate them to a clearly specified, but subordinate role in the technique of the examination; the category of the 'nurse' then appears; while the hospital itself, which was once little more than a poorhouse, was to become a place of training and of the correlation of knowledge; it represented a reversal therefore of the power relations and the constitution of a corpus of knowledge. The 'well-disciplined' hospital became the physical counterpart of the medical 'discipline'; this discipline could now abandon its textual character and take its references not so much from the tradition of author-authorities as from a domain of objects perpetually offered for examination. (Foucault 1979, p. 185)

If it is possible to determine accurately the historical moment when specific nursing functions emerge that play a "clearly specified, but subordinate role in the technique of the examination" in the hospital, then the fact can be recognized that the nursing staff as well as the "dominating" physician enter by virtue of their roles into complicity with disciplinary power; at the same time however, the potential *fracture point* of the medical-nursing, or in a word, of the therapeutic solidarity, is also recognizable, a fracture point that becomes virulent at the moment the consensus crumbles regarding the power-knowledge nexus, which makes possible and guarantees the hospital, and that the nursing staff become aware that what they do must become the object of a specific knowledge that does not play a merely supplementary role in the techniques of producing medical knowledge.

3. Disciplinary power demands a permanent register, it is essentially a "power of writing" (Foucault 1979, p. 189) and inspires entirely new recording and documentation methods whose function consists in enabling comparative fields to be organized—. . . making it possible to classify, to form categories, to determine averages, to fix norms: The hospitals of the eighteenth century, in particular, were great laboratories for scriptuary and documentary methods. The keeping of registers, their specification, the modes of transcription from one to the other, their circulation during visits, their comparison during regular meetings of doctors and administrators, the transmission of their data to centralizing bodies (either at the hospital or at the central office of the poorhouse), the accountancy of diseases, cures, deaths, at the level of a hospital, a town and even of the nation as a whole formed an integral part of the process by which hospitals were subjected to the disciplinary régime. (Foucault 1979, p. 190)

Through maximum individualization of the individual to a "case," a comparative system was created "that made possible the measurement of overall phenomena, the description of groups, the characterization of collective facts, the calculation of the gaps between individuals, their distribution in a given 'population'" (Foucault 1979, p. 190). Individualization in the normalist sense is a quasi-police function that consists in ascertaining small and even smaller differences between individuals, thereby constituting them to objects of knowledge that can be further and further broken down into components. In the context of disciplinary power, individualization means as much as unrestrained mass production of data. The hospital that is disciplined this way is the most important pivot between disciplinary power aiming at the individual body and the global regulation of the collective body (the population) undertaken by bio-power. The hospital attains such outstanding significance for the development of the human sciences because for the first time the "small techniques of notation, of registration, of constituting files, of arranging facts in columns and tables that are so familiar to us now," which were tested in its space, have transformed the individual (and not just the species) in his irreducible uniqueness into an object of knowledge and of a science that could be rightfully called "clinical science": "the problem of the entry of individual description, of the cross-examination, of anamnesis, of the 'file' into the general functioning of scientific discourse" (Foucault 1979, p. 191).

Disciplinary power functions in an individualizing way and thus reinforces deviations in two ways:

- First of all, in contrast with traditional power it is concerned with "ordinary individuality," which for a long time "remained below the threshold of description." In the age of disciplinary power, the chronicle becomes fundamental and loses its classic heroizing function: "It is no longer a monument for future memory, but a document for possible use" (Foucault 1979, p. 191).
- Second, it is an active individualizing power that makes the "individual difference" it is interested in perceptible in the first place or else produces it. The individual difference is not already "present" before the intervention of the power and only in need of representation; it is rather that disciplinary power creates the individual difference, namely, to the extent in which it is successful in giving it a means of articulation.

FROM CONTROL TO SELF-CONTROL

There are many indications that we are in a period of transition from one power regime to another. It is not by chance that Foucault's analytics of disciplinary power concentrate on the nineteenth century, the period when this power type receives its classic stamp, "but it is obvious that in the future we will have to divorce ourselves from the disciplinary society of today" (Foucault 1994b, p. 533). It appears that we are now in the middle of this future in which the crisis of disciplinary society is taking place. However, the transformation we are witnessing must not be imagined as happening according to the convenient pattern of a surgical incision. The strengths of the inventions of disciplinary power were demonstrated above all in the way these inventions became connected with a series of already existing important social institutions, to which they gave a completely new meaning, as we could observe in the example of the transformation from the classical to the modern hospital. The disciplinary power does not possess an essence of its own; it is thoroughly operative and therefore cannot be equated with one of the institutions that it uses as its milieu of realization. And what if the future of the disciplinary society, that is to say our future, consists in the disciplines, the procedures, for producing the "individual difference," becoming increasingly *deinstitutionalized* when they take their milieus piggy-back, so to speak, in order to be even more variable and adaptable than they could ever be within the framework of the classic fundamental institutions (army, factory, school, clinic, prison)? To what forces is the fully evolved disciplinary power exposed in our time?

To answer this question, or more modestly put, to contribute elements to its answer, it should be remembered that Foucault links his analytics of the disciplines to the problem of space in a fundamental way: The disciplines replace the impenetrable "mixed spaces" (remember the function of the "old" hospital as a collecting basin of poverty) with living tableaus, "which transform the confused, useless or dangerous multitudes into ordered multiplicities" (Foucault 1979, p. 148). The creation of a serial space is the prerequisite for the individualizing effect of normalizing power: every element in its place, no roving around or vagabonding. The main thing is to measure distances, to determine levels, to record exceptional features and harmonize the differences with each other beneficially. In the age of disciplinary power, the individualizing effect of normality can only be achieved within a closed space, a "milieu of confinement," which lends it its specifically repressive character. The dissolving or individualizing effects of the disciplines develop systematically within the already existing milieus of confinement, in which "abnormalities" are concentrated.

Although it was characteristic for predisciplinary power—as can be seen from the exclusion rituals with which leprosy was responded to—that it invariably worked with a massive and dichotomizing boundary drawn between the one and the other and that it excluded spatially or simply eliminated by force what was deviant instead of comprehending it as an object of potential knowledge and therapeutic intervention (the sword as the symbol of power in the "sovereignty societies"), the disciplines respond to disorder by including the "source of trouble" into the order, or more precisely: They respond with a strategy of forming enclaves rather than exclaves. The "dangerous mixtures" are confined (rather than forcefully expelled)—albeit at the price of subjecting them to a more intense and, as it were, more branched power, a power that replaces the friend/enemy distinction, the "massive and binary distinction between one set of people and another" with different kinds of separations and individualizing distributions: differentiation instead of exile-enclosure (Foucault 1979, p. 198). However, the decomposition of evil does not come about without exclusion, which now takes place within society and is localized institutionally and not least architecturally. It is as if the new power did not trust itself for a minute and therefore adopts the familiar milieus of confinement from the old power.

However, it is precisely these milieus of confinement that are at stake in modern times. The power of the norm(alization) is becoming radical to the same extent that it is gaining faith in itself and getting along without the walls of the milieus it has functioned within up to this time. For the future of the deinstitutionalized disciplines, Gilles Deleuze, the French philosopher and friend of Michel Foucault, has suggested the term control societies. Controls are virtually disciplines in the state of vagabondage. We must remember in connection with this term that Foucault had already pointed out *control*—the examining of behavior with a microscope—as an essential characteristic of the "monitoring" power that operates within the milieus of confinement. What is happening now is that this element is virtually being set free and its function changed: Control is separating from the architecture of the hierarchy to which it is still tied in the age of disciplinary power; it is ceasing to be a vertical privilege. Despite all preferences for circular architectures, disciplinary power was not able to manage without the model of the pyramid, the centralization at the top (Foucault 1979, p. 174). Control in the age of "control societies" is being subjected on the other hand to a decentering and deterritorializing movement that can no longer be restricted to the space of a "total institution" (Goffman, 1963). Even before Goffman it was thought to be true that surveillance does not come only from above, but also from below and from the side: a network that pervades the institution, as Foucault wrote, with the effects of power: "supervisors, perpetually supervised" (Foucault 1979, p. 177).

> We are in the process of entering "control" societies that, strictly speaking, are no longer disciplinary societies. It is not seldom that Foucault is regarded as a philosopher of disciplinary societies and their fundamental technique, confinement (not only hospital and prison, but also school, factory, barracks). In reality, though, he is among the first who say that we are in the process of departing from disciplinary societies, that they are no longer our reality. We are entering control societies that no longer function by internment but rather by constant control and direct communication. . . . Certainly, there is constant talk of the prison, school, and hospital: these institutions are in a state of crisis. They are indeed in a state of crisis, but this is precisely because they are anachronistic. New types of sanctioning, education and nursing are gradually developing. Open hospitals, home nursing etc. are no longer new. And it is foreseeable that education will not remain a closed milieu that distinguishes itself from the closed milieu of the working world, but that both will disappear and a terrible kind of permanent further education will appear in their place, a continuous control to which the worker—secondary school pupil or the executive—university student will be subjected. . . . In a control regime you are never finished with anything. (Deleuze 1990a, p. 236f.)

The control societies, whose dawn we are now experiencing, are freeing the disciplines from the corset of the milieus of confinement and enabling them to penetrate all of society. This expansion of their area of activity requires, however, a change in their mode of action. Deleuze expressed the difference in how controls are exerted using the following image: "The confinements are different kinds of molds, casting molds, whereas the controls are a modulation, they are like a self-forming mold that changes from one moment to the next or a sieve whose meshes vary from one point to another." (Deleuze 1990b, p. 242). Foucault, we remember, had said of disciplinary power that it has a "normalizing" effect, that it does not simply separate what is permitted from what is forbidden, but ascertains the individual's respective position differentially in a system of "degrees of normality" (and what is more, ascertains it again and again) (Foucault 1979, p. 184), and judges it according to its distance from the norm, which is a statistically obtained and temporary average value.

In his *Essay on Normalism (Versuch über den Normalismus)*, Jürgen Link (1997a) deals with the possible reasons for Foucault's unresolved ambivalence with regard to his own use of the theoretical term. Normalism, as it in the nineteenth century comes to comprehend central sectors of modern society, is not a uniform phenomenon; it appears in the form of two rivaling strategies that try to form fields of normality in different ways, but become effective always jointly. Normalism is namely itself a part of the problem that it is supposed to solve: If Broussais's principle of the fundamental continuity between normal and abnormal phenomena is really valid, the fear that basically anyone can cross the boundary, which is no longer ontologically established, that is, no longer perceptible for everyone to the same extent, must become virulent. The *protonormalists,* as Link calls them, react to this typically modern anxiety of an irreversible denormalization by employing the strategy of maximum compression of the zone of normality and a correspondingly "strict" semantic and symbolic marking of the boundaries of normality; the *flexible-normalist* strategy on the other hand, which became extremely prevalent in Western societies after the Second World War ("permissive society"), strives for a maximum expansion and dynamic quality of the zone of normality, for which purpose it always fixes a temporary boundary of normality; that is, keeps it reversible and, figuratively speaking, does not constitute it as a wall, but as a transitional space or "passage." This tug-of-war situation between the two strategies is taken into account by Foucault—without his conceptualizing it—insofar as his description of the new power order constantly oscillates between dynamic-open and repressive categories (disciplines, training, etc.).

The Janus-facedness of the normalizing societies is founded upon the paradoxical status of the boundary: Namely, if normalism is characterized on the one hand by the fact that its boundaries are invariably precarious and provisional because it presupposes a fundamental continuity between normal and abnormal phenomena and does not tolerate any qualitative (that is, anything not fundamentally within reach of the normalizing influence) differences or antagonisms, then it cannot on the other hand be separated from a boundary politics. This is because the activity of normalism has precisely the purpose of providing protection against the risk of irreversible denormalization (that is, of absolute abnormalities), a risk associated with the normal reproduction modus of modern societies. Although normalism has thus lost all respect for inviolable, qualitative boundaries (which possess to a certain degree the status of tabus), because it recognizes only flexible limits in a continuum it is still thoroughly convinced that there must be boundaries somewhere and they may only be transgressed at the cost of sociocultural catastrophes. For protonormalism, the "productive chaos" of the modern age can only be restrained by a clear specification of order, which demands in particular also from the subjects a strictly conforming behavior, and if need arise, even a confirmation of those norms on which the existence of the social order is made dependent. "The protonormalist strategies," writes Jürgen Link, "invariably tend to 'lean on' a prenormalist, 'qualitative' setting of boundaries and exclusions" (Link 1997b, p. 238). The (French) title of Foucault's famous study of the genealogy of the modern disciplinary power can be understood virtually as the motto of this authoritarian strategy: *Surveiller et punir (Control and Punish).*

The flexible-normalist strategy, however, does not rely on a control from outside or even on its subjects being educated, but on their willingness to continue the self-normalization process in view of uncertain and frequently blurred boundaries of normality. "Let things happen," is their motto, occasional "excursions" ("trips") away from the center of normality into the zones of beginning deviation or even into the region of abnormality keeps society from becoming rigid. It is demanded of individuals that they offset the risk of an undesired, possibly irreversible drifting into abnormality against the opposite risk of an obsessive-compulsive orientation towards rigid and fixed norms that promise maximum security, but exhibit as their price a tendency towards self-immobilization. The flexibility of normalist subjects does not consist then in the "subjects' being permanently 'located' on the periphery," but "in an area which has a relatively large 'oscillation range,' but which oscillates around the average and for that reason remains fixed to it (e.g., sexual variability as sporadic 'outings' within the defined limits of a 'permanent relationship' or as 'serial monogamy' with different 'phase timing' etc.)" (Link 1997a, p. 339).

What is changing during the transition to control societies is the status of the actual norm and the normalities from which the individual's position is measured. The norm no longer functions as a fixed reference for normalizing activity, but itself varies during the process of normalization; it is, paradoxically speaking, virtually the average of all deviations from a prescribed norm (regulation) imagined to be stable and resistant to time. Deviation is the normal thing. The (average) norm only exists so that deviations can continue to be recognized as deviations and they remain exposed to a gravitational force that hinders their floating around freely and uncontrolled proliferation. If it is no longer possible to establish a relation between deviation and a concept of perfection or the ideal type of "nature," then at least the statistics should create a substitute for the lost social framework of reference.

We must learn to think in terms of the *immanence of the norm* (in relation to the activity that undergoes its normative influence) and also the *immanence of the resistance to the norm.* Only then will we truly stop viewing its work "as restrictive, as 'repression' cast in prohibition formulas and practiced on a subject who exists before this exertion of influence and who can free himself from such a control or be freed from it" (Macherey 1991, p. 183). The norm does not precede its field of application, nor does it precede its own action, and this is what distinguishes it from ideals, laws, imperatives, regulations, and standards. Its normative function is only ordered to the extent that it is applied and the results of its intervention in a social field are continuously evaluated. This is why Deleuze emphasizes the variability of controls: self-forming molds that change from one moment to the next. As was explained in the beginning, statistical procedures and prognosis based on mathematical probability play a central role in this process of giving the norm a liquid character.

The self-forming molds are a precise image for the strategy of flexible normalism as defined by Jürgen Link. The norm loses its terrorist quality, which manifests itself by forcefully imposing itself upon the spontaneous will—depreciated by philosophers such as Kant as the sphere of inclination and subject to practical reason. The connection between moral concepts (guilt, conscience, obligation, sanctity of the obligation) and *cruelty* was revealed by Nietzsche in his *Genealogie der Mora (Genealogy of Morals).* These concepts, wrote Nietzsche, have "never really lost a certain savour of blood and torture," and he adds as an explanation, "not even in old Kant: the categorical imperative reeks of cruelty . . ." (Nietzsche 1887/1913, pp. 72–73). In Link's so-called *protonormalism* cruelty is not dispensed with and therefore the new power techniques are given the task of defending a boundary of normality that surrounds the normal field as a protective barrier if necessary, and this even possibly by force, yet no boundary is sacred in flexible normalism. Above all, no boundaries are set a priori, so that the need of having to resort to any possible means to ensure their future observance in the case of their transgression is avoided; boundaries are only set, with a bad conscience as it were, because there is a fundamental sympathy with the dynamics of modern society and its productive chaos should not be strangled by force, but only protected from irreversible effects of denormalization (abrupt breaks or antagonisms). Normalism, to modify a term of Gilles Deleuze's and Félix Guattari's, "is in a permanent state of pushing its boundary away and approaching it" (Deleuze & Guattari, 1981, p. 45), it oscillates, so to speak, equally between the spontaneous tendency towards social and cultural deinstitutionalization, or more precisely, to the largest possible expansion of the spectrum of normality and the opposite certainty that there must be a boundary somewhere. Instead of setting boundaries by authority and marking these symbolically and semantically as impermeable, flexible normalism—as is characteristic for the "control societies" described by Deleuze—relies on the willingness of individuals to make the scope of their behavior an object of permanent "risk evaluation."

For this reason it would be completely missing the point to associate control societies with the black utopias of permanent surveillance by an Orwellian Big Brother: Control, as Deleuze describes it, means essentially self-control and refers to a certain type of subject whose style of behavior is not shaped by external guidance and education (the authoritarian character) but by self-normalization and self-adjustment. Although the protonormalists, that is, the normalists against their will, pretend in their uncertainty about the course of the boundary of normality that they are in a maximum safety zone and try to contain the fluctuations that arise from permanent denormalization and renormalization processes by definite removal of certain "minus variants" to special material territories (prison, insane asylum), a more flexible mode of dealing with the "fundamental anxiety of the modern age," that is, not being normal, has been establishing itself in Western societies since 1945, primarily in the U.S.:

> The participating subjects devise imaginary axes of normality or areas of normality with center lines, tolerance zones, boundaries of normality and zones of abnormality, in short, symbolic normalist *landscapes* for very different kinds of proceedings, interactions, events and processes in very different cultural sectors. They are constantly placing themselves and other subjects in such *landscapes,* comparing their own imagined position with that of other subjects, and determining *distances* between. (Link, 1997a, p. 337)

Instead of being conditioned to strictly programmed, reflexlike responses, the subjects develop the ability for self-normalization by subjecting themselves to a continuous test to find out how far they can go without toppling over the edge of the spectrum of normality and losing contact to the reassuring normality within. Deleuze hints at this aspect of a kind of flexible psychomanagement that tries to guarantee the subjects' stability not at the cost of dynamics but based on them when he contrasts the discontinuous individual who was subjected to the disciplines, occupied a plotted space, and was in this sense truly fenced in with the individual who is subjected to control, that is, self-control, and more likely to be "wavelike" (Deleuze, 1990b, p. 244), a quality that connotes the inevitable rolling course of this non-ascertained subjectivity type who only feels sure of himself when constantly comparing his own life journey with alternative courses.

Jürgen Link shows in his *Essay on Normalism* (1997a) that what he calls the "mass therapy culture" of the United States draws the most radical consequences from the principle of continuity between normality and abnormality. If there is no intrinsic, qualitative boundary that is clearly marked between normal and abnormal phenomena, then it follows that the protonormalist strategy of externalizing what is abnormal (that is, definitively separating it from normality) must be abandoned and that we have always been living in a realm that manifests both normal and abnormal aspects. The emergence of a "culture of 'therapy for the normal'" in the U.S., as described by Robert and Françoise Castel in a collaboration with Anne Lovell (1982), leads consequently to a state in which there is a development of complete flexibility of all the stigmata used by a culture to distinguish between the healthy and the sick. Erving Goffman (1963), who dealt in a classic study with the contemporary forms of stigma management, shifts the perspective from normality to abnormality: how much of the abnormal is still found in what is thought to be pure normality? Not only the realm of abnormality but also that of normality has a high resolution, is differentiated, and finely graduated. What is even more significant, however, is that the differentiation within the spectrum of normality is not compact, but "flexible-continuous" (Link, 1997a, p. 80), so that in the end Goffman only speaks of "roles" in which the healthy/normal and sick/abnormal stand in opposition to each other: "One can therefore suspect that the role of normal and the role of stigmatized are parts of the same complex, cuts from the same standard cloth" (Goffman, 1963, p. 130). Stigma management is therefore "a general component of society" because in tendency there is no individual who does not participate in both roles and who is not capable of playing both roles. Goffman therefore also replaces the strict, qualitative opposition of normality and abnormality with the paradoxical "normal abnormality": "If, then, the stigmatized person is to be called a deviant, he might better be called a normal deviant" (Goffman, 1963, p. 162).

The *normal deviant* is the hero of the modern therapy culture as it was first invented in the United States—to a considerable extent under the influence of psychoanalysis, which by the turn of the twentieth century had already brought about what was considered by many contemporaries to be shocking normalization of sexual perversions. The stigma or normality management of contemporary American society now views the curing of illnesses as a "special case within an all-embracing system of 'early diagnosis' and life-accompanying normalization (readaption)." Link gives a detailed account of the institutional arrangements that lend expression to this strategy towards normalization of the abnormal or "abnormalization" of the normal as follows:

> As a result of the founding of community mental health centers under Kennedy, this trend towards flexible normalism was even given an institutional core of its own, which was followed by the tendency to transform elementary schools into de facto parallel community mental health centers (continuous testing and diagnosis of the children). A final decisive factor turned out to be the "takeover" of Sixty-Eight (which began in the USA much earlier). The culture revolution (counter-culture) radically tore down the boundaries of normality (e.g. with regard to sexual minorities). The official culture then "adopted" (as far as the legal level) some of these openings of boundaries. (Link, 1997a, p. 380)

The flexible normalism typical of control societies, as Goffman clearly illustrates, repeatedly verges on a *transnormalist realm,* a realm that functions according to the logic of "free proliferation" and no longer yields to the force of normalist mapping. If there is no reason to exclude abnormal or stigmatized individuals because abnormal tendencies are latently present in everyone, then it seems an obvious conclusion that the process of determining a particular positional value in the normality-abnormality continuum could be dispensed with entirely for every individual. However, precisely this consequence is not found in normalism. In flexible normalism the abandonment of permanent exclusion is compensated by constituting "risk classes," whose operativeness is dependent on the individual's willingness to make self-revelations on a kind of permanent basis. The fact that this "compulsion to confess" can be experienced as actually pleasurable by those who are subject to it is proven by the existence of a certain type of literature, which luxuriates in biographical self-exposure and intimate confessions and supplements the active mass production of data evaluated by medical and psychiatric experts. However, the pleasure gained from revealing one's most intimate wishes (the *coming-out* effect) cannot be separated from a specific stress connected with permanent production of data pertaining to others and of that pertaining to oneself because the production of this data invariably has the function of manifesting a still acceptable, still tolerable normality, that is, with reference to the always provisional average values. "The individual is no longer confined, but indebted" (Deleuze, 1990b, p. 246). This means that he pays for his "liberation" from the horrors of abnormality by committing himself to maintaining a book-keeping perspective towards his own small abnormalities or risk factors, which as a result must be constantly observed so that they do not develop into solid, compact abnormalities.

ILLNESS AS RISK—THE CURRENT ANXIETY

The crisis of the closed milieus, one could also say, is that their structural change cannot be welcomed as progress or even liberation without an effort, as Deleuze shows with the example of the hospital, unless progress is generally identified with the development of more flexibility:

> In the crisis of the hospital as a closed milieu, sectoring, day hospitals or home care nursing, for example, were at first a mark of new freedoms, but then became a component of the new control mechanisms, which are not inferior in any way to the harshest confinements. There are no reasons for fear or hope, but only for seeking new weapons (Deleuze, 1990b, p. 241).

The criterion for what Deleuze calls the "new forms of resistance against control societies" would be to avoid at all events that the fear of development of new flexibilities, which always also produce new impenetrabilities, ends up in a nostalgic perspective towards the relative security and clarity of the classic milieus of confinement. Responses to the most varied kinds of new flexibilities made possible by the normality complex of this century—such as the protonormalist affect that a boundary has now irrevocably been transgressed and "that it cannot continue like this" —have occurred all too often. Rather than erecting dams against the floods of permanent reforms, the willingness to resist should be made dependent on whether these reforms contain elements suitable for continuing to destigmatize the realm of pathologies or whether, on the contrary, they allow the regime of the great dichotomizations to be resurrected in a new guise.

The "new medicine which exists 'without doctor and patients' and ascertains potential patients and risk groups" cited by Deleuze (1990b, p. 247) appears at first glance to be the realization of an old dream by those who have so far been structurally underprivileged in the healing and nursing process. François Ewald (1986) has shown how the increasing penetration of the social fabric by risk technologies is also revolutionizing the conception of illness. Illnesses are now essentially "illnesses of solidarity" and are viewed according to the tuberculosis model, because "the other is a potential carrier of an evil that can strike me, it is for my own benefit that I monitor him, correct him, ensure his further development, provide for his hygiene and his sterilization" (Ewald, 1986, p. 361). Any person can pose a risk to another, so everyone is obliged to do his [or her] part in helping to reduce the risk, which means first and foremost being willing to perceive oneself as a risk. "There is risk everywhere. Germs spread, and there is the threat of their continued spread without check" (Ewald, 1986, p. 362). The paranoiac eccentricities that have resulted from risk thinking introduced into our perception of illness in this century do not have to be mentioned separately. They should be a warning to us not to overestimate the human benefits of a flexible normalism. It can lead from one moment to the next to the hysteria of a general mobilization against the omnipresent evil, even in times of peace.

NURSING CONCEPTUALIZATIONS
OF HEALTH AND ILLNESS

Nursing conceptualizations of health and illness, against the dichotomizing conceptualization of normal/abnormal and pathologizing of illness, emerged as a response to demedicalization of nursing in the United States beginning in the early 1970s. Within various nursing theories, health and illness are conceptualized in terms of individual adaptations (Roy & Andrews, 1991), constantly fluctuating processes of experiencing and evolving in concert with the environmental changes (Newman, 1994; Parse, 1992; Rogers, 1989), or as a continuum that bypasses the notion of normality. Such conceptualizations often maintain illness as personal experiences, not framed within the notion of "deviation from the given norm," which Foucault considers the basis for the normalizing processes of modern medicine. However, nursing work has been very much tied to the institutional base of normalizing processes remnants of the nineteenth-century hospital dynamics, which are structured around the disciplinary power of medicine. Hence, there had to exist a form of disillusion in nursing between how it proposes to conceptualize health/ illness and how it must carry on with its work within health care institutions.

In addition, the transition to control societies from disciplinary societies that Deleuze suggests for the current scene imposes an important issue to nursing, as it must shift its positioning from its earlier institutionalization within what Foucault calls "the milieu of confinement" to "open milieu." Nursing must address how it would need to conceptualize health/illness and "patient" in the context of open milieu and deinstitutionalization of control that emerges in the form of self-control and self-normalization. The conceptualization of illness as risk elevates the concept of health/illness as a continuum to another level at which all is healthy/none is healthy and all is ill/none is ill. What is important for nursing is to propose how nursing as an organized system and a culture of knowledge must address deinstitutionalization of health and health care.

Notes

1. In Bernard's work, the real identity—should one say in mechanisms or symptoms or both?—and continuity of pathological phenomena and the corresponding physiological phenomena are more a monotonous repetition than a theme (Canguilhem, 1978, p. 30).

2. A process whose counterpart is found in the simultaneously occurring installations in the schools which became, a sort of apparatus of uninterrupted examination that duplicated along its entire length the operation of teaching (Foucault, 1979, p. 186).

References

Canguilhem, G. (1978). *On the normal and the pathological* (C. R. Fawcett, Trans., with an introduction by Michel Foucault). Dordrecht, The Netherlands: D. Reidel. (Original work published in 1966).

Castel, R., Castel, F., & Lovell, A. (1982). *The psychiatric society* (A. Gold-hammer, Trans.). New York: Columbia University Press. (Original work published in 1979).

Deleuze, G. (1990a). Contrôle et devenir [Control and becoming]. *Pourparlers 1972–1990* (pp. 229–239). Paris: Minuit.

Deleuze, G. (1990b). Post-scriptum sur les sociétés de contrôle [Post-script on the control societies]. *Pourparlers 1972–1990* (pp. 240–247). Paris: Minuit.

Deleuze, G., & Guattari, F. (1981). *Anti-Ödipus. Kapitalismus und Schizophrenie 1 [Anti-Oedipus. Capitalism and schizophrenia]*. Frankfurt, Germany: Suhrkamp.

Ewald, F. (1986). *L'état providence [The state of providence]*. Paris: Grasset.

Foucault, M. (1973). *The birth of the clinic. An archaeology of medical perception* (A. M. Sheridan Smith, Trans.). London: Tavistock Publications. (Originally published in 1963).

Foucault, M. (1979). *Discipline and punish. The birth of the prison* (A. Sheridan, Trans.). Harmondsworth, UK: Penguin. (Originally published in 1975).

Foucault, M. (1981). *The history of sexuality. Volume I: An introduction.* (R. Hurley, Trans.). Harmondsworth, UK: Penguin. (Originally published in 1976).

Foucault, M. (1994a). Qui êtes-vous, professeur Foucault? Entretien avec P. Caruso [Who are you, Professor Foucault? An interview with P. Caruso]. In *Dits et écrits. 1954–1988* (Vol. 1, pp. 601–620). Paris: Gallimard.

Foucault, M. (1994b). La philosophie analytique de la politique [The philosophical analysis of politics]. In *Dits et écrits. 1954–1988* (Vol. 3, pp. 534–551). Paris: Gallimard.

Goffman, E. (1963). *Stigma: Notes on the management of spoiled identity.* Englewood Cliffs, NJ: Prentice-Hall.

Link, J. (1997a). *Versuch über den Normalismus. Wie Normalität produziert wird [Attempt on normalism. How normality is produced]*. Opladen, Germany: Westdeutscher.

Link, J. (1997b). Von Karl Kraus zu Rainald Goetz: Zwei Stadien der Medienkritik—Zwei Stadien des Normalismus [From Karl Kraus to Rainald Goetz: Two phases of media critiques—Two phases of normalism]? In F. Balke & B. Wagner (Eds.), *Vom Nutzen und Nachteil historischer Vergleiche. Der Fall Bonn—Weimar* (pp. 235–255). Frankfurt/New York: Campus.

Luhmann, N. (1997). *Die Gesellschaft der Gesellschaft [The society as social system]*. 2 volumes. Frankfurt, Germany: Suhrkamp.

Macherey, P. (1991). Für eine Naturgeschichte der Normen [In favor of a natural history of norms]. In F. Ewald & B. Waldenfels (Eds.), *Spiele der Wahrheit. Michel Foucaults Denken* (pp. 171–192). Frankfurt, Germany: Suhrkamp.

Newman, M. (1994). *Health as expanding consciousness* (2nd ed.). New York: National League for Nursing.

Nietzsche, F. (1913). The genealogy of morals: A polemic (H. B. Samuel, Trans.). In O. Levy (Ed.), *The complete works of Friedrich Nietzsche* (Vol. 13, pp. 72–73). Edinburgh, Scotland: T. N. Foulis (Originally published in German in 1887).

Nietzsche, F. (1968). The will to power (W. Kaufmann & R. J. Hollingdale, Trans.). New York: Vintage.

Parse, R. R. (1992). Human becoming: Parse's theory of nursing. *Nursing Science Quarterly, 5,* 35–42.

Roy, C., & Andrews, H. A. (1991). *The Roy adaptation model: The definitive statement.* Norwalk, CT: Appleton & Lange.

Rogers, M. E. (1989). Nursing: A science of unitary human beings. In J. Riehl-Sisca (Ed.), *Conceptual models for nursing practice* (3rd ed., pp. 181–188). Norwalk, CT: Appleton & Lange.

CHAPTER 16

Postscript*

Ingrid Kollak and Susanne Wied

S ome sciences seem to be devoid of any practice. People who learn and teach in these sciences are not infrequently questioned about the purpose and usefulness of what they do. Nursing, by contrast, is acknowledged as having a purpose and a social mission to fulfill, yet it possesses only the rudiments of science. Some people think that nursing does not have to be a science, while others actively contribute towards establishing a theory of nursing.

Those who have read our book as far as this Postscript presumably must be interested in building up a science of nursing. We therefore provide neither a justification for nursing theories nor any absolute definitions of the pertinent terms because inquiry into them and discussion of them are not supposed to end with the preceding essays but are intended to be initiated by them. Neither is it our intention to make our peace with nursing theories and their terms, but on the contrary, to examine their contents for improvements in nursing practice, teaching, and research.

Which terms, first of all, are we talking about? We are referring to those that appear in various nursing theories but are not specific to nursing, such as nursing diagnoses. We also mean terms that are familiar in everyday language, such as needs, scope, care, adaptation, and others. Because they are so practical and so widely and generally accepted, they are increasingly deprived of their specific meaning, even though—imperceptibly—they determine the way we think and

---

*Translated from German by Gerald Nixon.

act. The result is that to a large extent they are subjected to the personal interpretation of the reader and are never subsequently questioned. However, we insist that these terms be given a critical appraisal and considered in their proper context.

In this book, authors have expressed views they currently hold about certain terms and concepts of nursing theories or about neighboring sciences against the background of their education and study as well as their experience of nursing. In various ways they have pointed out the historical and contextual significance of nursing concepts and have outlined both the possibilities and the limitations. They have done this from a diachronic point of view, by inquiring into the origin and history of a term, or by examining the various contexts from which these terms are borrowed, or both. The interpretation of these terms has always been a matter of controversy and their meanings have undergone continual change. Of course, it is possible to introduce these terms unquestioningly into a given nursing context, but we cannot pretend they do not have a history of their own. The authors have also presented their studies from a synchronic perspective, showing that terms are not neutral and denote a certain fact or a set of facts. Terms like *interaction, adaptation, system, self-care, holism*, and others are put into many different contexts that we cannot simply ignore. Occasionally, without any intention on our part and without our even being aware, these terms by association link us to a certain social and cultural context and its sometimes controversial implications.

Terms thus possess a dynamic of their own, a power over meaning and interpretation on which, far from being able to avoid, we are forced to take up a position. But we can also harness this power for our own ends if we learn how to handle the terms properly and use them in a creative and purposeful (i.e., knowledge enhancing) way. This book wishes to motivate its readers to indulge in theoretical reflection and enter a productive association with terms. Moreover, a prerequisite of science is unequivocal terminology, for if an object of inquiry cannot be clearly named and described, no further research step is possible.

Because our book is a coproduction of American and German-speaking authors, it may be helpful to inquire into the different conditions that exist in these countries with regard to the education and training as well as the politics of nursing.

Nursing in the United States is envied all over the world for having dealt with the question of the academic and scientific status from the very beginning of this century. In Germany, as well as in Austria and Switzerland, we are still in the very early stages of such a development.

In German-speaking countries, even today, part of the nursing profession is still closely linked to Christian institutions, which is a result of historical development, reflected in, among other things, the divisions in nursing federations. The "mother house" system of training in the Lutheran Church, for example, functioned very efficiently until the 1980s, but this also meant that nursing was understood as a service in Christ's name rather than as a profession with special competence. The "free helpers"—nonregistered nurses not belonging to the deaconry, which supervised the Lutheran Church's charitable work—were instrumentalized (poorly paid with no career prospects; compare the confidential reports of the Kaiserswerther Verband) by the leading administrators of the church training institutions. These institutions were always headed by a pastor, never a deaconess, in such a way as to meet existing staff requirements but not to jeopardize deaconesses' willingness to work without pay. The deaconesses' high social standing was associated with virtues such as serving, the Christian ethic of "love thy neighbor," sacrifice, performing one's duty, and unconditional obedience to one's superiors—(male) doctors and clergymen. Free nursing organizations, such as the Agnes Karll Federation, sprang up as a countermovement, but they received scarcely any public attention. Nursing was instrumentalized militarily with the rise of the Red Cross, which borrowed its canon of values from those of Christian nursing associations. Under the National Socialist regime in Germany, the different nursing movements were merged into a monolithic structure of fascist orientation; it took years to recover from this devastation and the development of nursing as a profession was set back decades.

The growing trend towards the municipal administration of hospitals forced the Christian virtues of nurses into the background. Because no new virtues came to take their place, nursing the sick turned into a relatively unspecific, auxiliary occupation in medicine without any profile of its own. The rapid achievement of academic status, which gained ground in the 1990s thanks to the untiring efforts of a number of pioneers, can do little to conceal the lack of scientifically trained personnel. Overcoming structures that are deeply rooted in history is an arduous task. And even the present generation of academically trained teachers, researchers, and managers of nursing has gone through the practical phase of having to deal with the conditions that are associated with the pervasive structures of health care and the profession.

American and Canadian nurses, on the other hand, become familiar with nursing concepts right from the beginning of their training because they study to become nurses. Study courses begin immediately after the end of high school and general knowledge learning continues in the first terms of study. Thinking conceptually about nursing, drawing up concepts together with their lecturers and evaluating them with the rest of the course is the method preferred in the whole profession.[1]

In German-speaking countries, by contrast, those who leave school intending to take up a nursing career are first of all required to enroll in a training course; this entails signing a contract with a clinic, for example, and attending the health care training school belonging to it. Here, depending on the country, they must decide from the start either the area in which they wish to work in future (caring for the elderly, with children, in psychiatry, etc.) or the length of the training course or the qualification they are aiming for. The training itself is split into two quite separate spheres as far as both institutions and personnel are concerned (although there may be close connections at the institutional level): the clinic, home for the elderly. or other location of practical training on the one hand, and the corresponding school on the other.

The clinic, with its colleagues, mentors, and supervisors (if they exist) who either work with them or are in charge of their practical training, constitutes the practical side of their training. The corresponding school, with its lecturers and tutors, provides the theoretical knowledge that is necessary. This old principle of the hospital school places the focus on the needs of the training institution and does not represent part of the general educational system. It is no longer the norm but, in Germany at least, one can still find almost everywhere a system that teaches lessons on one day of the week, or in blocks of several weeks, in which the trainees are taught by doctors, psychologists, dieticians, and nursing teachers in the individual subjects. On the other days of the week, the trainees go about their work in accordance with the shift schedules of the training institution.

Should trained nurses decide to study further, they can do so only after their 3- or 4-year training course (the length depending on the country, which is considered the basic education for nursing) and, in addition, the required number of years' experience in health care. They then enter quite unfamiliar territory of higher education regarded as postgraduate, with a possibility of advancing to study for a doctoral degree upon having received excellent grades in their final examinations. Nursing concepts may be completely new to them at the beginning of their advanced study. An understanding of nursing based on the most recent state of nursing knowledge and practice is not necessarily the starting point of nursing studies at this level.

If we were to evaluate the different paths followed in nurses' education and training and their effect on kindling an awareness for theoretical reflection, we can certainly say that because of their college education American and Canadian nurses will be quite familiar with texts on nursing concepts. From the very beginning of their study they are used to inquiring into different concepts and theories that soon no longer overwhelm them. That nursing science is offered as a college or university course is taken for granted in the United States and Canada by teachers and students alike. All the more unconstrained, then, is the students' reception of nursing concepts, which, moreover, are not gauged purely against the standard of nursing practice. Theory and practice are two perfectly normal and equal components of training. And there lies the advantage.

Students in Germany, on the other hand, have often had to wait several years for an opportunity to study and they have greater misgivings and apprehension about texts and discussions on nursing theory. These students must first of all learn to take a detached view of the practical experience they have gained in their previous work. If they succeed in this, they have a great advantage over others: years of practical experience, the fact that they have mastered difficult situations in nursing as well as the task of cooperating with other professional groups, and the fact that they have a precise idea and understanding of the extent to which certain theoretical concepts are valid and of how these stand in relation to the theory and practice of other disciplines.

We can thus hope in our future work together for a mutual widening of perspectives, which will ultimately have a positive effect on the development of theory as well as practice. Learning from one another can take the form of direct human exchange, as provided by student and teacher exchanges with foreign countries. Anyone who has experienced this kind of direct contact knows how inspiring and encouraging it is. And sometimes the result is to be seen in projects like this book. If similar encouragement is given to readers of this book for ideas, plans, and projects of their own, this would naturally be a great success.

From a social point of view, too, it is essential that we look further than our own backyard, as the saying goes. For as the social need for individualized forms of care grows, nurses will have to be able to integrate different, even contrary concepts into their nursing strategies in the course of their careers. To this end, however, the pluralism of nursing concepts will also have to be taken for granted in the development of theory. (This view is not to be confused with a call for eclecticism or a system of "anything goes.") Only an understanding that is emancipatory with regard to both theory and practice will be able to meet a society's need for nurses, and to achieve this, the one-sided, self-sealing view of many nurses and nursing theorists will have to broaden.

Last but not least, it is worth raising the question of the price a society is ready to pay for nursing in its practical and theoretical forms. Whereas in the U.S. the public funding of nurses' education and research has been considerable, albeit still insufficient, the financing of nurses' training and nursing research in German-speaking countries can only be described as meager. Even today, training for a career in nursing is not part of general education, and unlike all other teachers, trainers at hospital schools do not necessarily have a university degree. With few exceptions, advanced nursing study courses are limited to higher education colleges and here, too, human and financial resources are insubstantial. Furthermore, the development of nursing theory will depend to a considerable extent on which projects are promoted and funded. Moreover, although winning academic status and adopting scientific standards may be great steps forward, this process must be accompanied by one of effectively raising awareness of nursing as a political issue. Here, too, theoretical concepts might variously provide a useful contribution.

Our inquiry into the benefits of cooperation in theoretical work against the background of the different conditions prevailing in nursing practice, teaching, and research can perhaps be summed up as follows: The common goal of our theoretical reflections on nursing is oriented towards recognizing and acting. Here, we can learn with and from each other to inquire into nursing concepts—confidently and bearing in mind the benefits to our respective fields of work—in order to understand which discussions and which movements these concepts are capable of sparking.

NOTE

1. A detailed account of nurses' education and training in the United States and the present state of nursing politics is given by Ingrid Kollak and Penny Powers in: Kollak & Powers (1998),. *Pflege-Ausbildung im Gespräch. Ein internationaler Vergleich [Nurses' Training Under Discussion. An International Comparison]* (pp. 219–237). Written by a team of international authors, the book describes the educational, training, and working conditions of nurses in 14 countries.

Synopsis of Selected Nursing Theories and Conceptual Models

Hesook Suzie Kim

ABDELLAH, FAYE G.

Abdellah proposed a classificatory framework for identifying nursing problems, based on her idea that nursing is basically oriented to meeting an individual client's total health needs. Her major effort was to differentiate nursing from medicine and disease orientation. Abdellah's framework identifies 21 nursing problems around which nurses must organize patient care. Although these problems refer to specific aspects of patients' needs, they point to what nurses should do in meeting these needs. She did not offer specific general assumptions to guide the identification of these needs, but included among them needs associated with physical, psychological, spiritual, communicative, interpersonal, and social aspects of individuals' well-being associated with health.

[*Sources:* Abdellah, F. G., Beland, I. L., Martin, A., & Matheney, R. V. (1960). Patient-centered approaches to nursing. New York: Macmillan; Abdellah, F. G., Beland, I. L., Martin, A., & Matheney, R. V. (1973). *New directions in patient-centered nursing.* New York: Macmillan.]

HENDERSON, VIRGINIA

Henderson was one of the pioneers who tried to identify the unique contributions of nursing within the health care arena. She identified 14 components of basic nursing care in association with her definition of nursing that supports the major goal of nursing as assisting individuals to gain independence in relation to the performance of activities "contributing to health or its recovery (or to peaceful death)." These components refer to basic human needs and humans' everyday functioning, including bodily needs; the need for safety in relation to environment; communication; and human activities associated with worship, occupation, enjoyment of life, and continuous learning. To Henderson, nursing's role is in being substitutive, supplementary, or complementary to patients who lack "knowledge, physical strength, or the will" to be independent in their daily lives.

[*Sources:* Henderson, V. (1960). *Basic principles of nursing care.* Geneva, Switzerland: International Council of Nurses; Henderson, V. (1966). *The nature of nursing.* New York: Macmillan; Henderson, V. (1991). *The nature of nursing—Reflections after 25 years.* New York: Macmillan.]

KING, IMOGENE M.

King presented a systems-oriented conceptual framework for nursing and proposed a theory of goal attainment. The conceptual framework representing knowledge that is essential for nursing consists of three interacting systems—the personal, the interpersonal, and the social—and encompasses goal, structure, function, resources, and decision making. The theory of goal attainment is the essential theoretical component of the interpersonal system within this conceptual framework. King considers the theory of goal attainment critical for nursing because interaction between clients and nurses is the essential process through which clients can be assisted to attain and maintain health in order to function in their roles. Several concepts are introduced in the theory of goal attainment: action, reaction, interaction, transaction, perception, judgment, role, growth and development, and goal attainment. Three specific propositions linking perceptual accuracy, role congruence, communication, transaction, goal attainment, growth and development, and satisfaction are advanced in the theory. The key to this theory is that the outcome of nursing care is influenced by client and nurse transaction.

[*Sources:* King, I. M. (1971). *Toward a theory for nursing: General concepts of human behavior.* New York: Wiley; King, I. M. (1989). King's general systems framework and theory. In J. Riehl-Sisca (Ed.), *Conceptual models for nursing practice* (3rd ed., pp. 149–158). Norwalk, CT: Appleton & Lange; King, I. M. (1990). *A theory for nursing: Systems, concepts, process.* Albany, NY: Delmar. (Originally published in 1981)]

LEININGER, MADELEINE

Leininger's culture-care diversity and universality theory is based on two major concepts: care and transculturality. She believes that care is the core of nursing and is essential to healing. When care is combined with the understanding that human beings' lives are grounded within unique cultures from birth to death, nursing can engage in universal and culture-specific practices to help people with their lives related to health and well-being. Culture care in Leininger's theory stands for various modes by which culture influences how people deal with their lives and conditions, and includes both folk and professional health-care practices. This is articulated in Leininger's "sunrise enabler" that specifies various dynamics among cultural and social structures, care expressions, and transcultural care decisions and actions. In this theory of culture care, both diversity and universality are emphasized, oriented to culture-care preservation and maintenance, culture-care accommodation and negotiation, and culture-care repatterning and restructuring, which would result in culturally congruent care for health, well-being, and dying.

[*Sources:* Leininger, M. M. (1984). Transcultural nursing: An overview. *Nursing Outlook, 32*(2), 72–73; Leininger, M. M. (1991). *Culture care diversity and universality: A theory of nursing.* New York: National League of Nursing; Leininger, M. M. (1995). *Transcultural nursing: Concepts, theories, research, and practice* (2nd ed.). New York: McGraw-Hill; Leininger, M. M., & McFarland, M. (2002). *Transcultural nursing: Concepts, theories, research and practice* (3rd ed.). New York: McGraw-Hill.]

NEUMAN, BETTY

The Neuman systems model is based on the systems perspective within which clients are viewed to be open systems responding to environmental stressors in order to maintain system stability and integrity. The client system is identified by the core component of basic structure and energy resources, which are protected by lines of resistance, normal line of defense, and flexible line of defense organized in a concentric circle. These lines of resistance and defense and the dynamic relationships among five variables of the system (physiological, psychological, sociocultural, developmental, and spiritual) determine how the client responds to stressors. Nursing's role is to help the client system in relation to stressors, reactions, or reconstitution in the modes of primary, secondary, and tertiary prevention.

[*Sources:* Neuman, B. (1998). *The Neuman systems model* (4th ed.). Norwalk, CT: Appleton & Lange.]

NEWMAN, MARGARET

Newman developed her theory of health as an expanding consciousness, drawing ideas from Rogers' holistic and unitary view of humans, David Bohm's notion of implicate and explicate orders of universe, and Young's idea of the acceleration of evolution of consciousness. Newman conceptualized consciousness as pertaining to all information of a system that specifies the system's capacity to interact with its environment. Consciousness as the essence of all things that exist, including humans, is embedded within time, reflected in movement. Health as expanding consciousness is manifested in human experiences in time and space, and is expressed as transformation to a more highly organized pattern of the whole. Newman proposed a hermeneutic, dialectic approach to study health and nursing aimed at pattern recognition, and a participatory research engagement that is itself a human experience of transformation.

[*Sources:* Newman, M. A. (1990). Newman's theory of health as praxis. *Nursing Science Quarterly, 3,* 37–41; Newman, M. A. (1994). *Health as expanding consciousness* (2nd ed.). New York: National League for Nursing.]

OREM, DOROTHEA E.

Orem's general theory of self-care consists of three interrelated subtheories: the theory of self-care, the self-care deficit theory, and the theory of nursing systems. These theories are founded upon the concept of self-care, which refers to "the practice of activities that individuals initiate and perform on their own behalf in maintaining life, health, and well-being." The theory of self-care is structured about the concepts of self-care agency; three areas of self-care requisites identified as universal, developmental, and health deviation; and therapeutic self-care demand. The theory of self-care deficit identifies the connection between nursing and individuals in need of "help" due to self-care deficit. Orem delineates five modes of helping in this theory. The theory of nursing systems describes three forms of nursing systems, that is, wholly compensatory, partly compensatory, and supportive educative systems, through which nursing agency is exercised to meet self-care requisites of patients.

[*Sources:* Orem, D. E. (1991). *Nursing: Concepts of practice* (4th ed.). St. Louis, MO: Mosby.]

ORLANDO, IDA JEAN

Orlando developed her theoretical ideas about nursing based on her work related to the *dynamic nurse-patient relationship,* and extended it to encompass the unique contribution of nursing to patient care. She introduced four terms to categorize nurses' responses to patients needs: automatic, deliberative, "disciplined professional," and "nursing process disciplined." The *disciplined professional and nursing process disciplined* actions and reactions are viewed to be the major processes through which nurses can deliberately address patients' immediate needs by investigating patients' immediate experiences and associated thoughts, feelings, and perceptions and responding to them interactively. To Orlando, nursing is unique in addressing patients' "immediate" situational needs through communicative and interactive processes so that patients will be relieved of distress or gain greater sense of adequacy or well-being.

[*Sources:* Orlando, I. J. (1961). *The dynamic nurse-patient relationship: Function, process and principles.* New York: Putnam; Orlando, I. J. (1972). *The discipline and teaching of nursing process.* New York: Putnam; Orlando, I. J. (1990). *The dynamic nurse-patient relationship: Function, process and principles.* New York: National League for Nursing. (Reprinted from Putnam 1961 publication)]

PARSE, ROSEMARY RIZZO

Parse cited Rogers' science of unitary human beings and the existential phenomenology of Heidegger, Sartre, and Merleau-Ponty as providing the core assumptions that undergird her theory of "human becoming." Her theory is based on the view that humans are evolving, unitary entities in constant mutual interrelationship with the universe. Health is the expression of this evolving, experienced by humans as a process of becoming and negentropic "unfolding" characterized by meaning, rhythmicity and co-transcendence. Key concepts of the theory are imaging, valuing, languaging, revealing-concealing, enabling-limiting, connecting-separating, powering, originating, and transforming. These nine concepts are structured into three theoretical statements, which are the basis for Parse's research and practice methodology.

[*Sources:* Parse, R. R. (1992). Human becoming: Parse's theory of nursing. *Nursing Science Quarterly, 5,* 35–42; Parse, R. R. (Ed.). (1995). *Illuminations: The human becoming theory in practice and research.* New York: National League for Nursing; Parse, R. R. (1996). The human becoming theory: Challenges in practice and research. *Nursing Science Quarterly, 9,* 55–60; Parse, R. R. (1997). The human becoming theory: The was, is, and will be. *Nursing Science Quarterly, 10,* 32–38.]

PEPLAU, HILDEGARD E.

The focus of Peplau's theory is interpersonal processes in nursing, especially those pertaining to relationships between patients and nurses. Her theory of interpersonal relations is generative, as she believes that encounters between patients and nurses influence the development and maturing of both participants. She identified four phases of interpersonal relations: orientation, identification, exploitation, and resolution. Within these phases, nurses are believed to assume the roles of teacher, resource, counselor, leader, technical expert, and surrogate, according to the needs of the patient during the interpersonal process. To Peplau, nursing is a "maturing force and an educative instrument" and a therapeutic process that involves interpersonal relations between patients and nurses.

[*Sources:* Peplau, H. (1952). *Interpersonal relations in nursing.* New York: Putnam; Peplau, H. (1988). The art and science of nursing: Similarities, differences, and relations. *Nursing Science Quarterly, 1,* 8–15.]

ROGERS, MARTHA E.

Rogers' theory is founded on the basic assumption that human beings are unitary beings engaged in evolutionary life processes that are unidirectionally oriented and involve mutuality with one's environment.

The major concepts of the theory are human and environmental energy fields, which define humans and environment and are irreducible and indivisible, signified as single-wave patterns, existing pandimensionally. Humans and their environment as energy fields are in constant, mutual interaction and interpenetrate with each other. Three principles of homeodynamics are specified as governing life processes and energy field patterns: The principle of integrality accounts for the mutual and simultaneous changes that occur in the interaction between human and environmental energy fields, and the principle of resonancy refers to dynamic, rhythmic changes in wave patterns that accompany the mutual process of human and environmental energy fields. The third principle, helicy, focuses on the nature of change in energy fields through mutual processes identified as innovative, moving toward increasing complexity and diversity, rhythmic, and unpredictable. Rogers viewed her theory as a science of unitary human beings, providing the foundation for developing theories in nursing.

[*Sources:* Rogers, M. E. (1970). *The theoretical basis of nursing.* Philadelphia: Davis; Rogers, M. E. (1989). Nursing: A science of unitary human beings. In J. Riehl-Sisca (Ed.), *Conceptual models for nursing practice* (3rd ed., pp. 181–188). Norwalk, CT: Appleton & Lange; Rogers, M. E. (1990). Nursing: Science of unitary, irreducible, human beings: Update 1990. In E. A. M. Barrett (Ed.), *Visions of Rogers' science-based nursing* (pp. 5–11). New York: National League for Nursing; Rogers, M. E. (1992). Nursing science and the space age. *Nursing Science Quarterly, 5,* 27–34.]

Roy, Callista

The Roy adaptation model was developed based on key ideas in von Bertalanffy's general system theory and Helson's adaptation level theory. Roy conceptualized persons as adaptive systems that handle inputs of stimuli—identified as focal, contextual, and residual stimuli—through two sets of control processes in relation to presenting adaptation level. The control processes are designated as regulator and cognator subsystems. Through such processing, adaptive systems exhibit behavioral responses as outputs that are either adaptive or maladaptive (or ineffective). Within the model, four adaptive modes are identified as the specific areas in which adaptive responses would be observed. These are physiological, self-concept, role function, and interdependence modes, which are oriented to specific goals for, and the needs of, the adaptive system. As an additional foundational idea for her theory, Roy introduced the concept of veritivity, which refers to the common purposefulness of human existence.

[*Sources:* Roy, C. (1984). *Introduction to nursing: An adaptation model* (2nd ed.). Englewood Cliffs, NJ: Prentice-Hall; Roy, C., & Andrews, H. A. (1991). *The Roy adaptation model: The definitive statement.* Norwalk, CT: Appleton & Lange; Roy, C. (1997). Future of the Roy model: Challenge to redefine adaptation. *Nursing Science Quarterly, 10,* 42–48; Roy, C., & Andrews, H. A. (1999). *The Roy adaptation model* (2nd ed.). Stamford, CT: Appleton & Lange; Roy, C., & Roberts, S. (1981). *Theory construction in nursing: An adaptation model.* Englewood Cliffs, NJ: Prentice-Hall.]

WATSON, JEAN

Watson based her theory of caring and human care on the assumption that health refers to harmony within the mind-body-spirit as a whole being and is expressed by the congruency between the perceived and experienced self. To Watson, her theory is a humanistic approach to nursing that emphasizes human-to-human responsiveness rooted in upholding humanistic values. Caring as the central component of nursing is oriented to health promotion and growth. Watson identified ten carative factors as the basis from which caring can be operationalized in nursing. These factors are the essential characteristics, attitudes, and processes through which nurses can promote health and growth in individuals. Watson expanded her model by embracing the existential ethics of Levinas and Løgstrup, and specifies caring for self and others through *caritas and comunitas.*

[*Sources:* Watson, J. (1979). *Nursing: The philosophy and science of caring.* Boston: Little, Brown; Watson, J. (1988). *Nursing: Human science and human care,* New York: National League for Nursing; Watson, J. (1988). New dimensions of human caring theory. *Nursing Science Quarterly, 1,* 175–181; Watson, J. (1997). The theory of human caring: Retrospective and prospective. *Nursing Science Quarterly, 10,* 49–52; Watson, J. (2003). Love and caring: Ethics of face and hand—An invitation to return to the heart and soul of nursing and our deep humanity. *Nursing Administration Quarterly, 27,* 197–202; Watson, J. (2004). Caritas and communitas: A caring science ethical view of self and community. *Journal of Japan Academy of Nursing Science, 24,* 66–71.]

Selected Middle-Range Theories in Nursing

Hesook Suzie Kim

Auvil-Novak, S. E. (1997). A middle-range theory of chronotherapeutic intervention for postsurgical pain. *Nursing Research, 46,* 66–71.

Beck, C. T. (1993). Teetering on the edge: A substantive theory of postpartum depression. *Nursing Research, 42,* 42–48.

Bengton, V. L., & Roberts, E. L. (1991). Intergenerational solidarity in aging families: An example of formal theory construction. *Journal of Marriage and the Family, 53,* 856–870.

Chinn, P. (2001). Toward a theory of nursing art. In N. L. Chaska (Ed.), *The nursing profession: Tomorrow and beyond* (pp. 287–298). Thousand Oaks, CA: Sage.

Colling, K. B. (2003). A taxonomy of passive behaviors in people with Alzheimer's disease. *Journal of Nursing Scholarship, 32,* 239–244.

Cooley, M. E. (1999). Analysis and evaluation of the trajectory theory of chronic illness management. *Scholarly Inquiry for Nursing Practice, 13,* 75–95.

Dorsey, C. J., & Murdaugh, C. L. (2003). The theory of self-care management for vulnerable populations. *Journal of Theory Construction and Testing, 7,* 43–49.

Dunn, K. S. (2004). Toward a middle-range theory of adaptation to chronic pain. *Nursing Science Quarterly, 17,* 78–84.

Eakes, G. G., Burke, M. L., & Hainsworth, M. A. (1998). Middle-range theory of chronic sorrow. *Image: Journal of Nursing Scholarship, 30,* 179–184.

Engerbretson, J., & Littleton, L. Y. (2001). Cultural negotiation: A constructivist-based model for nursing practice. *Nursing Outlook, 49,* 223–230.

Estabrooks, C. A., & Morse, J. M. (1992). Toward a theory of touch: The touching process and acquiring a touching style. *Journal of Advanced Nursing, 17,* 448–456.

Finfgeld, D. L. (1999). Courage as a process of pushing beyond the struggle. *Qualitative Health Research, 9,* 803–814.

Good, M., & Moore, S. M. (1996). Clinical practice guidelines as a new source of middle-range theory: Focus on acute pain. *Nursing Outlook, 44,* 74–79.

Huth, M. M., & Moore, S. M. (1998). Prescriptive theory of acute pain management in infants and children. *Journal of Society of Pediatric Nursing, 3,* 23–32.

Jenny, J., & Logan, J. (1996). Caring and comfort metaphors used by patients in critical care. *Image: Journal of Nursing Scholarship, 28,* 349–352.

Jezewski, M. A. (1995). Evolution of a grounded theory: Conflict resolution through culture brokering. *Advances in Nursing Science, 17,* 14–30.

Jirovex, M. M., Jenkins, J., Isenberg, M., & Baiardi, J. (1999). Urine control theory derived from Roy's conceptual framework. *Nursing Science Quarterly, 12,* 251–255.

Kearney, M. H. (2001). Enduring love: A grounded formal theory of women's experience of domestic violence. *Research in Nursing and Health, 24,* 270–282.

Kim, H. S. (1983). Collaborative decision making in nursing practice: A theoretical framework. In P. Chinn (Ed.), *Advances in nursing theory development* (pp. 271–283). Washington, DC: Aspen Systems.

Lenz, E. R., Suppe, F., Gift, A. G., Pugh, L. C., & Milligan, R. A. (1995). Collaborative development of middle-range nursing theories: Toward a theory of unpleasant symptoms. *Advances in Nursing Science, 17,* 1–13.

Lenz, E. R., Pugh, L. C., Milligan, R. A., Gift, A., & Suppe, F. (1997). The middle-range theory of unpleasant symptoms: An update. *Advances in Nursing Science, 19,* 14–27.

Meleis, A. I., Sawyer, L. M., Im, E. O., Messias, D. K. H., & Schumacher, P. (2000). Experiencing transitions: An emerging middle-range theory. *Advances in Nursing Science, 23,* 12–28.

Mishel, M. H. (1988). Uncertainty in illness. *Image: Journal of Nursing Scholarship, 20,* 225–232.

Mishel, M. H. (1990). Reconceptualization of the uncertainty of illness theory. *Image: Journal of Nursing Scholarship, 22,* 256–262.

Morse, J. M. (2001). Toward a praxis theory of suffering. *Advances in Nursing Science, 24,* 47–59.

Morse, J. M., Havens, G. A. D., & Wilson, S. (1997). The comforting interaction: Developing a model of nurse-patient relationship. *Scholarly Inquiry for Nursing Practice, 11,* 321–347.

Olson, J., & Hanchett, E. (1997). Nurse-expressed empathy, patient outcomes, and development of a middle-range theory. *Image: Journal of Nursing Scholarship, 29,* 71–76.

Polk, L. V. (1997). Toward a middle-range theory of resilience. *Advances in Nursing Science, 19,* 1–13.

Reed, P. G. (1991). Toward a nursing theory of self-transcendence: Deductive reformulation using developmental theories. *Advances in Nursing Science, 13,* 64–77.

Ruland, C. M., & Moore, S. M. (1998). Theory construction based on standards of care: A proposed theory of the peaceful end of life. *Nursing Outlook, 46,* 169–175.

Sanford, R. C. (2000). Caring through relation and dialogue: A nursing perspective for patient education. *Advances in Nursing Science, 22,* 1–15.

Scambler, G., & Hopkins, A. (1990). Generating a model of epileptic stigma: The role of qualitative analysis. *Social Science and Medicine, 30,* 1187–1194.

Schmidt, S., Nachtigall, C., Wuethrich-Martone, O., & Strauss, B. (2002). Attachment and coping with chronic illness. *Journal of Psychosomatic Research, 53,* 763–773.

Smith, A. A., & Friedemann, M. L. (1999). Perceived family dynamics of persons with chronic pain. *Journal of Advanced Nursing, 30,* 543–551.

Smith, M. J., & Liehr, P. (1999). Attentively embracing story: A middle-range theory with practice and research implications. *Scholarly Inquiry for Nursing Practice, 13,* 187–204.

Swanson, K. M. (1991). Empirical development of a middle range theory of caring. *Nursing Research, 40,* 161–166.

Thomas, S. P. (1991). Toward a new conceptualization of women's anger. *Issues in Mental Health Nursing, 12,* 31–49.

Whittemore, R., & Roy, C. (2002). Adapting to diabetes mellitus: A theory synthesis. *Nursing Science Quarterly, 15,* 311–317.

Woods, S. J., & Isenberg, M. A. (2001). Adaptation as a mediator of intimate abuse and traumatic stress in battered women. *Nursing Science Quarterly, 14,* 215–221.

Wuest, J. (2001). Precarious ordering: Toward a formal theory of women's caring. *Health Care Women International, 22,* 167–193.)

Index

Need(s)
    as a concept, 71–72, 77, 85
    claims, 75–77, 82
    definition of, 13
    identifications, 81–82
    meaning of, 73
    satisfaction, 13, 81–83
    science of, 80
Need statement(s), 73, 77, 79, 85
    as claim-grounds statement,
        74
    differentiation from want
        statement, 76
    thick, 73–74
    thin, 73–74
Need theories, nursing, 17–22,
    77–78
Need theorists, 17
Neopragmatism, 187, 193, 196
Normal, 44
    and abnormal, 50, 282
    and pathological, 45, 262–263
    deviant, 282
Normalism (normalist), 44, 52, 261,
    273, 277, 280
    flexible, 44, 277–279, 282
    one-dimensionality of, 261
Normality, 44, 277
    and abnormality, 280, 282
Normalization, 44, 52, 265, 275
Normalizing, 265, 276
Nosology of continuity, 262
Notes on Nursing, 171
Nursing clients, 4
Nursing: Human Science and Human Care, 173
Nursing: The Philosophy and Science of Caring, 172
Nursing theories,
    analysis of, 4–5
    categorization of, 2
    comprehension of, 5–6
    conceptual focus of, 3
Nursing theory development, 2

On the Normal and Pathological,
    262
Organicism, 92, 93, 95
Organizations, 132

Parse's Human Becoming theory,
    149–152
Parson's systems theory,
    113–114
Phenomenological
    method, 144
    reduction, 144–145
Phenomenology, 56, 60, 143
    Heideggerian, 146, 163
    Husserlian, 143
    interpretive, 153
    of Merleau-Ponty, 147
Poetry therapy, 208
Practice domain, 3, 28
Pragmatics of Human Communication, 55
Pragmatic
    bioethics, 196
    ethos, 188–189
    method, 192–193
Pragmaticism, 185
Pragmatism, 164–167, 184–199
    and epistemology, 192–194
    and human conduct, 194–196
    and instrumentalism, 185
    and reality, 191–192
    and truth, 188–190
    clinical, 196
    in nursing, 197
    major tenets of, 187
Protonormalism (protonormalist),
    44, 277–279
Professionalism, 84

Reductionism, 92
Reminiscence training, 208
Risk, 260, 280, 284
Rogerian science of unitary human
    beings, 64–66, 101–105

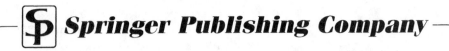
Springer Publishing Company

Dictionary of Nursing Theory and Research, *3rd Edition*

Bethel Ann Powers, PhD, RN
Thomas R. Knapp, EdD

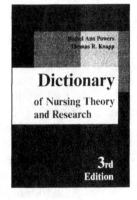

"The exceptional readability and convenient size of this dictionary make it a wonderful companion for any nurse seeking to demystify the phenomena of nursing theory and research."

—**Nursing Research,** praise for previous edition

"An excellent collection of information essential to all nurses, not only those involved in research but also practicing nurses interested in innovation and change. Students at all academic levels will find it particularly useful. The definition of terms are clear and accurate and the range of topics is comprehensive, with frequent cross-referencing and citations given from relevant literature..."

—**Nursing Times,** praise for previous edition

The new edition of this concise reference includes updated terminology and the addition of many new terms with examples and references that reflect current nursing practice. With the inclusion of research, theory, statistical, and epidemiological definitions and cross-reference notes at the end of each entry, this compilation is a handy and up-to-date dictionary for students, clinicians, and researchers.

Partial Contents:
- Preface to the Third Edition
- Explanatory Notes
- Alphabetical Listing of Research and Theory Terms
- References
- About the Authors

August 2005   224pp   0-8261-1774-0   softcover

11 West 42nd Street, New York, NY 10036-8002 • **Fax: 212-941-7842**
Order Toll-Free: 877-687-7476 • **Order On-line: www.springerpub.com**

Springer Publishing Company

Encyclopedia of Nursing Research
2nd Edition

Joyce J. Fitzpatrick, PhD, RN, FAAN
Editor-in-Chief
Meredith Wallace, PhD, RN, APRN-BC
Associate Editor

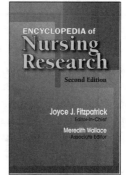

The push toward evidence-based practice makes it crucial for all nurses to be familiar with basic research terminology, methods, databases, and seminal research in specific clinical areas. This comprehensive reference is a "one-stop" resource for everything you need to know about nursing research and its utilization. Compiled by the world's leading authorities in nursing research, this thoroughly updated new edition presents key terms and concepts by over 200 contributors, with nearly 30% newly added terms. It is written for nurse researchers, graduate students, and clinicians. Extensive cross references assist in the information-seeking process.

Over 300 articles include topics such as: nursing services, electronic networks and technology, nursing education, nursing care, specialties in nursing, patients' reactions and adjustments, historical, philosophical, and cultural issues, nursing organizations and publications.

Partial Contents:

- Advanced Practice Nursing
- Clinical Nursing Research
- Computer-Based Documentation
- Data Management
- Ethics of Research
- Family Caregiving to Frail Elderly
- Geriatrics
- Henderson's Model

- Internet
- Journals in Nursing Research
- Measurement and Scales
- Nursing Theoretical Models
- Qualitative and Quantitative Research
- Research Utilization
- Statistical Techniques

September 2005   837pp (est.)   0-8261-9812-0   hardcover

11 West 42nd Street, New York, NY 10036-8002 • Fax: 212-941-7842
Order Toll-Free: 877-687-7476 • Order On-line: www.springerpub.com

3

Springer Publishing Company

Theory-Directed Nursing Practice

2nd Edition

Shirley Melat Ziegler, PhD, RN, Editor

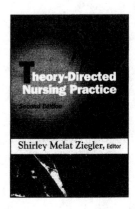

This popular textbook demonstrates the application of theory to nursing practice. Nearly 10 middle-range theories are presented, along with their clinical applications. Each chapter follows a common format: a case is presented, along with several possible theories to use. Finally one theory is selected for use and is described in depth. New to this edition is a selection in each chapter on research supporting the theories discussed.

Partial Contents

- Introduction to Theory-Directed Nursing Practice, *S.M. Ziegler*
- Aguilera's Theory of Crisis Intervention, *T.L. Jones*
- Bandura's Social Cognitive Theory, *S.M. Ziegler, W.K. Arnold, S. Chaney, L. Hough, O. Hughes, R. Nieswiadomy,* and *G.W. Watson*
- Beck's Cognitive Theory of Depression, *S.M. Ziegler*
- Bowen's Family Theory, *W.K. Arnold, R. Nieswiadomy* and *G.W. Watson*
- Erikson's Theory of Psychosocial Development, *C.E. Mobley* and *J. Johnson-Russell*
- Lazarus' Theory of Coping, *K.M. Baldwin*
- Peplau's Theory with an Emphasis on Anxiety, *W. K. Arnold* and *R. Nieswiadomy*
- Lewin's Field Theory with Emphasis on Change, *Susan Chaney* and *L. Hough*
- Thomas's Conflict Theory, *L. Hough* and *S. Chaney*
- Strategy for Theory-Directed Nursing Practice, *S.M. Ziegler*
- Appendix A: Glossary of Nursing Process Terms
- Appendix B: Glossary of Theory Terms
- Appendix C: Rationale for the Level of Theory and Specific Theories Selected

2005   304pp   0-8261-7632-1   hardcover

11 West 42nd Street, New York, NY 10036-8002 • **Fax: 212-941-7842**
Order Toll-Free: 877-687-7476 • **Order On-line: www.springerpub.com**